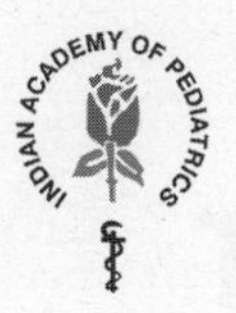

PRACTICAL PEDIATRIC DIGEST

Publication of IAP Chennai City Branch

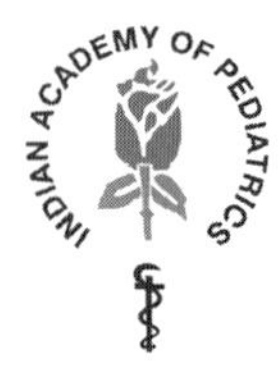

PRACTICAL PEDIATRIC DIGEST

Editor-in-Chief

A Parthasarathy
Senior Consultant Pediatrician
AP Child Care, Chennai
Former Distinguished Professor of Pediatrics
The Tamil Nadu Dr MGR Medical University, Chennai
Retired Senior Clinical Professor of Pediatrics
Madras Medical College, Chennai
Deputy Superintendent
Institute of Child Health and Hospital for Children, Chennai, Tamil Nadu
apartha2030@gmail.com

Executive Editor

A Somasundaram
Consultant in Developmental Pediatrics
Kanchi Kamakoti CHILDS Trust Hospital
Consultant Pediatrician, Sabari Child Care Clinic and Center for Child Development
Formerly, Senior Assistant Professor of Pediatrics
Institute of Child Health and Hospital for Children
Madras Medical College, Chennai, Tamil Nadu
drsoma2001@yahoo.com

Publication Editor

P Sudhakar
Senior Assistant Professor of Pediatrics
Institute of Child Health and Hospital for Children
Madras Medical College, Chennai
Consultant Pediatrician and Development Pediatrician
BFCC Child Care Center, Chennai, Tamil Nadu
drsudhakar2001@gmail.com

Forewords

Pramod Jog
Anupam Sachdeva
S Sachidananda Kamath
Major K Nagaraju
R Somasekar

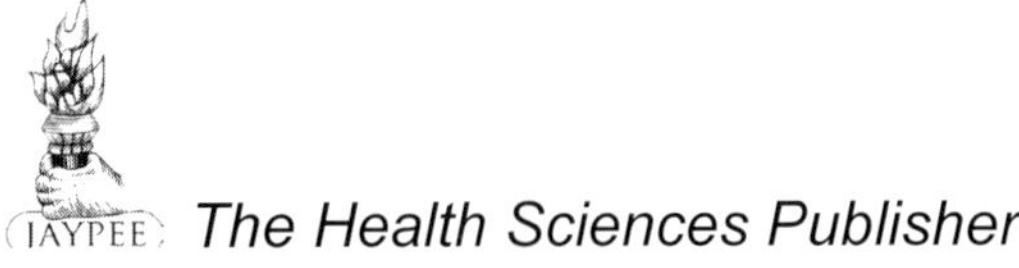

New Delhi | London | Philadelphia | Panama

Editorial Board

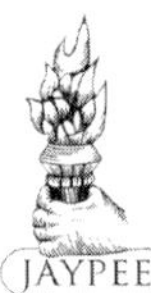

JAYPEE **Jaypee Brothers Medical Publishers (P) Ltd.**

Headquarters
Jaypee Brothers Medical Publishers (P) Ltd.
4838/24, Ansari Road, Daryaganj
New Delhi 110 002, India
Phone: +91-11-43574357
Fax: +91-11-43574314
E-mail: jaypee@jaypeebrothers.com

Overseas Offices

J.P. Medical Ltd.
83, Victoria Street, London
SW1H 0HW (UK)
Phone: +44 20 3170 8910
Fax: +44 (0) 20 3008 6180
E-mail: info@jpmedpub.com

Jaypee-Highlights Medical Publishers Inc.
City of Knowledge, Building 235, 2nd Floor
Panama City, Panama
Phone: +1 507-301-0496
Fax: +1 507-301-0499
E-mail: cservice@jphmedical.com

Jaypee Medical Inc.
325, Chestnut Street
Suite 412, Philadelphia
PA 19106, USA
Phone: +1 267-519-9789
E-mail: support@jpmedus.com

Jaypee Brothers Medical Publishers (P) Ltd.
17/1-B, Babar Road, Block-B, Shaymali
Mohammadpur, Dhaka-1207
Bangladesh
Mobile: +08801912003485
E-mail: jaypeedhaka@gmail.com

Jaypee Brothers Medical Publishers (P) Ltd.
Bhotahity, Kathmandu, Nepal
Phone: +977-9741283608
E-mail: kathmandu@jaypeebrothers.com

Website: www.jaypeebrothers.com
Website: www.jaypeedigital.com

Inquiries for bulk sales may be solicited at: jaypee@jaypeebrothers.com

Practical Pediatric Digest

First Edition : **2017**

ISBN : 978-93-86150-86-8

Printed at Rajkamal Electric Press, Plot No. 2, Phase-IV, Kundli, Haryana.

Dedicated to

The parents and their suffering children whose valuable history and clinical presentation have contributed to enrich our knowledge.

Contributors

Alok Gupta
Pediatrician and Counselor
Pediatric Specialties Clinic
Jaipur
Former Assistant Professor
Pediatric Medicine
Mahatma Gandhi Medical
College and Hospital
Jaipur, Rajasthan
docalok@hotmail.com

A Parthasarathy
Senior Consultant Pediatrician
AP Child Care, Chennai
Former Distinguished Professor
of Pediatrics
The Tamil Nadu Dr MGR Medical
University, Chennai
Retired Senior Clinical Professor
of Pediatrics
Madras Medical College
Chennai
Deputy Superintendent
Institute of Child Health and
Hospital for Children
Chennai, Tamil Nadu
apartha2030@gmail.com

A Somasundaram
Consultant in Developmental
Pediatrics
Kanchi Kamakoti CHILDS
Trust Hospital
Consultant Pediatrician
Sabari Child Care Clinic and
Center for Child Development
Formerly Senior Assistant
Professor of Pediatrics
Institute of Child Health and
Hospital for Children
Madras Medical College
Chennai, Tamil Nadu
drsoma2001@yahoo.com
9841676097

Balakrishnan Natarajan
Senior Civil Surgeon
Assistant Professor of Radiology
Institute of Child Health and
Hospital for Children
Madras Medical College
Chennai, Tamil Nadu
nirmalanatarajan89@gmail.com
9840180283

B Bhaskar Raju
Former Professor
Department of Pediatric
Gastroenterology
Institute of Child Health and
Hospital for Children
Madras Medical College
Chennai, Tamil Nadu
drbhaskarraju@yahoo.com
9841017164

C Amarnath
Associate Professor and Head
Department of Radiology
Stanley Medical College
Chennai, Tamil Nadu
amarrd02@yahoo.co.in
9884877622

Dheivamani Nirmala
Professor, Department of
Pediatric Gastroenterology
Institute of Child Health and
Hospital for Children
Madras Medical College
Chennai, Tamil Nadu
nirmalanatarajan89@gmail.com
9840151024

Ethiraj Prabhu
Senior Consultant and Head
Institute of Nuclear Imaging and
Molecular Medicine
Tamil Nadu Government
Multi-Super Specialty Hospital
Chennai, Tamil Nadu
dreprabhu@gmail.com
9382730296

Ganga Devi Rajapandian
Associate Consultant
Department of Radiology
Government Tamil Nadu
Multi-Super Specialty Hospital
Chennai, Tamil Nadu
gangasundarkumar@yahoo.co.in
9444311305

G Duraiarasan
Associate Professor
Department of Pediatrics
Government Medical College
Tiruvannamalai, Tamil Nadu
drdurai_07@yahoo.com
9381014773

Giridhar Sethuraman
Associate Professor
Department of Neonatology
Chettinad Hospital and Research
Institute
Chennai, Tamil Nadu
giridharsethu@gmail.com
9841027228

Gnanasambandam Subramaniyan
Professor and Head
Department of Pediatric Cardiology
Institute of Child Health and
Hospital for Children
Madras Medical College
Chennai, Tamil Nadu
gnanams68@gmail.com
9566833339

Gopala Krishnan
Assistant Professor
Department of Pediatric
Cardiology
Institute of Child Health and
Hospital for Children, Egmore
Chennai, Tamil Nadu
drgkcardio@gmail.com
9841651277

G Vijayalakshmi
Professor and Head
Department of Pediatric Radiology
Institute of Child Health and Hospital for Children
Madras Medical College
Chennai, Tamil Nadu
drviji.rad@gmail.com
9840045520

Hemchand K Prasad
Consultant and Head
Department of Pediatric Endocrinology and Diabetes
Dr Mehta's Children's Hospital
Chennai, Tamil Nadu
hemchan82@gmail.com
09884984280

Janani Sankar
Senior Consultant
Kanchi Kamakoti CHILDS Trust Hospital,
Chennai, Tamil Nadu
janani.sankar@yahoo.com
9841078101

Jaydeep Choudhury
Associate Professor
Department of Pediatrics
Institute of Child Health
Kolkata, West Bengal
drjaydeep_choudhury@yahoo.co.in

J Ritchie Sharon Solomon
Assistant Professor
Department of Pediatric Cardiology
Institute of Child Health and Hospital for Children
Madras Medical College
Chennai, Tamil Nadu

Karnan Sudha
Consultant
Department of Radiology
Scans World
Chennai, Tamil Nadu
sudhadav08@gmail.com

Kathirvelu Gopinathan
Associate Professor
Department of Radiology
Government Kilpauk Medical College and Government Royapettah Hospital
Chennai, Tamil Nadu
drgopinathanmdrd@gmail.com
9841356950

K Nedunchelian
Senior Consultant and Head (Research and Academics)
Dr Mehta's Children's Hospital
Chennai, Tamil Nadu
drknedunchelian@gmail.com

Mahesh Janarthanan
Consultant
Department of Pediatric Rheumatology
Sri Ramachandra University
Chennai, Tamil Nadu
maheshjanarthanan@hotmail.com
9952552330

M Deenadayalan
Consultant
Department of Pediatric Hematology, Oncology and Bone Marrow Transplantation
Global Cancer Institute
Chennai, Tamil Nadu
drdeenadayalanm@gmail.com
9841089345

MKC Nair
Vice-Chancellor
Kerala University for Health Sciences, Thrissur
Founder Director
Child Development Center
Government Medical College
Thiruvananthapuram, Kerala
cdcmkc@gmail.com

M Prabakaran
Former Professor
Department of Radiology
Madras Medical College
Chennai, Tamil Nadu
drm.prabakaran@gmail.com
9444051419

Mugil Varman Rajasekaran
Pediatric Radiology Fellow
Department of Radiodiagnosis
Christian Medical College and Hospital
Vellore, Tamil Nadu
mugilmbbs@gmail.com

MVN Malleswari
Registrar in Pediatrics
Kanchi Kamakoti CHILDS Trust Hospital
Chennai, Tamil Nadu

NC Gowrishankar
Pediatric Pulmonologist and Bronchoscopist
Head (Pediatrics—Clinical Operations and Quality)
Dr Mehta's Children's Hospital
Chennai, Tamil Nadu
cugowri@yahoo.com
9444047740

N Thilothammal
Former Professor
Department of Pediatric Neurology
Institute of Child Health and Hospital for Children
Madras Medical College
Chennai, Tamil Nadu
dr.n.thilothammal@gmail.com
9444985005

Palani Gunasekaran
Director
King Institute of Preventive Medicine and Research Center
Guindy, Tamil Nadu
gunzking@gmail.com
9840960225

P Ramachandran
Professor and Head
Department of Pediatrics
Sri Ramachandra Medical College and Research Institute
Chennai, Tamil Nadu
ramachandran_dr@rediffmail.com
9840471901

PSN Menon
Consultant and Head
Department of Pediatrics
Jaber Al-Ahmed Armed Forces
Hospital, Kuwait
Former Professor
Department of Pediatrics
All India Institute of
Medical Sciences
New Delhi
psnmenon@hotmail.com

P Sudhakar
Senior Assistant Professor
of Pediatrics
Institute of Child Health and
Hospital for Children
Madras Medical College
Chennai
Consultant Pediatrician and
Development Pediatrician
BFCC Child Care Center
Chennai, Tamil Nadu
drsudhakar2001@gmail.com
9443620861

P Thirumal
Consultant
Department of Pediatric
Gastroenterology
Sri Manakula Vinayagar
Medical College and Hospital
Puducherry
thirumaal777@yahoo.co.in

Ramamurthi Palaniraman
Child Health Consultant
CR Women and Child
Health Center
Tindivanam, Tamil Nadu
amvarsh@gmail.com
9345033079

R Ezhilarasu
Senior Assistant Professor of
Pediatrics
Institute of Child Health and
Hospital for Children
Madras Medical College
Chennai, Tamil Nadu
elilarasu74@gmail.com
9841021018

R Remesh Kumar
Medical Superintendent and
Chief Pediatrician
NSS Medical Mission Hospital
Pandalam, Pathanamthitta
Kerala
drremesh2006@yahoo.com

R Somasekar
Professor
Department of Pediatrics
Institute of Child
Health and Hospital
for Children
Madras Medical College
Chennai, Tamil Nadu

RV Dhakshayani
Assistant Professor
Department of Pediatrics
Institute of Child Health
and Hospital for Children
Madras Medical College Chennai,
Tamil Nadu
dhaksh357@yahoo.com

R Velmurugan
Professor
Department of Pediatric Surgery
Institute of Child Health and
Hospital for Children
Madras Medical College
Chennai, Tamil Nadu
velsurgeon@ymail.com
9840271700

Sampath Santhosh
Junior Consultant
Institute of Nuclear Imaging and
Molecular Medicine
Tamil Nadu Government
Multi-Super Specialty Hospital
Chennai, Tamil Nadu

Sangeetha
Assistant Professor
Department of Pediatric
Medicine
Sri Ramachandra Medical
College and Research Institute
Chennai, Tamil Nadu
sangeethaperungo@gmail.com
9843086986

Satish Datla
DM Resident
Department of Neonatology
Chettinad Hospital and
Research Institute
Chennai, Tamil Nadu
satishddr@rediffmail.com

S Babu
Consultant Pediatrician
VeeCare Sundar Hospital,
Poonamallee
Chennai, Tamil Nadu

S Kirupa
Consultant Microbiologist and
Infection Control Officer
CSI Kalyani Multispeciality
Hospital
Chennai, Tamil Nadu
drkirupa@yahoo.co.in
9841327605

S Mangalabharathi
Associate Professor
Department of Neonatology
Institute of Child Health and
Hospital for Children
Madras Medical College
Chennai, Tamil Nadu
drmangalabharathi@gmail.com
9840786836

S Muralinath
Senior Consultant
Department of Radiology
Kanchi Kamakoti CHILDS
Trust Hospital
Chennai, Tamil Nadu
muralinath_sonic@yahoo.co.in
9841020675

S Narmada
Director and Consultant
Pediatrician
Nalam Medical Center
and Hospital
Vellore, Tamil Nadu
dr.narmadhaashok@gmail.com
9443098899

Somu Sivabalan
Senior Consultant Pediatrician and Pulmonologist
Kanchi Kamakoti CHILDS Trust Hospital
Chennai, Tamil Nadu
sivabalan.somu@gmail.com
9444720233

S Shanthi
Professor of Pediatrics
Institute of Child Health and Hospital for Children
Madras Medical College
Chennai, Tamil Nadu

S Thangavelu
Former Reader
Department of Pediatrics
Institute of Child Health and Hospital for Children
Madras Medical College
Chennai
Senior Consultant and Director
Department of Pediatrics
Dr Mehta's Children's Hospital
Chennai, Tamil Nadu
thangavelu.dr@gmail.com
9790970772

Sumathi Bavanandam
Assistant Professor
Department of Pediatric Gastroenterology
Institute of Child Health and Hospital for Children
Chennai, Tamil Nadu
drbsumathi@rediffmail.com
9841371490

S Vasanth Kumar
Visiting Consultant
Kanchi Kamakoti CHILDS Trust Hospital
Anna Nagar
Chennai, Tamil Nadu

T Muthusamy
Senior Consultant Pediatrician
Apollo Clinic
Chennai, Tamil Nadu

TN Manohar
Senior Consultant Pediatrician
Chennai, Tamil Nadu

TS Ekambaranath
Senior Assistant Professor
Institute of Social Pediatrics
Stanley Medical College
Chennai, Tamil Nadu
eknath_dr@yahoo.com
9944021679

T Sivaraman
Senior Assistant Professor of Pediatrics
Institute of Child Health and Hospital for Children
Madras Medical College
Chennai, Tamil Nadu
drmani_76@yahoo.com
9884238721

Umamaheshwari B
DNB Pediatrics Trainee
Dr Mehta's Children's Hospital
Chennai, Tamil Nadu

U Umadevi
Professor
Institute of Microbiology
Madras Medical College
Chennai, Tamil Nadu
umakarthik89@gmail.com
9884075862

Vadavil Suhas Das
Resident in Pediatrics
Kanchi Kamakoti CHILDS Trust Hospital
Chennai, Tamil Nadu
realsuhas@gmail.com

Vasumathy Vedantham
Consultant Ophthalmologist
Pediatric Retina Specialist and Medical Director
Radhatri Nethralaya Eye Hospital
Chennai, Tamil Nadu
drvasumathy@gmail.com
9442631370

V Poovazhagi
Professor
Department of Pediatrics
Chengalpattu Medical College
Chengalpattu, Tamil Nadu
poomuthu@yahoo.com
9840033020

VV Varadarajan
Hon Director
Department of Pediatrics
Sooriya Hospital, Chennai
Senior Visiting Consultant
Kanchi Kamakoti CHILDS Trust Hospital, Chennai, Tamil Nadu
drvvvaradarajan@gmail.com
9840037076

Foreword

Pediatrics made **P**alatable and **D**igestible

It is the tragedy of the world that no one knows what he doesn't know—and the less a man knows, the more sure he is that he knows everything!

– Jouce Cary, British Author (1888–1957)

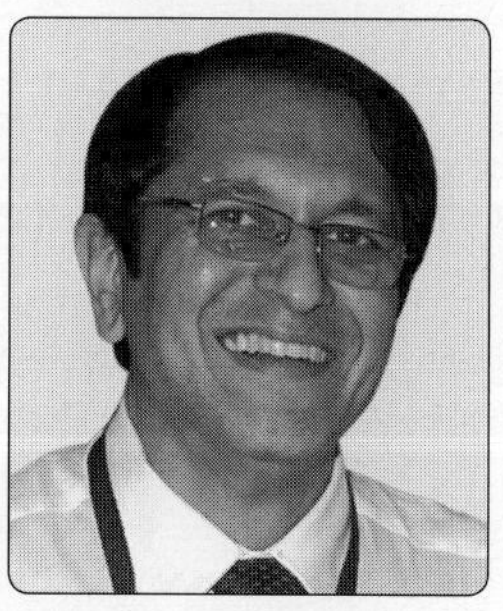

Theory and practice are the two hands of any clinician. Practicing with just one leaves the doctor and the patient with a handicap. Our increasing knowledge will benefit child care, only if the 'right' knowledge combines with the 'left' out.

Practical Pediatric Digest is a bridge between what needs to be known and what needs to be done.

Dr Parthasarathy (Editor-in-Chief) has set on our (study) tables, a variety of dishes, cooked with intelligent technique by masterchefs of their field, to give us **P**ediatrics in a **P**alatable and **D**igestible form. I congratulate all the authors for their hard work, knowledge and thoughtfulness.

If a little knowledge is dangerous, where is the man who has so much to be out of danger!

– TH Huxley

The Indian Academy of Pediatrics (IAP) has always promoted ethical and rational pediatric care, and this publication will keep our members *out of danger* for years to come.

I am confident that the digest, a flagship project of IAP, Chennai will become extremely popular among students and doctors over the years, and guides all those caring for neonates, children and adolescents in India and abroad.

Pramod Jog
President IAP, 2016

Foreword

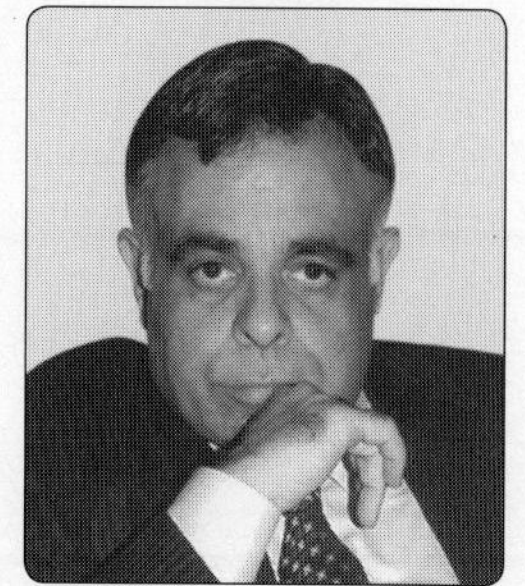

It is my pleasure to write a foreword for *Practical Pediatric Digest*. The editors of the book are very well-known authors and have been the forefront of producing excellent manuscripts for the Indian Academy of Pediatrics (IAP). The contents of the book show how well thought out the chapters are. I am sure with the group of wisemen, writing and editing this book it will be a part of the library of each pediatrician.

I congratulate the editors in this effort.

Anupam Sachdeva
National President
Elect IAP, 2016

Foreword

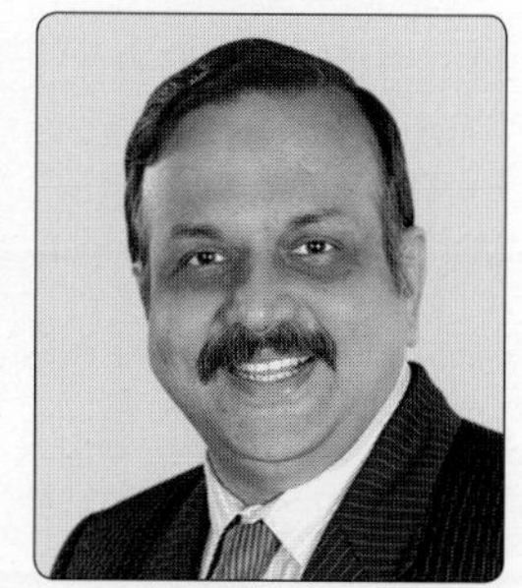

It is both a pleasure and a privilege to write a foreword for *Practical Pediatric Digest* published under the aegis of Chennai-City Branch of Indian Academy of Pediatrics (IAP), Tamil Nadu State Chapter (IAP–TNSC). The book with 14 chapters covering 42 topics has relevant clinical and significant diagnostic information, and can be comparable to the best available currently in the global market. As a digest, it reflects the intensive effort by contributors and reviewers, assuring the user of a broad and collective expertise.

I congratulate Dr A Parthasarathy (Editor-in-Chief), Dr A Somasundaram (Executive Editor), Dr P Sudhakar (Publication Editor), Drs PSN Menon, MKC Nair, K Nedunchelian, P Ramachandran (Chief Academic Editors) and the dedicated contributors for their magnanimous and magnificent effort in bringing out this remarkable book.

I also commend the office bearers of Chennai-City Branch of IAP–TNSC for their brilliant initiative in bringing out the book.

I am sure that this will become an indispensable tool for practicing pediatricians, neonatologists, undergraduates and postgraduates of pediatrics and academicians.

S Sachidananda Kamath
National President, IAP 2015

Foreword

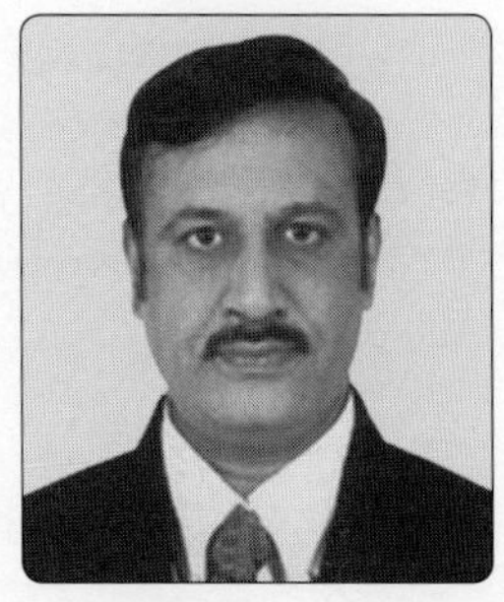

I am delighted to write this foreword for *Practical Pediatric Digest* brought out by Indian Academy of Pediatrics (IAP), Chennai-City Branch.

Going through the contents of the book, I am convinced that this book is useful for the practicing pediatricians as a desktop reference. All chapters are relevant and authors have taken great pains to present the recent advances in their respective fields.

I congratulate Dr A Parthasarathy (Editor-in-Chief), appropriately supported by Dr A Somasundaram, Dr P Sudhakar, and other editors for bringing this beautiful book.

I appreciate the publishers, M/s Jaypee Brothers Medical Publishers (P) Ltd, New Delhi, India, for bringing the book in a beautiful format.

Major K Nagaraju
President
Indian Academy of Pediatrics–Tamil Nadu State Chapter (IAP–TNSC), 2016
President, Pediatric Allergy Association of India
Professor
Allergy and Clinical Immunology
Saveetha Medical College and Hospital, Chennai
Director
VN Allergy and Asthma Research Center
Chennai, Tamil Nadu

Foreword

Ignited minds are the most powerful resource on earth.

– Dr APJ Abdul Kalam

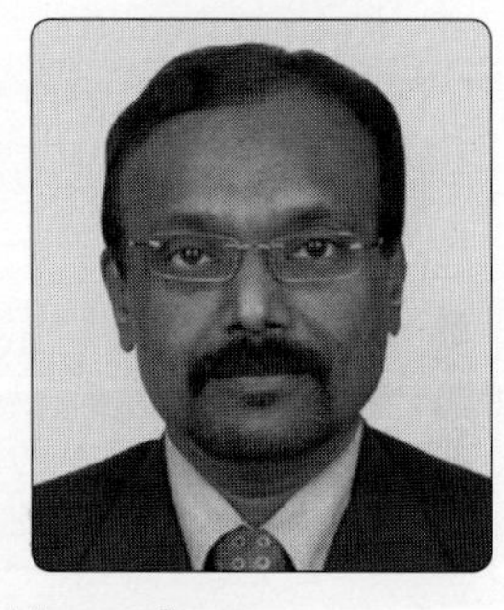

True to these thoughts, the *Practical Pediatric Digest* designed to be a practical and easy-to-use ready-reckoner, providing a plethora of knowledge and information in a simple-lucid format to the busy practicing pediatricians in their day-to-day practice. It is not an exhaustive reflection, instead it provides a concise summary of the most common disorders in children.

Practical Pediatric Digest stands proud with the focus on applications and exercises, and discussion of all pediatric problems that call for retrieval and integration of prior knowledge. I am sure that this book will be very useful for undergraduates, postgraduates, and also to busy consultants to give the much-needed confidence in each field written by various competitive authors.

The articles contributed by experts in their respective fields are written in a simple and easy-to-understand format, and have taken pains to give updated information in the reader-friendly manner. I congratulate the various editors for having done the excellent job in choosing the right topics in the related field. I also deeply appreciate their extraordinary efforts, their dedications and commitments to excellence under the noble leadership of its Editor-in-Chief, Dr A Parthasarathy.

I thank one and all involved in this venture and bringing out the book on the eve of MAMMALLA PEDICON 2016, this honor at this stage the *Indian Academy of Pediatrics (IAP)–Chennai City Branch.*

R Somasekar
Professor
Department of Pediatrics
Institute of Child Health and Hospital for Children
Madras Medical College, Chennai, Tamil Nadu
President
Indian Academy of Pediatrics–Chennai City Branch (IAP–CCB)

Preface

Medical learning is a continuous process. Apart from the theory we learnt during our undergraduate and postgraduate trainings, we gain our own experience and practical knowledge during subsequent office/hospital practice, and also through various continuing medical educations (CMEs) about the latest trends in the diagnosis and management of common and uncommon pediatric illnesses, and update ourselves with new knowledge. Thus 'we learn to unlearn only to re-learn and thus continue to learn.'

With this objective in mind of educating the practicing and upcoming pediatricians, faculties and medical students, the Chennai-City branch of the Tamil Nadu State Chapter of Indian Academy of Pediatrics (IAP) regularly organizes at least one CME a month and an annual mega CME every year to benefit the delegates who attend them. Many who could not attend felt that they should also get the experts' views and update themselves. None other than our Editor-in-Chief gave the idea of coming out with a book containing all the topics discussed. And that is how the *Practical Pediatric Digest* is born with selected topics of practical guidelines.

This book contains 14 chapters with 42 topics discussed during the three annual mega CMEs conducted during the years 2013, 2014 and 2015 in about 300 pages presented in a 'reader-friendly' format, which have undergone 3 levels of reviews and edited by 'eagle-eyed' expert editors. It is our fervent hope that the topics presented will benefit you in your day-to-day practice. Kindly pass on your feedback to us so that we can improve upon the contents in the future editions of the book.

A Parthasarathy
A Somasundaram
P Sudhakar

Acknowledgments

The editorial board would like to place on record its appreciation and gratitude to all editors who responded with their fine-tuned manuscripts on time enabling the publishers to bring out the book on schedule.

The Editor-in-Chief thanks all members of the editorial board—the Associate, Academic and Chief Academic Editors for their 'eagle-eye' review and edit remarks at the 3 levels of reviews and editing process which have been incorporated with author approval. In particular, the services rendered by the Executive Editor and the Publication Editor in getting the manuscripts from authors on time and the production department of M/s Jaypee Brothers Medical Publishers (P) Ltd (Health Sciences Publishers), New Delhi, India, for formatting and obtaining approval for the proofs from respective authors within a short span of time.

For secretarial and correspondence assistance, the Editor-in-Chief would like to thank Mrs Nirmala, Dr (Mrs) Pathibha, Mrs Kavitha, Dr (Ms) Shruthi Pavana, Miss Swathi Pavana, Miss Kavya, Miss Mahiya, Mr R Janardhanan, Mr P Balaji, (Late) Mr A Sriramulu, Chennai and Mr R Asokan, Thiruvananthapuram, Kerala, India. The Executive Editor is indebted and grateful to the services of Dr (Mrs) Kirupa Somasundaram.

The editorial board is indebted to Dr R Somasekar (President, IAP-CCB) and Dr S Babu (Secretary, IAP-CCB) for kind permission to publish the book and to all the National Presidents and the TNSC State President for their encouraging *Forewords*.

Our grateful thanks to Shri Jitendar P Vij (Group Chairman); Mr Ankit Vij (Group President); Mr Tarun Duneja (Director-Publishing); Mr KK Raman (Production Manager); Mrs Samina Khan (Executive Assistant to the Director-Publishing); Heena Gogia (Project Coordinator); Mohit Bhargava (Production Coordinator); and the team of M/s Jaypee Brothers Medical Publishers (P) Ltd, New Delhi, India, for printing and publishing the book at record time.

Contents

Plate 1

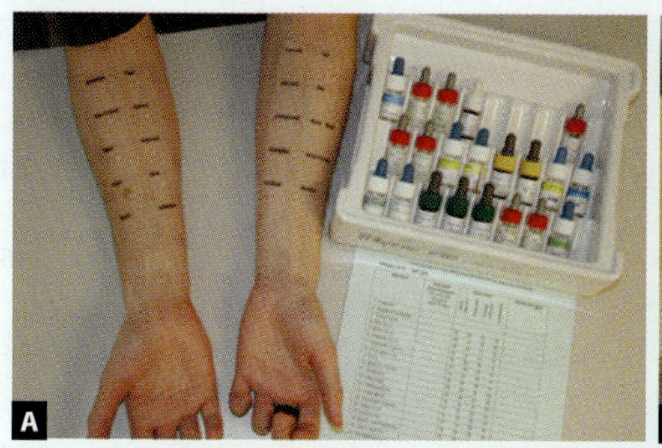

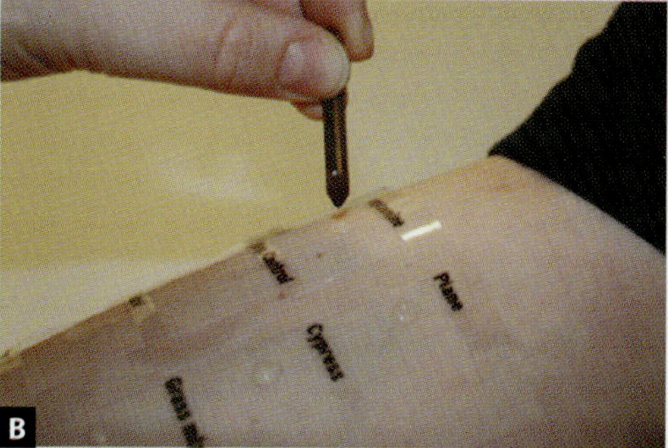

Figs 3.1.2A and B: Methodology of skin testing

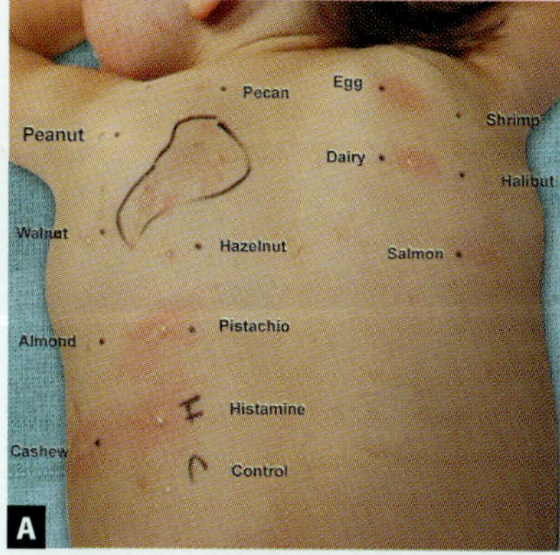

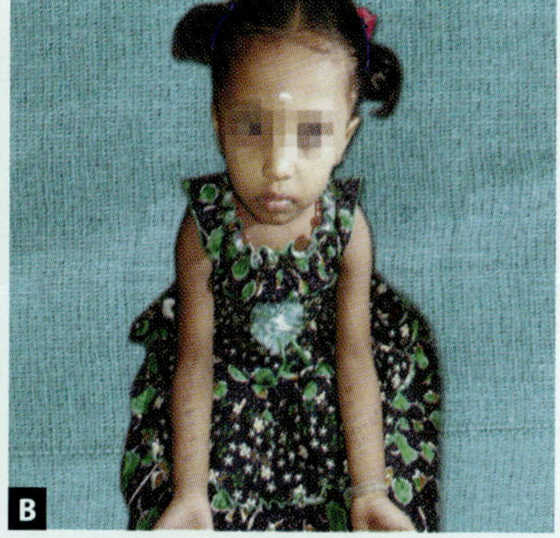

Figs 3.1.3A and B: Allergy skin testing in children

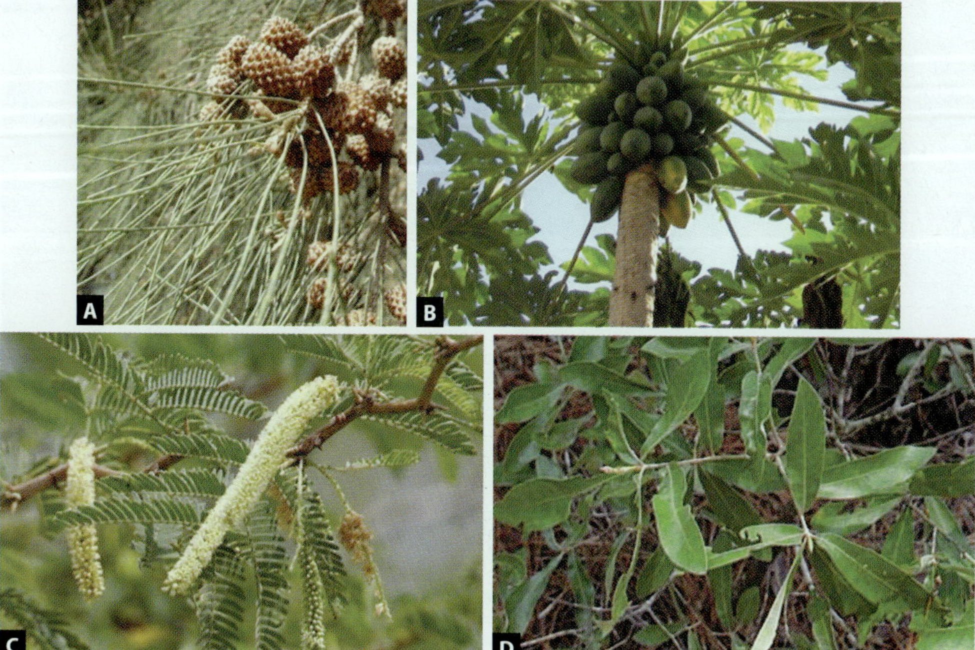

Figs 3.1.4A to D: (A) Casuarina; (B) Carica papaya; (C) Prosopis; (D) Quercus incana (Blue jack oak)

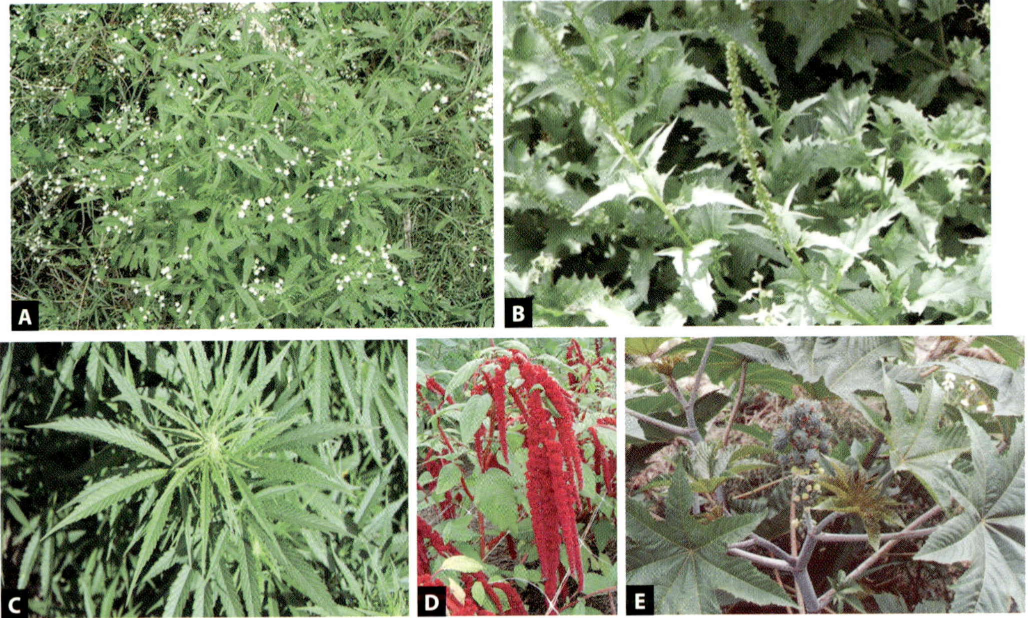

Figs 3.1.5A to E: (A) Parthenium; (B) Chenopodium; (C) Cannabis sativa; (D) Amaranthus; (E) Ricinus communis

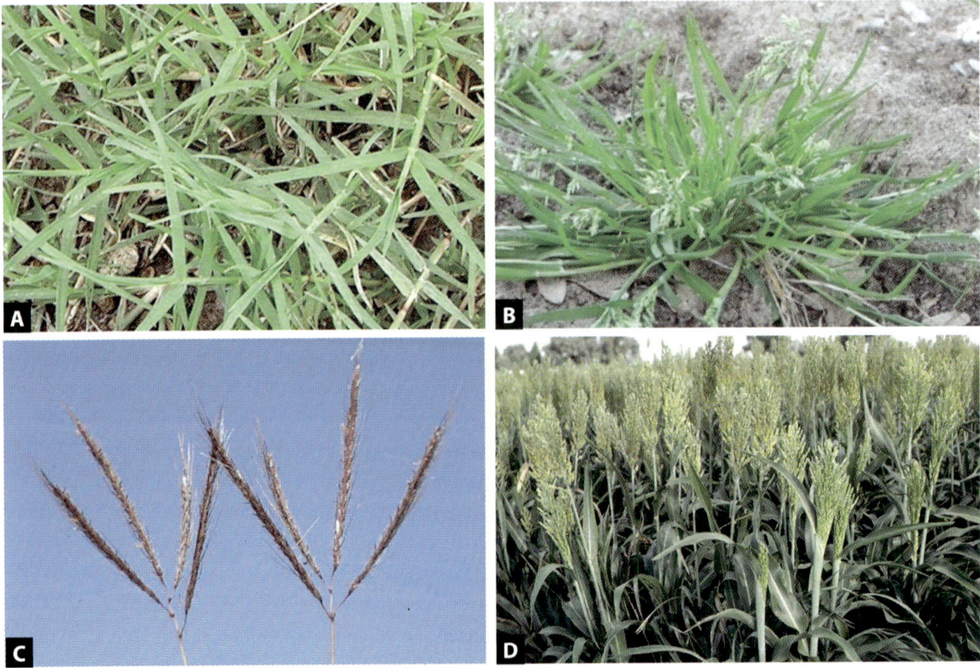

Figs 3.1.6A to D: (A) Cynodon; (B) Poa annum; (C) *Dicanthium annulatum*; (D) *Sorghum*

Plate 3

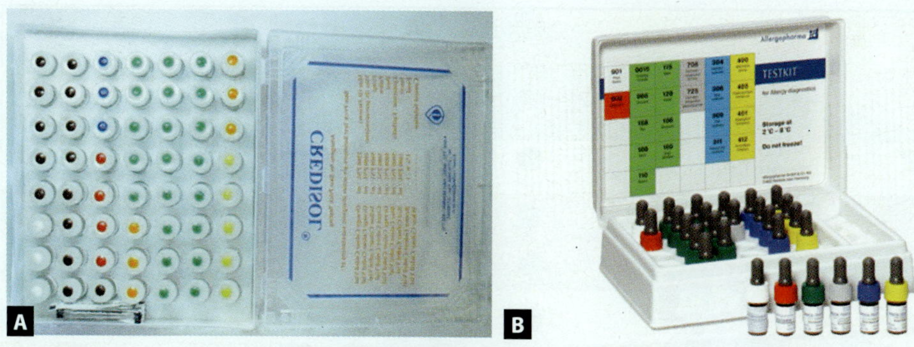

Figs 3.1.7A and B: Allergen skin testing kits available in India

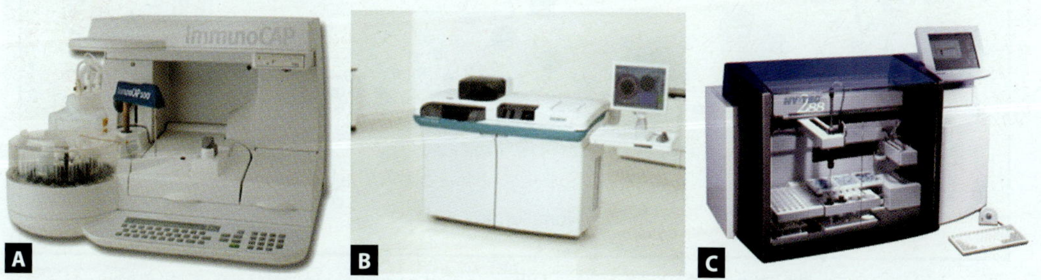

Figs 3.1.8A to C: Various systems with different techniques for doing allergen panel

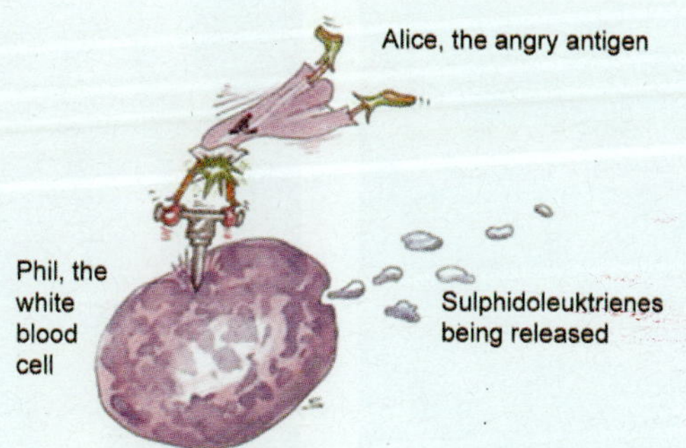

Fig. 3.1.9: Pictorial representation of CAST

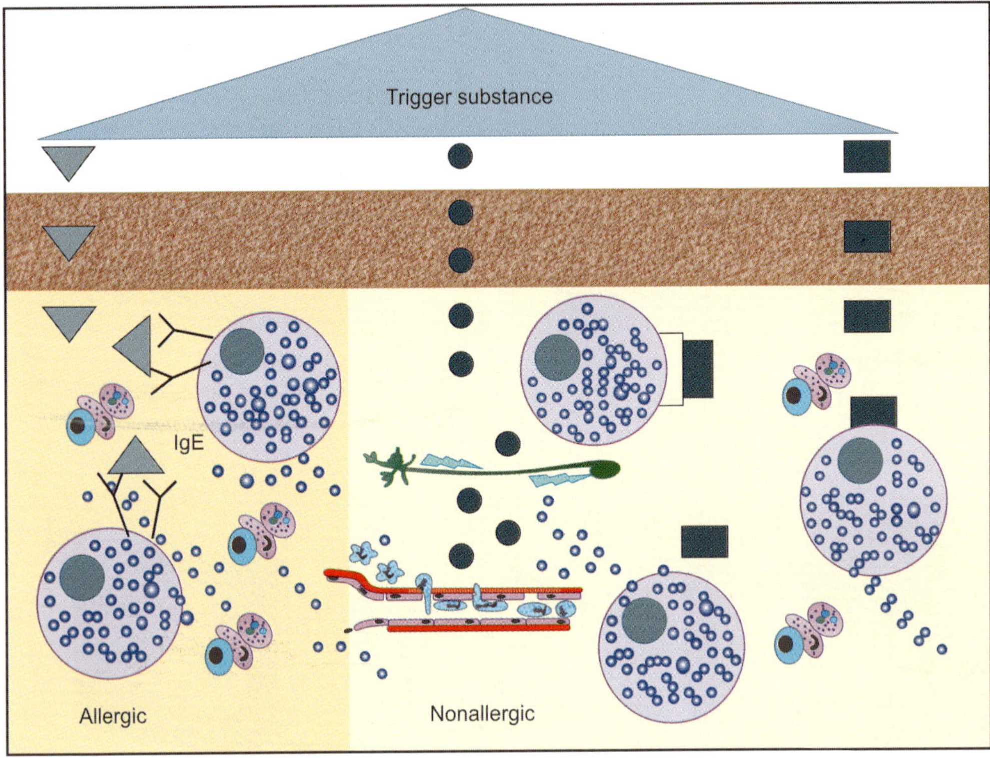

Fig. 3.2.1: Pathogenesis of allergic and non allergic urticaria

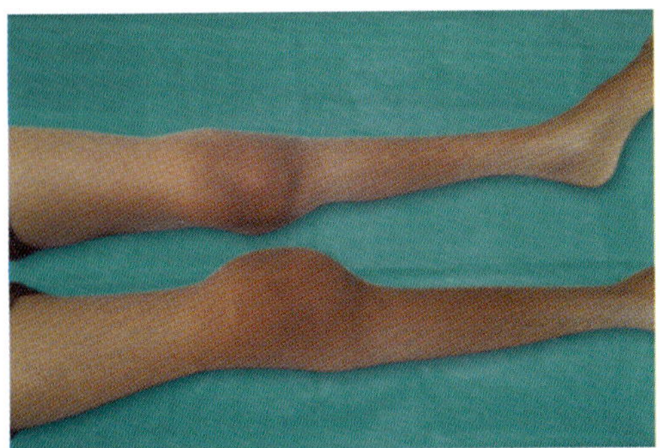

Fig. 3.3.1: Oligoarthritis right knee. The diagnosis in this scenario is most likely Oligoarticular JIA

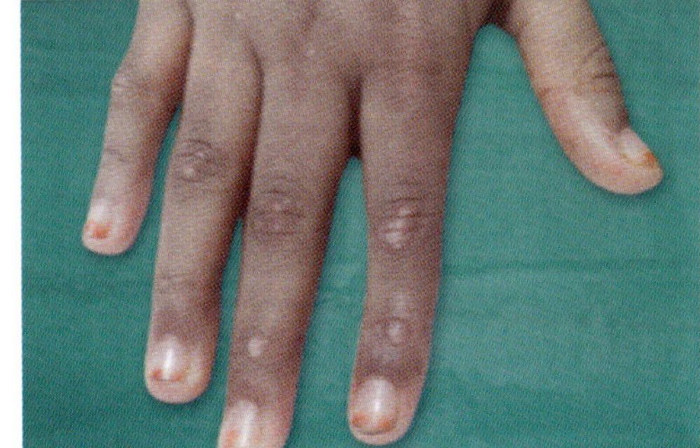

Fig. 3.3.2: Gottron's papules. The diagnosis is juvenile dermatomyositis

Plate 5

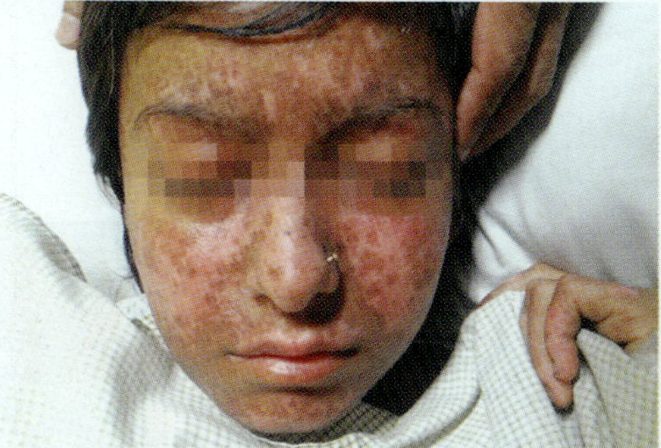

Fig. 3.3.3: SLE-malar rash. The diagnosis in this case is SLE

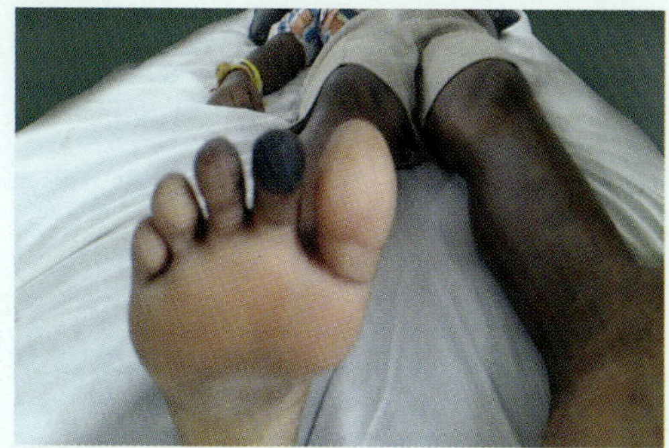

Fig. 3.3.4: Gangrene of right second toe in a child with suspected vasculitis (Discolored toe)

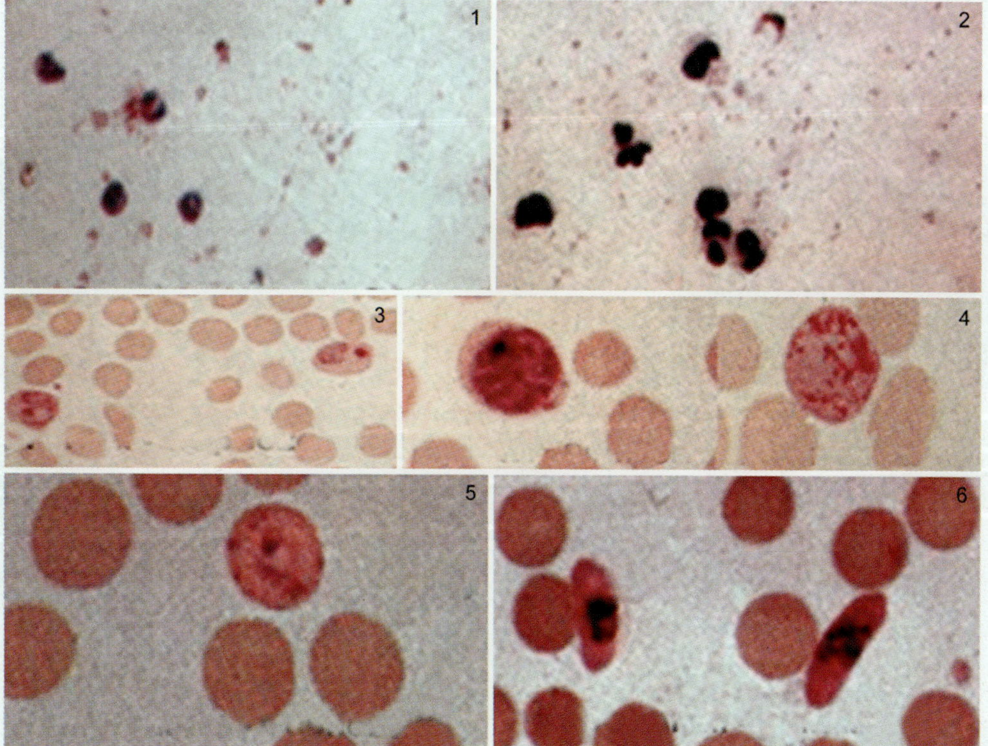

Fig. 4.1.1: Malarial parasites in light microscopy. (1) *P. vivax*—trophozoites and gametocytes, (2) *P. falciparum*—rings and gametocytes, (3) *P. vivax*—trophozoites, (4) *P. vivax*—schizont *P. vivax* gametocytes, (5) *P. falciparum*—trophozoites, (6) *P. falciparum*—gametocytes
Source: Approach to Malaria Diagnosis, TAG Archives: Rapid Diagnosis of Malaria. Srinivas/Feb.25.2015/Diagnosis. *www.malariasite.com*

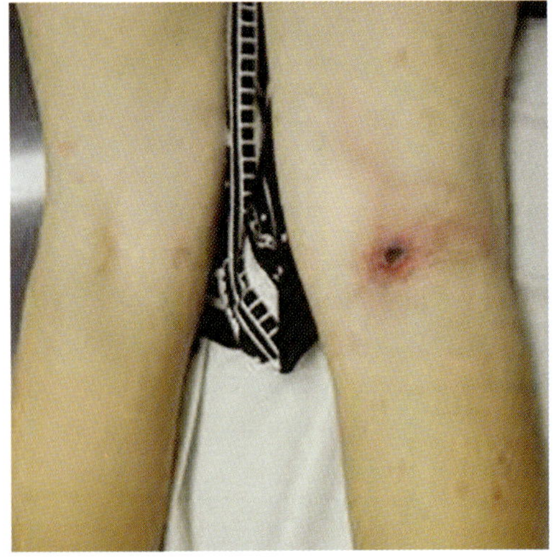

Fig. 4.2.4: Eschar in scrub typhus

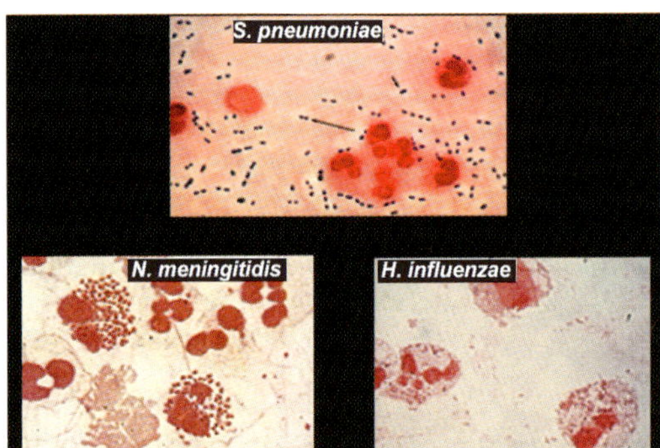

Fig. 5.3.1: Gram's staining (Direct Smear)

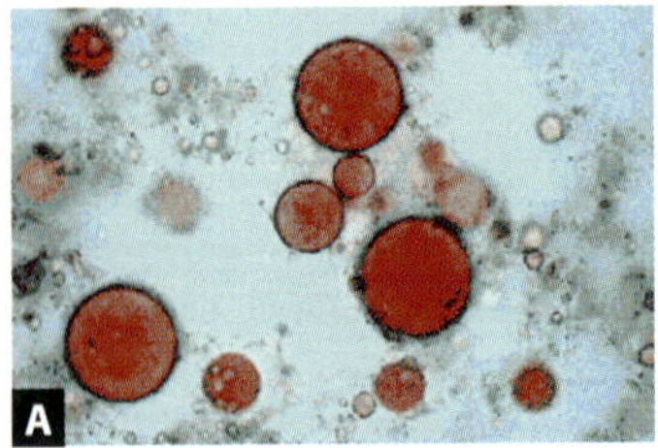

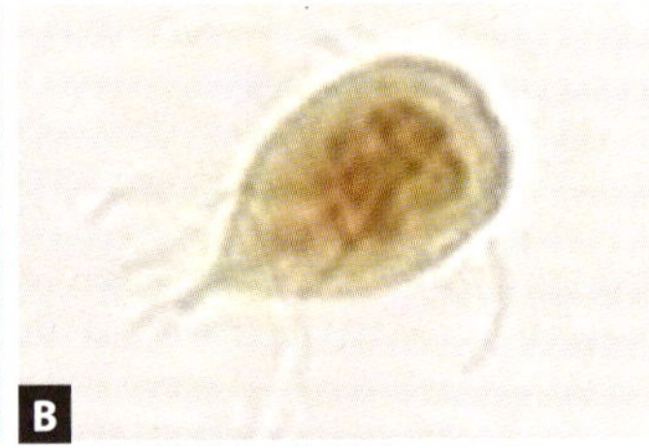

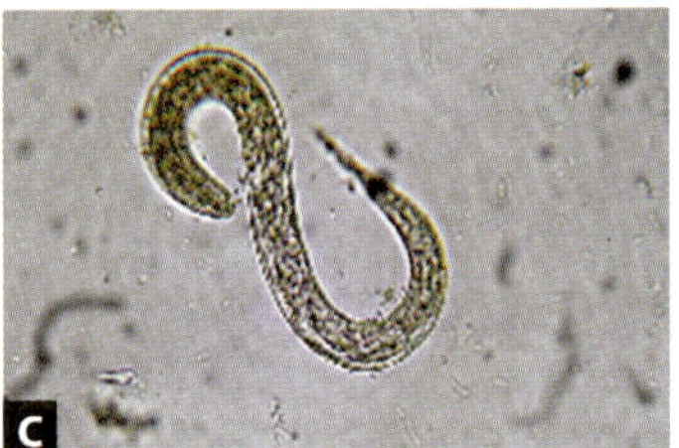

Figs 8.2.1A to C: Stool examination. (A) Stool fat globules; (B) *Giardia lamblia* trophozoite in stool; (C) Strongyloides stercoralis larva

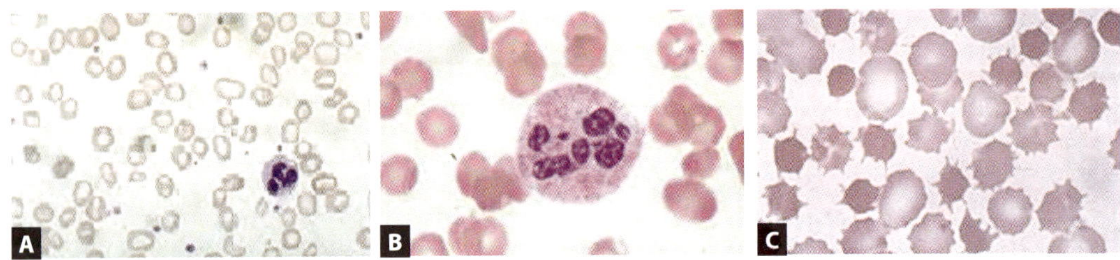

Figs 8.2.2A to C: Peripheral blood smear study. (A) Hypochromic microcytic anemia; (B) Macrocytic anemia; (C) Acanthocytes

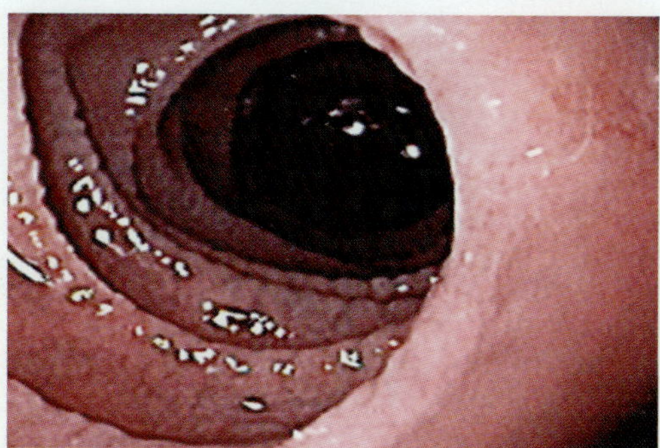

Fig. 8.2.3: Upper endoscopic view showing scalloping of duodenal folds

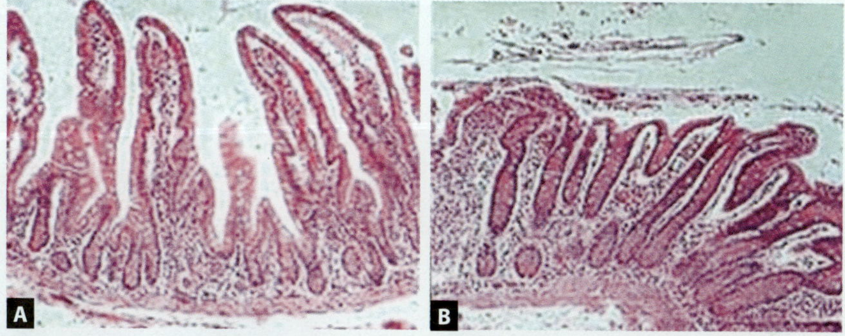

Figs 8.2.4A and B: Small bowel histology snowing normal and mucosal changes in celiac disease. (A) Normal mucosa; (B) Celiac disease

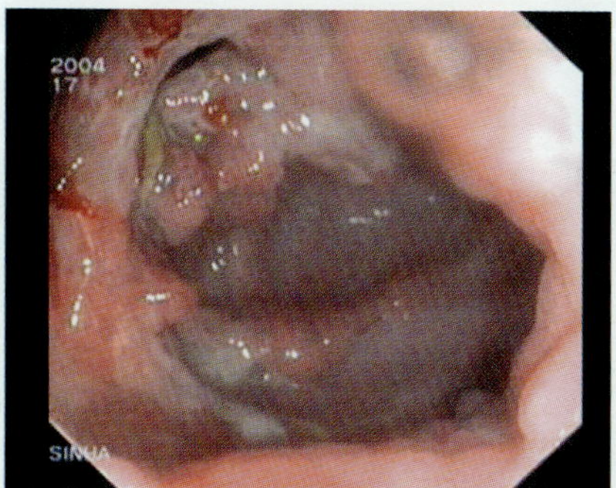

Fig. 8.2.5: Colonoscopy showing ulcer and nodularity of ileum

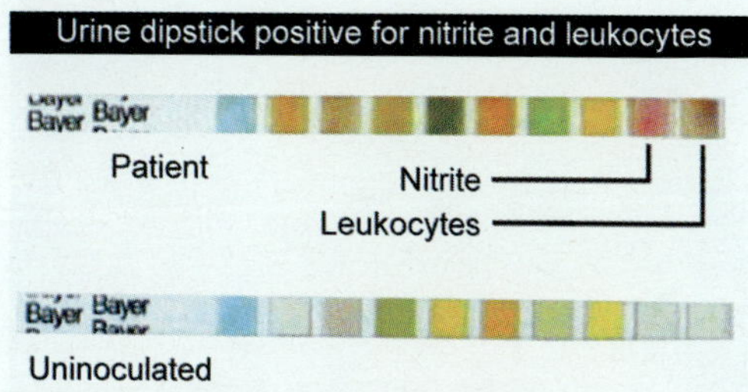

Fig. 9.2.1: Urine dipstick

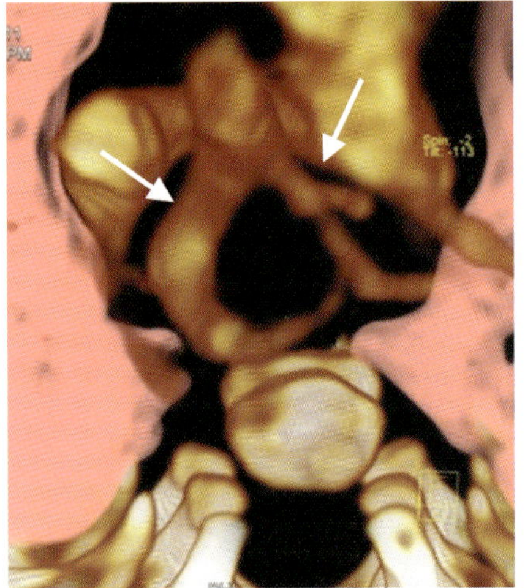

Fig. 13.3.22: 3D-VRT: Complete vascular ring

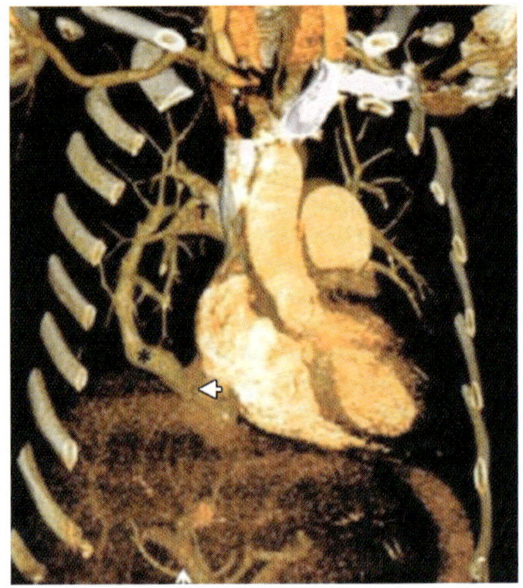

Fig. 13.3.23: 3D-VRT: Scimitar syndrome: Anomalous vein (arrowhead) draining the right lung into inferior vena cava (IVC)

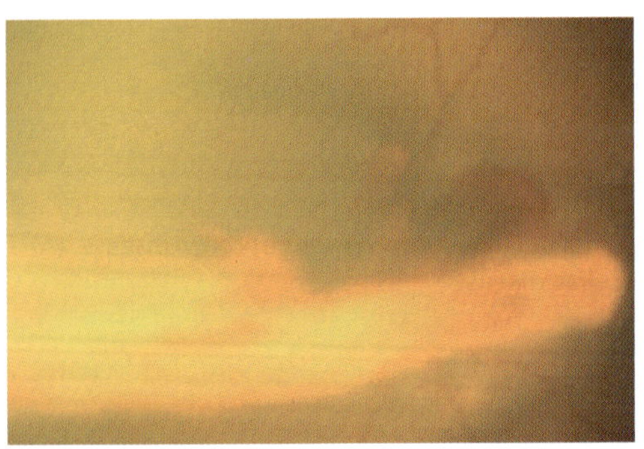

Fig. 14.2.2: Stage IVB ROP

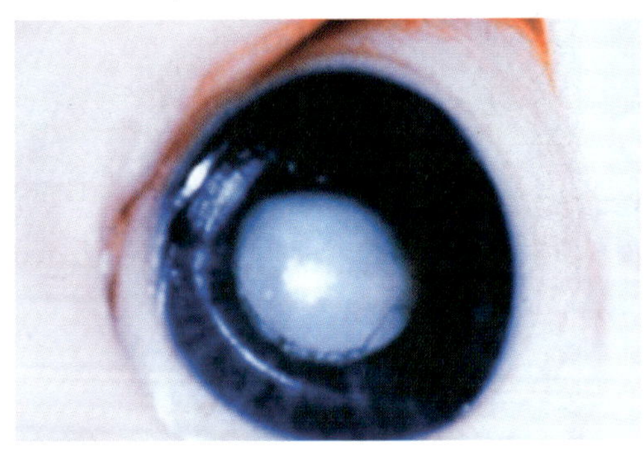

Fig. 14.2.3: Stage V ROP

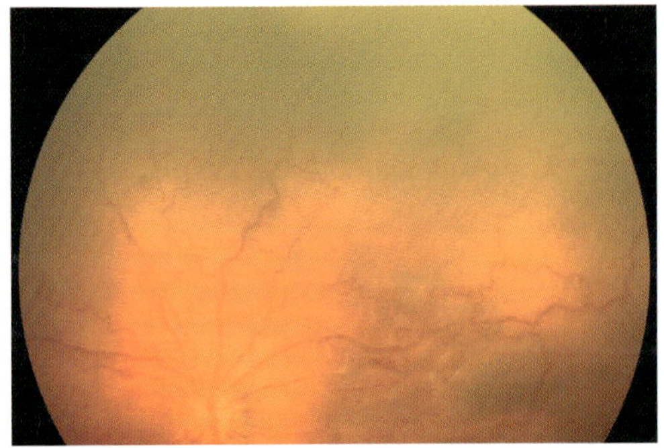

Fig. 14.2.4: AP ROP with plus disease and collaterals

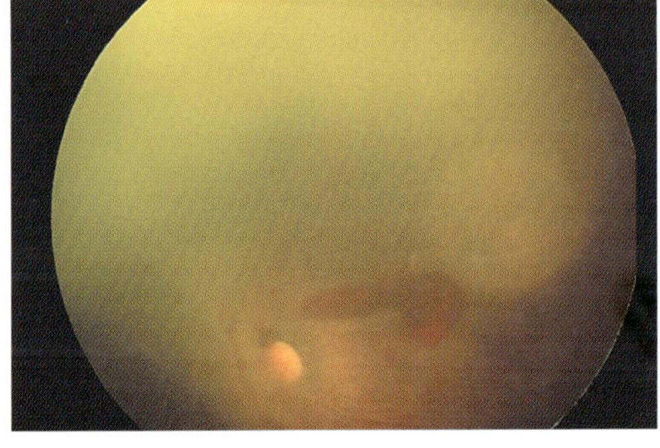

Fig. 14.2.5: Zone I ROP Stage III ROP involving all 12 clock hours with plus disease (Rush disease)

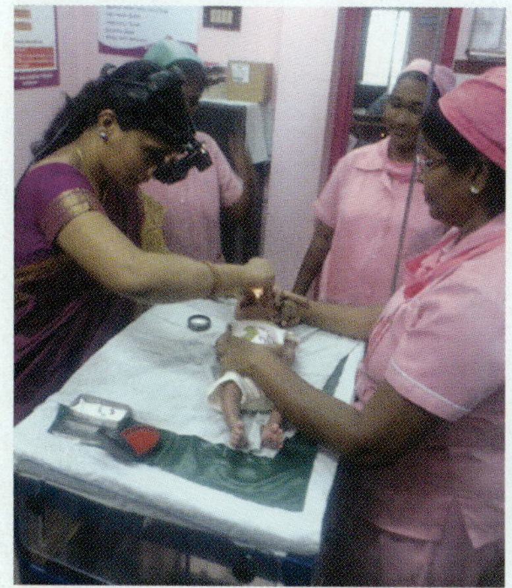

Fig. 14.2.6: ROP screening with indirect ophthalmoscope

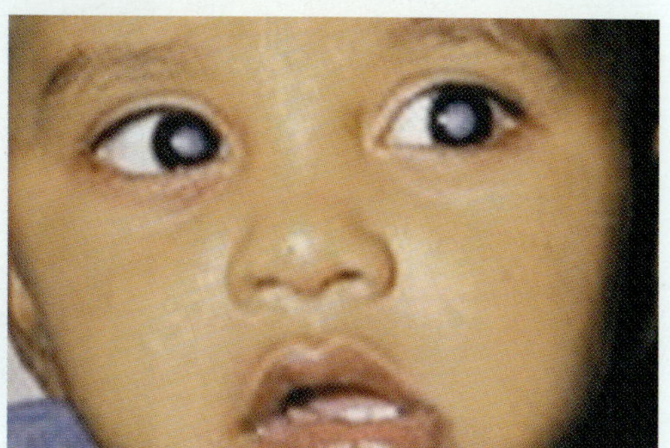

Fig. 14.2.7: Childhood cataract

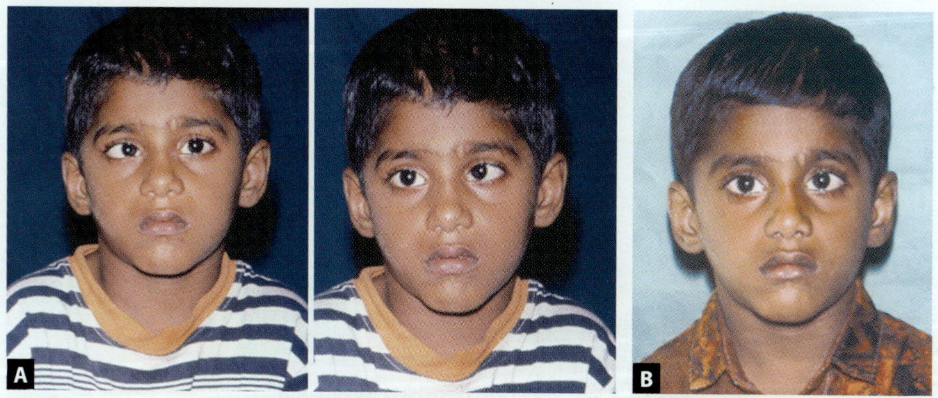

Figs 14.2.9A and B: Squint (A) Before surgery; (B) After surgery

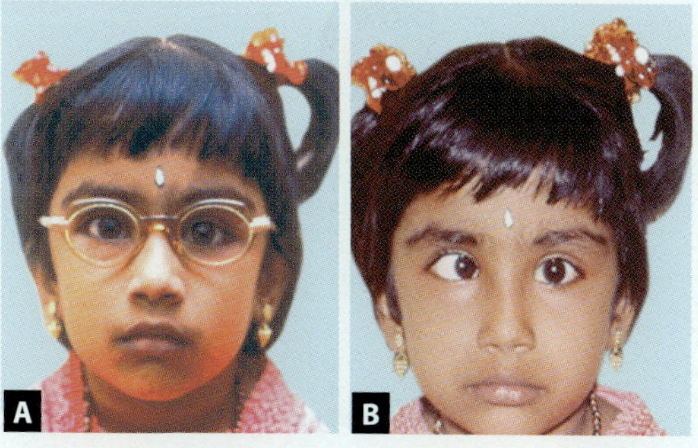

Figs 14.2.10A and B: Squint getting corrected with spectacles

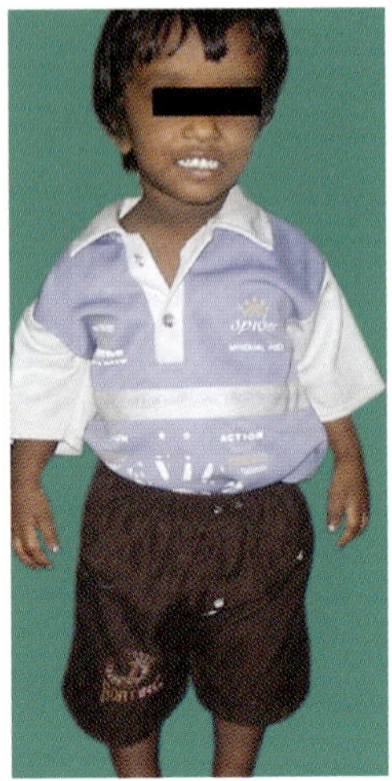

Fig. 14.3.1A: Achondroplasia showing the clinical features of rhizomelic short stature

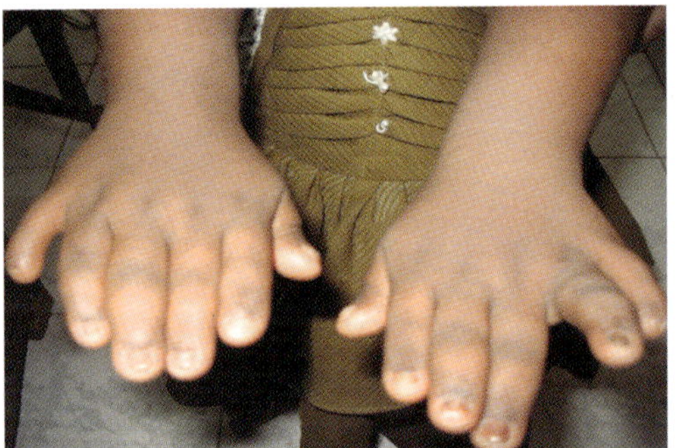

Fig 14.3.3A: Short-rib dysplasia group with polydactyly

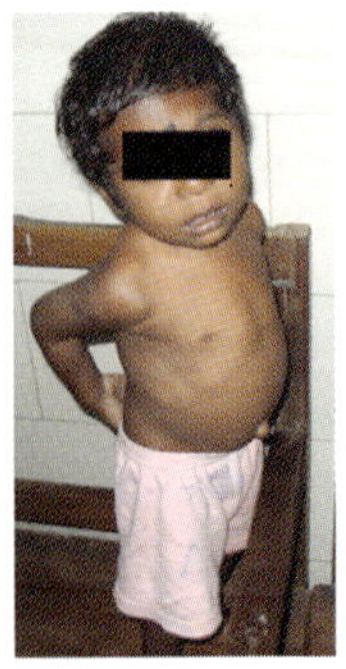

Fig. 14.3.6A: Dyggve-Melchior Clausen dysplasia

Newborn

Reviewers: *PSN Menon, Alok Gupta, R Remesh Kumar, K Nedunchelian, Jaydeep Choudhury, RV Dhakshayani*

1.1 Neonatal Sepsis Screen

Giridhar Sethuraman, Satish Datla
Reviewers: *PSN Menon, Alok Gupta, R Remesh Kumar*

INTRODUCTION

Neonatal sepsis is a common and dreaded cause of morbidity and mortality in newborns. As per the National Neonatal Perinatal Database (NNPD) 2002–2003, the incidence of neonatal sepsis in India was 30 per 1000 livebirths. It is 3% among intramural and 39.7% among extramural admissions. Early diagnosis of sepsis is vital for ensuring good short-term and long-term clinical outcomes.

Unfortunately, signs of neonatal sepsis are nonspecific and require a high index of suspicion. There is no single diagnostic test with 100% sensitivity and specificity. Blood culture or isolation of pathogenic organisms from normally sterile body spaces is the gold standard for diagnosis of neonatal sepsis. But the rate of culture positivity is low, which is influenced by factors such as intrapartum antimicrobial administration and low bacterial load. Conversely, positive cultures may be due to contamination. Supplemental diagnostic tests based on evaluation of immune response often can help resolve ambiguities in these situations. In this article, we review the role of conventional and commonly available diagnostic tests—cultures, blood counts, acute phase reactants, inflammatory mediator levels and molecular assays in the diagnosis of neonatal sepsis.

CULTURES

Blood Culture

A blood culture should be performed in all neonates with suspicion of sepsis (**Flow chart 1.1.1**). Blood can be drawn from peripheral vein or artery puncture. Sterilization of sampling site should involve cleansing for at least 30 seconds or two consecutive cleansings. Alcoholic solutions of chlorhexidine or povidone-iodine are preferred. Sampling from newly placed umbilical catheters can also be used. Always ensure a blood volume of at least 1 mL is sampled, in order to account for low level bacteremia. A single pediatric (not adult) blood culture bottle inoculated with adequate blood volume is sufficient. As anaerobic organisms are rarely implicated in neonatal sepsis, the entire specimen should be used for aerobic culture. Manual culture methods, relying on development of turbidity in broth, are adequate and yield 96% positivity after 48 hours and 98% positivity at 72 hours. Automated culture methods with a turnover time of ≤36 hours are acceptable alternatives, if available.

Cerebrospinal Fluid Culture

A lumbar puncture (LP) should be considered for examination of the cerebrospinal fluid (CSF) in any septic neonate before initiation of therapy. Up to 15% of infants with sepsis have accompanying meningitis. LP should be performed in infants with clinical signs of sepsis (except in preterm infants presenting with signs of RDS), in infants with positive blood culture, in infants whose clinical course and lab values strongly suggest bacterial sepsis, and in infants who clinically worsen even on antibiotics. Asymptomatic babies being investigated for maternal risk factors need not undergo LP. CSF evaluation can be deferred till the neonate is stable, if the neonate is critically ill or likely to suffer cardiovascular or respiratory compromise from the procedure.

CSF values indicative of meningitis are controversial. Until more data are available, it would appear prudent to consider meningitis

Flow chart 1.1.1: Evaluation of a neonate with sepsis

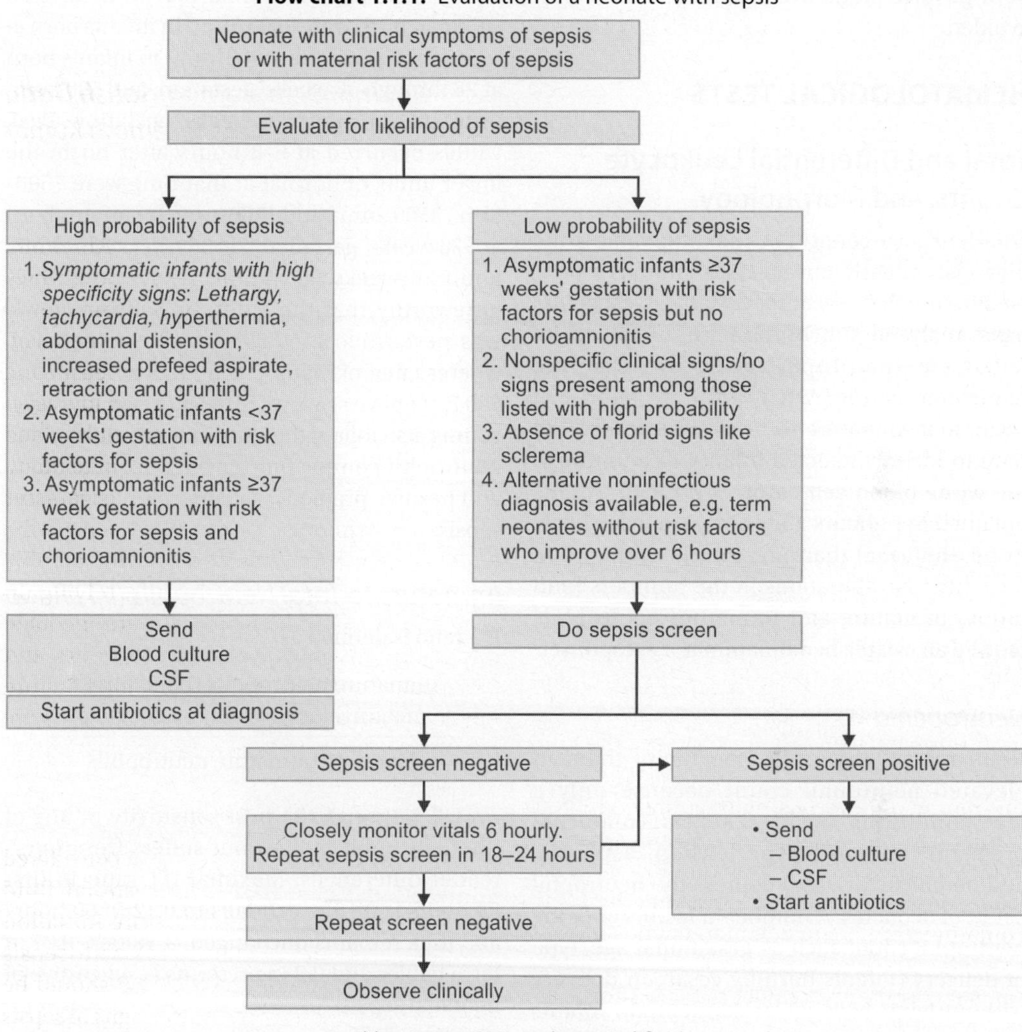

Abbreviation: CSF, cerebrospinal fluid.

in infants with white blood cells in excess of 20/mm^3 or a protein level in excess of 100 mg/dL in the CSF. In the normoglycemic newborn infant, glucose concentrations in CSF are similar to those in older infants and children (70–80% of a simultaneously obtained blood specimen). A low glucose concentration is the CSF variable with the greatest specificity for the diagnosis of meningitis. In case of a traumatic tap, one should send for culture as cell counts and biochemical analysis become unreliable, even with correction of CSF white blood cell count for the red blood cells.

Other Body Fluid Cultures

A suprapubic or catheterized urine sample should be cultured in case of late onset sepsis (>72 hours). The yield is very low in case of early onset sepsis. Neonates at risk for fungal sepsis and very low birth weight (VLBW) infants with poor weight gain should also have a urine culture. Cultures of tracheal aspirate specimens should be obtained immediately after endotracheal tube placement and not after 12 hours as the trachea quickly becomes colonized after intubation. Bacterial cultures of the axilla, groin, and the external ear canal have poor positive predictive accuracy and are best avoided.

HEMATOLOGICAL TESTS

Total and Differential Leukocyte Counts, and Morphology

Total leukocyte count (TLC) has little value in the diagnosis of early-onset sepsis and has a poor positive predictive accuracy. Many investigators have analyzed subcomponents of the white leukocyte (neutrophil indices)—absolute neutrophil count (ANC), absolute band cell count and immature to total neutrophil (I/T) ratio to identify infected infants. The timing of the white blood cell count is critical. Counts obtained 6–12 hours after birth are more likely to be abnormal than are counts obtained at birth because alterations in the numbers (and ratios) of mature and immature neutrophils require an established inflammatory response.

Neutropenia

Neutropenia has better specificity than an elevated neutrophil count because only a few conditions besides sepsis (maternal pregnancy-induced hypertension, asphyxia, and hemolytic disease) depress the neutrophil count of neonates. A number of factors alter the neutrophil count such as gestational age, type of delivery (infants born by cesarean delivery without labor have lower counts than infants delivered vaginally), site of sampling (neutrophil counts are lower in samples from arterial blood), and altitude (infants born at elevated altitudes have higher total neutrophil counts).

In late preterm and term infants, the definition for neutropenia most commonly used is that suggested by Manroe et al. (<1800/mm^3 at birth and <7800/mm^3 at 12–14 hours of age). In 1994, the same group published new information on neutrophil concentrations specifically from VLBW neonates. The range of counts differed from that of higher gestation neonates, with a wider range of distribution. Schmutz et al. reinvestigated these reference ranges using modern cell-counting instrumentation in 30254 infants born at 23–42 weeks' gestation. In this study, the lower limits of normal for neutrophil values at birth were 3500/mm^3 in infants born at >36 weeks' gestation, 1000/mm^3 in infants born at 28 through 36 weeks' gestation, and 500/mm^3 in infants born at <28 weeks' gestation. Peak values occurred at 6–8 hours after birth; the lower limits of normal at that time were 7500/mm^3, 3500/mm^3, and 1500/mm^3 for infants born at >36 weeks' gestation, 28–36 weeks' gestation, and <28 weeks' gestation, respectively. It is noteworthy that the study by Schmutz et al. was performed at 4800 feet above sea level, whereas that of Manroe et al. was performed at 500 feet above sea level. Absolute immature cell counts also follow the same pattern as absolute neutrophil counts, but have a poor sensitivity and positive predictive accuracy for early-onset sepsis.

Immature to Total Neutrophils (I/T) Ratio

I/T ratio is defined as:

$$\frac{\text{Immature neutrophils (band forms, metamyelocytes and myelocytes)}}{\text{Mature + Immature neutrophils}}$$

I/T ratio has the best sensitivity of any of the neutrophil indices but suffers from inter-reader differences. Maximal I/T ratio in first 24 hours is 0.16 which falls to 0.12 in 60 hours and then remains unchanged. A value > 0.27 in term babies and 0.2 in preterms is suggestive of neonatal sepsis.

Platelet Counts

Low platelet counts in infected infants are a nonspecific, insensitive and late indicator of sepsis. Platelet counts are not useful in clinical response to antimicrobial agents as they mostly remain depressed for days.

ACUTE PHASE REACTANTS (Figure 1.1.1)

Microerythrocyte Sedimentation Rate

Microerythrocyte sedimentation rate (μ-ESR) is a rapid bedside investigation for neonatal sepsis but suffers from low accuracy. In this

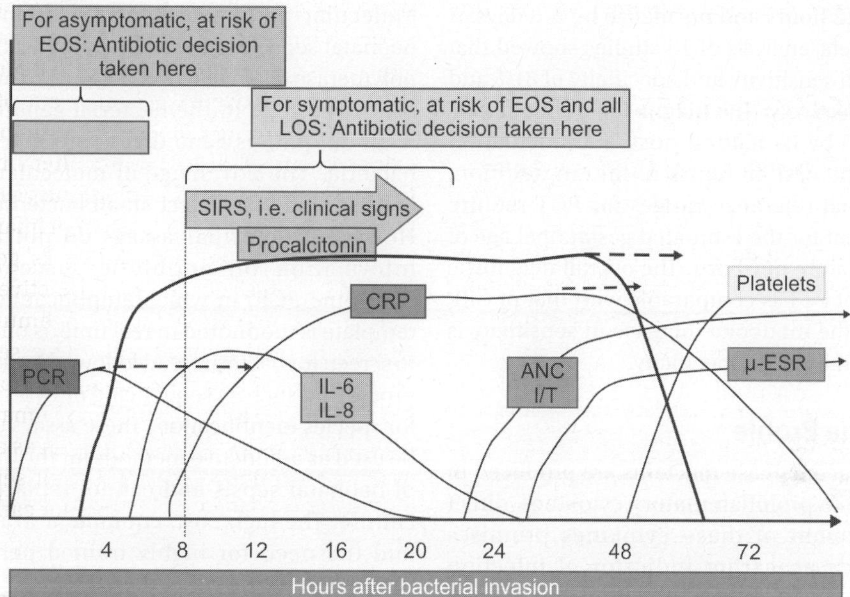

Fig. 1.1.1: Acute phase reactants and systemic responses to infection
Characteristic changes in acute phase reactants, hematological tests and other systemic responses after an inflammatory stimulus.
Abbreviations: ANC, absolute neutrophil count; CRP, C-reactive protein; EOS, early onset sepsis; ESR, erythrocyte sedimentation rate; IL-6, interleukin 6; IL-8, interleukin 8; I/T, immature to total neutrophil ratio; LOS, late onset sepsis; PCR, polymerase chain reaction; SIRS, systemic inflammatory response syndrome.

test, capillary blood is collected in a standard pre-heparinized micro-hematocrit tube (75 mm length, internal diameter 1.1 mm and outer diameter of 1.5 mm) and the fall of erythrocyte column after 1 hour is read. A 1-hour value more than the age of the baby in days + 3 in the first 2 weeks of life or >15 mm is suggestive of infection.

C-reactive Protein

Serum C-reactive protein (CRP) is one of the most useful of the acute phase reactants for assisting in the diagnosis of neonatal sepsis. CRP is synthesized within 6–8 hours of exposure to an infective process or tissue damage, peaks at around 36–48 hours and has a half-life of 19 hours. Most surveys have shown that CRP is a "specific" but "late" marker of neonatal infection. The cut-off value in neonates is 10 mg/L.

A number of factors are to be considered while interpreting CRP. Sensitivity of serial CRP testing is lower for bacteremia due to gram-positive than to gram-negative bacteria, with the sensitivity for detecting coagulase negative staphylococci being as low as 55%. CRP values can exceed 10 mg/L, especially after vaginal delivery that involves instrumentation. False-positive CRP elevation also occurs in infants born to women with chorioamnionitis as well as those with viral infections, birth asphyxia, respiratory distress syndrome, intracerebral hemorrhage and meconium aspiration pneumonia. Serial CRP values are better with negative predictive value of upto 99% indicating that if CRP determinations remain persistently normal, it is strong evidence that bacterial sepsis is unlikely and antibiotics can be safely discontinued.

Procalcitonin

Procalcitonin (PCT) is now available as another rapid diagnostic test for neonatal sepsis. PCT levels increase rapidly by 2 hours of an infection, peak by 12 hours and normalize by 2–3 days. A recent meta-analysis of 16 studies showed that PCT has a sensitivity and specificity of 81% and 79% respectively. The diagnostic utility of PCT is limited by its natural postnatal fluctuation during the first 48 hours of life. In addition, the normal reference ranges for PCT require adjustment for the estimated gestational age of the premature newborn. The overall diagnostic efficacy of PCT is comparable with that of CRP because the moderate increase in sensitivity is offset by the lack of specificity.

Cytokine Profile

Because acute phase reactants are produced in response to proinflammatory cytokines, direct measurement of these cytokines promises to provide an earlier indicator of infection than could be achieved by measurement of secondary responses. The levels of these cytokines, interleukin 6 (IL-6) and 8 (IL-8) increase rapidly with bacterial sepsis, but normalize early in serum within the first 24 hours, limiting their use as clinical markers. In our country, these tests are not routinely done outside research settings.

COMBINATION OF TESTS

Compared to a single test, a sepsis screen panel, containing a combination of tests provides improved diagnostic accuracy. Traditionally, the sepsis screen consists of four tests: CRP, ANC, I/T ratio and μ-ESR. The purpose of the sepsis screen is to *rule out rather than to rule in* sepsis. In other words, the panel might be of value in deciding which "high-risk" healthy-appearing neonates do not need antimicrobial agents or whether therapy can be safely discontinued.

MOLECULAR TECHNIQUES

Advances in molecular microbiology has brought us newer molecular assays with the potential to diagnose sepsis rapidly and reliably. Molecular pathogen detection methods for neonatal sepsis are based on amplification, e.g. polymerase chain reaction (PCR). PCR amplifies 16S rRNA gene in the bacterial genome. This is an ubiquitous gene that is preserved in all bacteria. The advantage of molecular assays is their ability to detect small bacterial loads. However, molecular assays do not provide information on antibiotic susceptibility. Real-time PCR, in which amplification of the template is monitored in real time, is often used to screen for bacterial load followed by post-PCR processing such as sequencing or hybridization for species identification. These assays can best be used as adjunctive methods for the diagnosis of neonatal sepsis and cannot replace blood culture. The high cost, equipment availability and the need for highly trained personnel, precludes routine use of these assays.

SUMMARY

Blood and sterile body fluid culture continues to remain as the gold standard test for diagnosing neonatal sepsis. A number of rapid diagnostic tests for neonatal sepsis have been evaluated. The hematological tests, especially neutrophil indices, are useful tests but suffer from low diagnostic accuracy when used singly. The acute phase reactants CRP and PCT are popular and have been evaluated across large studies. CRP has high specificity and serial CRP has good negative predictive value and has been demonstrated to be reliable marker for safe discontinuation of antibiotics. PCT has better sensitivity than CRP but its utility is complicated by the natural physiological rise after birth and the need for age-specific normative reference values. Molecular pathogen detection methods based on PCR have high sensitivity and specificity but do not have sufficient diagnostic accuracy to replace culture. Combination of tests including hematological indices and acute phase reactants has better diagnostic utility compared to individual tests.

BIBLIOGRAPHY

1. Benitz WE. Adjunctive laboratory tests in the diagnosis of early-onset neonatal sepsis. Clin Perinatol. 2010;37(2):421-38.
2. Benitz WE, Han MY, Madan A, Ramachandra P. Serial serum C-reactive protein levels in the diagnosis of neonatal infection. Pediatrics. 1998;102(4):e41.
3. National Neonatology Forum: Evidence-based Clinical Practice Guidelines. Management of neonatal sepsis. 2010. pp. 155-72.
4. Pammi M, Flores A, Leeflang M, Versalovic J. Molecular assays in the diagnosis of neonatal sepsis: a systematic review and meta-analysis. Pediatrics. 2011;128(4):e973-85.
5. Polin RA. Committee on Fetus and Newborn. Management of neonates with suspected or proven early-onset bacterial sepsis. Pediatrics. 2012;129(5):1006-15.
6. Schmutz N, Henry E, Jopling J, Christensen RD. Expected ranges for blood neutrophil concentrations of neonates: the Manroe and Mouzinho charts revisited. J Perinatol. 2008; 28(4):275-81.

1.2 Screening for Inborn Errors of Metabolism

S Mangalabharathi

Reviewers: *K Nedunchelian, Jaydeep Choudhury, RV Dhakshayani*

WHAT IS NEWBORN SCREENING FOR INBORN ERRORS OF METABOLISM?

Newborn screening is a set of blood tests done at birth to look for evidence of certain common endocrine and genetic disorders. It has the potential to identify risk of such diseases even before the appearance of clinical symptoms. Newborn screening (NBS) is conceived as a public health program in which every newborn is tested for early identification of a selective panel of disorders based on the premise that early intervention of the affected newborn before symptomatic disease sets in, will lead to a significant reduction in mortality and associated disabilities.

WHY IS NEWBORN SCREENING IMPORTANT?

- Inborn errors of metabolism (IEM) presentations are not straight-forward and often critical
- Initial symptoms are extremely nonspecific
- Untreated individuals have significant morbidity and/or mortality
- Early treatment improves the longevity and quality of life and reduces the financial burden.

IS NEWBORN SCREENING REQUIRED IN INDIAN SCENARIO?

While the individual diseases are rare, they collectively account for a significant proportion of neonatal and childhood morbidity and mortality. About 4% of the population in India suffer from mental retardation and 5–15% of the sick newborns have a metabolic problem. It is estimated that 1 in 2000 Indian newborns suffer at birth from some kind of metabolic disorder. Investigations are expensive. Cost of treatment is prohibitive and many modalities are not easily available. Late diagnosis and treatment takes its toll on the quality of life.

The thrust in India in the past decade was prevention of recurrence by prenatal diagnosis

(PND) and termination of affected pregnancies in families having an affected child. However, recently an increasing number of individuals with IEM especially lysosomal storage disorders (LSDs) are being treated. There is an urgent need in India to examine scope for newborn screening for IEM. Early detection and early treatment can prevent mental retardation, spasticity, serious illness, and premature death. The planning of prenatal diagnostic services and newborn screening should take into consideration the common disorders prevalent in the country.

WHAT ARE THE IEMs TO BE SCREENED?

Every country should design its own panel of screening tests. The decision depends not only upon the prevalence of IEMs but on many other factors. The criteria put forward by Wilson and Juegner is a very useful one.

Wilson and Juegner Criteria for Disease Screening

- The condition sought should be an important health problem.
- There should be an accepted treatment for patients with recognized disease.
- Facilities for diagnosis and treatment should be available.
- There should be a recognizable latent or early symptomatic stage.
- There should be a suitable test or examination.
- The test should be acceptable to the population.
- The natural history of the condition, including development from latent to declared disease, should be adequately understood.
- There should be an agreed policy on whom to treat as patients.
- The cost of case-finding (including diagnosis and treatment of patients diagnosed) should be economically balanced in relation to possible expenditure on medical care as a whole.
- Case-finding should be a continuing process and not a "once and for all" project.

Congenital hypothyroidism, congenital adrenal hyperplasia, galactosemia, G6PD deficiency, cystic fibrosis, etc. are some of the common disorders screened for in the basic metabolic screen. An extended screen for conditions like amino acid disorders, organic acid disorders and fatty acid disorders is possible from a heel-prick filter paper sample using tandem mass spectroscopy (TMS).

Amongst the single gene disorders, the common IEM are mucopolysaccharidosis (MPS), metachromatic leukodystrophy, oculocutaneous albinism, Wilson disease and amino acid disorders. The common amino acid disorders are hyperglycinemia, homocystinuria, alkaptonuria and maple syrup urine disease (MSUD). MPS (37%), LSDs (24%), Wilson disease (14%), galactosemia (5%) and glycogen storage disease (4%) were the most common disorders at KEM Hospital, Mumbai and AIIMS, New Delhi.

HOW DO IEMs PRESENT?

Inborn errors of metabolism (IEM) are an important cause of acute illness in newborns. Presentation may mimic common neonatal conditions like sepsis. Prompt detection requires high index of suspicion.

When we come to the type of presentation, it can be any one of the three types:

1. Intoxication type
2. Energy deficiency type
3. Storage type.

It can be explained by going through the basic biochemistry with the following illustration:

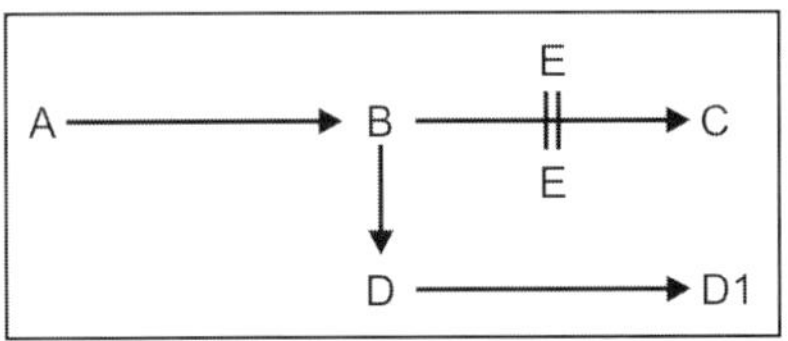

When a precursor "A" in the body is to be converted to product "C" through product "B" with one helping enzyme in the pathway, the inadequacy or absence of that particular enzyme (E) results in one of three things:

1. Absence of product "C"
2. Excess of substance "A" and "B"
3. A new pathway taken by product "B" to produce new products "D" and "D1".

WHAT TECHNOLOGY IS USED FOR IEM SCREENING?

The first generation technology was bacterial inhibition assay (BIA) pioneered by Dr Robert Guthrie. He also developed the dried blood spot (DBS) technique of collecting blood on a special filter paper from a heel prick. This process was manual and took up to 24 hours. With introduction of automation, second generation fluorometric or colorimetric assays were developed.

Alternative techniques are chromatographic (thin layer chromatography for amino acids or organic acids) or high pressure liquid chromatography (HPLC). Introduction of MS/MS for newborn screening was the third generation technology for simultaneous assays for aminoacidurias, organic acidemias and fatty acid oxidation defects. Its application for NBS analyses where multiple analytes in less than 3 minutes and has a sensitivity of 100% and specificity of 99% for some disorders. A relative disadvantage of MS/MS is that congenital hypothyroidism and galactosemia cannot be tested.

An elevated analyte concentration from the original specimen requires tracking the child to obtain a second DBS. If the analyte is abnormal in the second assay, the baby has to be referred for confirmatory tests and therapy. Thus, it should be understood that merely detecting an abnormal analyte from a DBS is not diagnostic and must be followed by confirmatory tests. Confirmatory tests would include amino acid measurement by a quantitative technique like HPLC or estimation of enzyme activity or genotyping.

Screening tests → Specialised tests → Specific tests → Diagnosis

WHAT ARE THE COMMON DISORDERS DETECTED BY NEWBORN SCREENING?

Congenital Hypothyroidism

Occurs in approximately 1 : 2000 to 1 : 4000 newborns and is one of the most common preventable causes of intellectual disability (mental retardation). Newborn screening programs allow for early identification and treatment of affected infants to minimize complications. Approximately, 85% of permanent cases of congenital hypothyroidism are sporadic, and most of these are caused by thyroid dysgenesis. The remaining 15% are caused by one of the hereditary inborn errors of thyroid hormone synthesis or secretion, and may present during or after the neonatal period. Newborn screening programs use one of the following strategies, each of which detects the majority of infants with primary congenital hypothyroidism:

- Initial blood thyroxine (T4) assay, with follow-up TSH assay, if the blood T4 value is below a certain concentration—This strategy also may detect infants with a delayed rise in blood TSH concentration and those with central hypothyroidism, but not those with subclinical primary hypothyroidism.
- Initial blood TSH assay—This strategy also detects infants with subclinical hypothyroidism, but not those with central hypothyroidism.
- Simultaneous T4 and TSH assay—This strategy has the potential to detect all the thyroid disorders described with the above two screening approaches.

Congenital Adrenal Hyperplasia

Congenital adrenal hyperplasia (CAH) is a disorder of adrenal cortex. This results in low concentration of aldosterone and cortisol and elevated 17-hydroxyprogesterone (17OHP). Over 95 % of the cases of congenital adrenal hyperplasia (CAH) are due to 21-hydroxylase deficiency. It is one of the most commonly known autosomal recessive disorders. Congenital adrenal hyperplasia (CAH) caused by steroid 21-hydroxylase deficiency occurs in 1:16,000-1: 20,000 births.

If not promptly diagnosed and treated, CAH can cause death in early infancy from shock, hyponatremia and hyperkalaemia. Affected girls usually have ambiguous genitalia but boys appear normal. By identifying babies with severe, salt-wasting CAH before they develop adrenal crises, screening reduces morbidity and mortality, particularly among affected boys.

Elevated 17-hydroxyprogesterone (17OHP) is the primary marker used when screening for CAH.

G6PD Deficiency

Glucose 6-phosphate dehydrogenase (G6PD) deficiency, an X-linked disorder, is the most common enzymatic disorder of red blood cells in humans, affecting 200–400 million people worldwide. The International Committee for Standardization in Hematology has recommended the Beutler Fluorescent spot test for screening of G6PD deficiency. However, this test requires an UV light source which poses a serious limitation to its use in mass screening programs in resource poor settings.

Recently, two new screening tests have been developed which are cheaper, easier to perform, do not require an UV light source and have a high sensitivity and specificity. One of them is the color reduction test involving reduction of a blue dye, dichlorophenol indophenol, to a colorless state and is produced by Sigma Diagnostics, USA. The other test is the modified Formazan ring test method which uses the principle of the MTT linked spot test.

Those neonates who will be identified as positive for G6PD deficiency on the screening test will need to undergo a definitive quantitative test.

Cystic Fibrosis

Cystic fibrosis is a multisystem disease affecting lungs, pancreas, intestine, liver and sweat glands. Cystic fibrosis was thought to be rare in India. However, published reports indicate that cystic fibrosis is probably more common than previously thought but is underdiagnosed or missed in majority of the cases. Newborn screening for cystic fibrosis (CF) is performed using the same dried blood spot sample obtained from the heel prick test.

Testing starts by measuring the IRT (immunoreactive trypsinogen) level. Detection of Cystic fibrosis in newborns depends on the presence of immunoreactive trypsinogen (IRT). IRT levels tend to remain raised for several months in babies with CF, whereas in false positive cases, values usually return to normal within first few weeks of life. A high IRT level triggers DNA tests that look for the most common CF gene mutations.

The diagnostic evaluation for CF involves sweat chloride testing and genetic testing.

Others Including Amino Acid Disorders

Newborn screening originated with phenylketonuria (PKU), which can be easily treated by dietary modifications, but causes severe mental retardation, if not identified and treated early. These disorders and the screening tests are summarized in the **Table 1.2.1**.

What Analytes are Measured by Tandem Mass Spectrometry?

- *Amino acids:* Building blocks of proteins
- *Carnitine:* Transportation system for fats in and out of mitochondria
- *Acylcarnitine:* Acyl carnitines are identified by the size of fat molecule attached to it and categorized simply as short, medium and long chain.

Which Disorders can be Detected by TMS?

- *Amino acid disorders:*
  - Urea cycle disorders
  - Homocystinuria
  - Hypermethioninemia

Table 1.2.1: Amino acid, lysosomal storage disorders and the screening tests

Condition	*Incidence*	*Type of test*	*Analytes tested*
Phenylketonuria, hyperphenylalaninemia	1:12000 to 1:15000	BIA, C, F, MS/MS	Phenylalanine, tyrosine
Maple syrup urine disease	1:250000	BIA, F, MS/MS	Leucine or valine and leucine/isoleucine
Homocystinuria	1:250000	BIA, C, MS/MS	Homocysteine or methionine
Tyrosinemia	1:150000	BIA, C, MS/MS	Tyrosine, methionine (type 1)
Galactosemia (classical)	1:60000	BIA, F	Galactose, galactose-1-phosphate
Biotinidase deficiency	1:250000	F	Biotinidase enzyme activity
Organic acidemias (Glutaric acidemia type I and II, isovaleric acidemia, propionic acidemia, methylmalonic acidemia, disorders of ketogenesis and ketolysis)		MS/MS	Respective target acylcarnitine concentration
Urea cycle defects		MS/MS	Respective target amino acid concentrations
Medium chain acyl-CoA dehydrogenase deficiency	1:14600	MS/MS	C6, C8, C10, C10:1, C8/C10 ratio
Lysosomal storage disorders (Pompe's, Gaucher, Fabry, MPS I, Krabbe, Niemann-Pick type A and B)	1:7000 (cumulative)	MS/MS	Respective enzyme activity

Abbreviations: BIA, bacterial inhibition assay; C, chromatography; F, fluorometric; MS/MS-Tandem, mass spectrometry.

- Non-ketotic hyperglycinemia
- Hyperammonemia, Hyperornithinemia, Homocitrullinuria
- MSUD
- PKU
- Tyrosinemia

• *Organic acid disorders:*
- Glutaric acidemia type 1
- Isovaleric acidemia
- 3-ketothiolase deficiency
- 3-Methylcrotonyl CoA carboxylase deficiency
- 3-Methylglutaconyl CoA hydratase deficiency
- Multiple carboxylase deficiency
- Beta-ketohexoses deficiency
- Methylmalonic acidemia
- Methylmalonic acidemia with homocystinuria
- Propionic acidemia

• *Fatty acid oxidation disorders:*
- Short chain acyl CoA dehydrogenase deficiency (SCAD)
- Medium chain acyl CoA dehydrogenase deficiency (MCAD)
- Mitochondrial trifunctional protein deficiency
- Long chain 3-hydroxy acyl CoA dehydrogenase deficiency (LCHAD)
- Very long chain acyl CoA dehydrogenase deficiency (VLCAD)
- Carnitine transport defect
- Carnitine palmitoyl transferase deficiency type 1 (CPT 1)
- Carnitine palmitoyl transferase deficiency type 2 (CPT 2)
- Glutaric acidemia type 2
- Carnitine acylcarnitine translocase deficiency

What is the Sensitivity and Specificity of TMS?

MS/MS-based neonatal screening showed sensitivity of 100% and specificity of 83–99% depending on the IEM.

What is the Screening Sample?

3–5 drops of blood are taken from the baby's heel. Baby's heel is pricked with a lancet and drops of blood are collected on special filter paper.

When should the Newborn Screening Sample be Collected?

Infant must be 48 hours of age or older in order to obtain a satisfactory sample for screening. Ideal time is 3-4 days of age. Sample should be taken prior to administering antibiotics or transfusing blood or blood products.

What is the Cut-off Age for an Infant when Accepting Sample for Newborn Screening?

Till one month of age except for disorders by TMS. Test methodologies for other tests are set to obtain valid values till 30 days of age. Result values of tests carried out beyond 30 days may overlap considerably making it difficult to distinguish presence or absence of disorders.

What are the Factors which Affect Results and Interpretation?

- Size of blood spot
- Blood for test aspirated from iv catheter
- Intravenous fluid hydration with dextrose prior to collection of sample can flush out short-lived active acylcarnitine metabolite from the intravascular bloodstream
- IV fluids
- Blood transfusion
- Low protein diet
- Supplemented with amino acids
- Drugs such as valproic acid, MCT oil, antibiotics.

How Long to Wait to Screen an Infant who has been Transfused?

Given the presumption that the mean age of RBCs of the transfused blood is 60–80 days, it is suggested that sample should be collected 60 days after discontinuation of transfusion.

What to do for an Infant who Needs Antibiotics Prior to 24 hours of Age?

Sample taken from infants receiving antibiotics at the time of collection may yield false results. Sample should be collected prior to starting antibiotic therapy or 24–36 hours after discontinuation of antibiotic therapy.

BIBLIOGRAPHY

1. CDC Grand Rounds. Newborn Screening and Improved Outcomes. Morb Mortal Wkly Rep. 2012;61:390-3.
2. Muranjan M, Agarwal S. Prenatal diagnosis and Newborn screening: Relevance in India. Indian J Practical Pediatr. 2010;12(2):131
3. Rama Devi AR, Naushad SM. Newborn screening in India. Indian J Pediatr. 2004;71:157-60.
4. Sanghvi U, Diwakar KK. Universal newborn screening for congenital hypothyroidism, Indian J Pediatr. 2008;45:331-2.
5. White PC. Neonatal screening for congenital adrenal hyperplasia. Nat Rev Endocrinol. 2009; 5(9):490-8.

2

CHAPTER

Fluid and Electrolyte

Reviewers: *K Nedunchelian, Jaydeep Choudhury, RV Dhakshayani, P Ramachandran, NC Gowrishankar, Hemchand K Prasad*

2.1 Approach to Arterial Blood Gas Analysis

R Ezhilarasu

Reviewers: *K Nedunchelian, Jaydeep Choudhury, RV Dhakshayani*

INTRODUCTION

The term arterial blood gas (ABG) analysis refers to a specific set of tests performed in an arterial blood sample.

- Acid-proton (H^+) donor
- Base-proton (H^+) acceptor.

Buffers are substances that limit changes in hydrogen ion concentration (pH) when hydrogen ions are added or removed from solution. Two important buffers in the body are bicarbonate (HCO_3) and carbonic acid (H_2CO_3). Bicarbonate production is regulated by kidneys. CO_2 is regulated by the lungs. Activation of the lung buffers starts within 1-3 minutes of the insult. Renal system may take from hours to days to correct the imbalance.

Nonbicarbonate buffers—plasma proteins, hemoglobin, organic and inorganic phosphates and oxyhemoglobin.

COMPONENTS OF ABG AND THEIR NORMAL VALUES

- pH—Arterial blood pH 7.35–7.45
- $paCO_2$—Arterial CO_2 tension 35–45 mm Hg
- paO_2—Arterial O_2 tension 70–100 mm Hg
- HCO_3—Serum HCO_3 concentration 22–26 mEq/L
- SBE—Standard base excess -2 to +2

PURPOSES OF ARTERIAL BLOOD GAS ANALYSIS

- To determine oxygenation
- To determine acid-base status.

DETERMINING OXYGENATION

- *Hypoxia:* Reduced oxygen pressure in the alveoli (pAO_2)
- *Hypoxemia:* Low arterial oxygen tension (paO_2)

Objective assessment of hypoxemia may be facilitated by:

- Alveolar arterial oxygen gradient estimation,
- Ratio between the arterial oxygen pressure (paO_2) and the inspired oxygen tension (FiO_2) estimation (paO_2/FiO_2) (Normal ratio >450–500).

ALVEOLAR ARTERIAL OXYGEN GRADIENT ESTIMATION ($AaDO_2$)

$pAO_2 = FiO_2\ (760–47) - (paCO_2/0.8)$;

where FiO_2—Fraction of inspired oxygen;

47—Water vapor pressure;

760—Atmospheric pressure;

0.8—Respiratory quotient;

$pACO_2 = paCO_2$ because there is no gradient;

$AaDO_2 = pAO_2 - paO_2$; where

pAO_2 is calculated from the above-mentioned formula.

paO_2 is read from blood gas.

Normal alveolar arterial O_2 gradient about 10–20 mm Hg.

Increased $AaDO_2$ signifies decreased O_2 in the arterial blood compared to O_2 in the alveolus. Normal $AaDO_2$ in the face of hypoxemia is due to hypoventilation and not due to underlying lung disease.

$AaDO_2$ increases with the age of the patient.

Normally, this gradient increases by 5–7 mm Hg for every 10% increase in the FiO_2.

ACID-BASE STATUS

Step1

- Look for a change in the pH
- pH <7.35 acidemia or >7.45 alkalemia

Step 2

Look for underlying pathological process:

- pH low-acidosis; look at the $PaCO_2$. If it is high (>45), then, there is respiratory acidosis. pH and $PaCO_2$ moves in opposite direction. If the $PaCO_2$ is within normal, then look for HCO_3. If it is low (<22), then it is metabolic acidosis. pH and HCO_3 move in the same direction.

- pH high-alkalosis; look at the $PaCO_2$. If it is low (<35), then, there is respiratory alkalosis. If the $PaCO_2$ is within normal, then look for HCO_3. If it is high (>26) then it is metabolic alkalosis.

Step 3

Look for the adequacy of compensation. This step will also find out whether it is primary disorder or it is a mixed disorder.

In metabolic acidosis, if the $paCO_2$ changes within expected compensation, it is called primary metabolic acidosis. If the $paCO_2$ changes is less than expected, then it is metabolic acidosis with respiratory alkalosis. If the $paCO_2$ changes is more than the expected, then it is metabolic acidosis with respiratory acidosis.

In metabolic alkalosis, if the $paCO_2$ changes within expected compensation, it is called primary metabolic alkalosis. If the $paCO_2$ level is less than expected, then it is metabolic alkalosis with respiratory alkalosis. If the $paCO_2$ level is more than expected, then it is metabolic alkalosis with respiratory acidosis.

In respiratory acidosis, if the HCO_3 changes within expected compensation, it is called primary respiratory acidosis. If the HCO_3 level is more than expected, then it is respiratory acidosis with metabolic alkalosis. If the HCO_3 level is less than expected, then it is respiratory acidosis with metabolic acidosis.

In respiratory alkalosis, if the HCO_3 changes within expected compensation, it is called primary respiratory alkalosis. If the HCO_3 level is more than expected, it is respiratory alkalosis with metabolic alkalosis. If the HCO_3 level is less than expected, then it is respiratory alkalosis with metabolic acidosis.

Step 4

In primary respiratory disturbance, is it acute or chronic?

In respiratory acidosis, the pH reduces by 0.08 in acute and 0.03 in chronic causes respectively for every 10 mm Hg increase in PCO_2.

In respiratory alkalosis, the pH increases by 0.08 in acute and 0.03 in chronic causes respectively for every 10 mm Hg decrease in PCO_2.

Step 5

Expected metabolic compensations in respiratory disorders:

- *Respiratory acidosis:* HCO_3 reduces by 1 in acute and 3.5 in chronic causes for every 10 mm Hg rise in PCO_2.
- *Respiratory alkalosis:* HCO_3 increases by 2 in acute and 4 in chronic causes for every 10 mm Hg decrease in PCO_2.

Step 6

Expected respiratory compensations in metabolic disturbances:

- *Metabolic acidosis:* Expected $PCO_2 = (1.5 \times [HCO_3]) + 8 +/-2$ or the expected PCO_2 is equal to last two digits of pH.
- *Metabolic alkalosis:* Expected PCO_2 = 7 mm for 10 mEq rise in HCO_3.

Step 7

For metabolic acidosis, to determine whether anion gap is present or not:

- Anion gap (Calculated difference between positively charged electrolytes and negatively charged electrolytes) = $Na^+ - (Cl^- + HCO_3^-)$
- Normal anion gap is 8 to 12 mEq/L if it is more than 12, it is called wide anion gap acidosis.

Base Excess

It is an estimate of the amount of strong acid or base needed to correct the metabolic component of an acid-base disorder (restore plasma pH to 7.40 at $paCO_2$ 40 mm Hg).

BIBLIOGRAPHY

1. Benjamin Abelow's Understanding Acid-base, 1998.
2. Nelson's Textbook of Pediatrics, 20th edition, Vol 1; 373-84.
3. Roger's Textbook of Pediatric Intensive Care, 4th edition.

2.2 Changing Concepts in Maintenance Fluid Therapy

S Thangavelu

Reviewers: *P Ramachandran, NC Gowrishankar, Hemchand K Prasad*

Intravenous fluid (IVF) is one of the commonly prescribed medications. It is a paradox that the most simple medication like intravenous fluid has to be explained by a complex theory. Holliday Segar's model on fluid therapy was the standard guideline used since 1957 and in the last ten years, this is being subjected to major criticism. Better understanding of the internal homeostasis makes this subject more clear and understandable. For making this intricate subject simpler, this article is presented in a question and answer format.

WHO NEEDS INTRAVENOUS FLUID THERAPY?

In general oral fluid is considered superior compared to IVF on scientific basis as well as for practical reasons. But there are four clinical situations where use of IVF scores over oral therapy:

1. *Correction of shock:* Whatever be the cause of shock, isotonic IVF bolus is the cornerstone of treatment. Volume and rate of administration differ according to the severity and cause of shock. Isotonic fluids like normal saline and Ringer lactate are the fluids of choice and dextrose containing fluids are not preferred for fluid boluses to correct shock.
2. *Correction of dehydration:* As per the current understanding, only isotonic fluid should be used for the correction of dehydration. Earlier no clear concept was there in the type of fluid used for correction of dehydration.
3. *Replacement of losses:* Pathological loss of fluid through various routes is to be replaced every 1–6 hours to prevent development of dehydration or shock. Type of fluid varies with the clinical situation, e.g. gastrointestinal losses such as vomiting and diarrhea have different fluids prescribed.
4. *Maintenance of fluid:* Major changes have been made in this area. The model prescribed by Holliday Segar was questioned with robust evidence in the recent years. Fluid suggested by them was one-fifth (0.18%) isotonic fluid and the rate of fluid administration was guided by the formula given in **Table 2.2.1**. These two factors are now modified to half isotonic fluid at the rate of 60–100% of the maintenance fluid volume calculated by Holliday Segar.

WHAT ARE THE INDICATIONS OF INTRAVENOUS MAINTENANCE FLUID THERAPY?

The maintenance fluids generally are used to maintain homeostasis when an individual with normal fluid and electrolyte balance is unable to take oral fluid.

Oral fluid cannot be taken by:

1. Child with altered level of consciousness. For example, meningoencephalitis, acute encephalopathy

Table 2.2.1: Maintenance fluid (water) requirement

Body weight in kg	Volume per 24 hours	Volume per hour
Up to 10 kg	100 mL/kg	4 mL/kg/hour
11–20 kg	1000 mL plus 50 mL/kg for each 1 kg>10	40 mL/hour plus 2 mL/kg for each 1 kg>10
21 kg	1500 mL plus 20 mL/kg for each 1 kg>20	60 mL/hour plus 1 mL/kg/hour for each 1 kg >20

Note: Maximum maintenance fluid is 100 mL/hr; In obese children take the 50th centile as the standard weight for fluid calculation (Weight for age? Weight for height?)

2. Child with tachypnea or respiratory distress. For example, bronchiolitis, bronchopneumonia
3. Child with recurrent vomiting of any cause.

Oral fluids should be avoided in:

1. Preoperative and postoperative states
2. Child with abdominal surgical pathology
3. Critically ill child after correction of shock and dehydration and after recovery from septic shock.

Intravenous maintenance fluid (IVMF) is given only for a short period till child recovers from critical illness and shows his readiness to take sufficient oral fluid.

WHAT IS THE NEED TO GIVE INTRAVENOUS MAINTENANCE FLUID?

There are physiological water losses through various routes. This is usually replaced by food and liquids consumed as part of diet by a normal person in a healthy state. These losses have to be replaced by IV maintenance fluid if a patient cannot take food or liquid. Volume of this fluid was calculated by Holliday Segar as per his formula **(Table 2.2.1)** based on the concept of calorie intake **(Table 2.2.2)**.

WHAT ARE THE NECESSARY CONSTITUENTS OF IVMF?

Intravenous maintenance fluid (IVMF) contains water, sodium, potassium and dextrose. Sodium and potassium are considered as essential electrolytes and including them is necessary to prevent serious deficit of these electrolytes. Others like calcium, magnesium, bicarbonate and phosphate are not routinely included. Dextrose is expected to provide at least 20% of the calorie requirements, so that basic energy need is provided and endogenous breakdown is prevented.

Table 2.2.2: Typical water losses per 100 kilocalories (kcal) of energy expended for a healthy 10 kg child

Source of water loss and estimated water loss (mL per 100 kcal/day). Data calculated according to Pickering and Winters.

Insensible	*Sensible*
Skin 20–30% Respiratory 15%	Stool 5% Minimal sweating 10% Urine 40–50%

WHAT IS THE EARLIER CONCEPT OF IVMF CALCULATION AND THE HISTORICAL BACKGROUND?

Holliday and Segar formulated a simplified method to calculate the maintenance fluid in 1957. They prescribed IVMF based on the belief that requirement of sodium is 3 mEq/kg/day and potassium 2 mEq/kg/day and hence 0.18 NS with 5% dextrose with 20 mEq of potassium per 100 mL of maintenance fluid. His concept on maintenance fluid was based on the research work done by great medical teachers and researchers like Claude Bernard, Darrow, Talbot and Gamble and other scholars during 1950s.

This was a simple formula based on caloric requirement which was well received by everyone and adopted in a global scale. But with current knowledge we realize the fact that this solution is hypotonic and the quality of this solution is the culprit causing hyponatremia, which was not realized at that time. Current concept favors usage of isotonic fluid to prevent unwanted fluid shifts ignoring the policy of calculating IVMF based on electrolyte requirement.

WHAT IS THE FOCUS OF CURRENT CONTROVERSY AND PITFALLS RECOGNIZED IN HOLLIDAY SEGAR FORMULA?

Main focus is using isotonic fluid replacing hypotonic IVMF. Since 1950s, 0.18% NS containing fluid (Isolyte P) has been used as IVMF in all children. Various studies have proved that hospital acquired hyponatremia is caused by use of such hypotonic fluid. Here the focus of controversy is two-folds and pitfalls identified in Holliday Segar (HS) model are excess water and less salt.

Excess Water

- Weight-based calculation method of HS model has overestimated the calorie requirement and thereby maintenance fluid requirement compared to surface area method.

- This was calculated in active healthy children and applying this calculation to critically ill sedated children in intensive care environment will overestimate the maintenance fluid volume, even though fever and sepsis may increase the metabolic rate.
- In acute illness or after surgery, the requirement may be only 50–60 mL/kg/day.

Less Salt

- Electrolyte requirement per kg body weight per day was arrived at calculating the urinary electrolyte excretion of breastfed children. Current evidence states that it may vary considerably.
- It also disregards the importance of maintaining plasma tonicity which will be modified by hypotonic IV fluid. For example, 0.18 NS (similar to Isolyte P) has 800 mL of electrolyte free water (EFW) resulting in hyponatremia and fluid shift into brain causing cerebral edema, seizures, encephalopathy and brain death due to cerebral herniation **(Fig. 2.2.1)**.
- Method of calculating physiological water losses such as insensible losses, urinary losses are also questioned and found to be overestimated in HS model.
- Overriding influence of antidiuretic hormone (ADH) was not recognized when Holliday Segar conceived his formula in 1957. Increased ADH secretion is commonly observed because of nonosmotic stimuli such as stress due to hospitalization, fever, vomiting, surgery, pain and use of nonsteroidal anti-inflammatory drug (NSAID). This reduces urine output and leads frequently to hyponatremia as the kidneys are unable to excrete the excess free water infused by the hypotonic fluids. ADH concentration was found to be reduced after usage of normal saline and not with 5% dextrose.

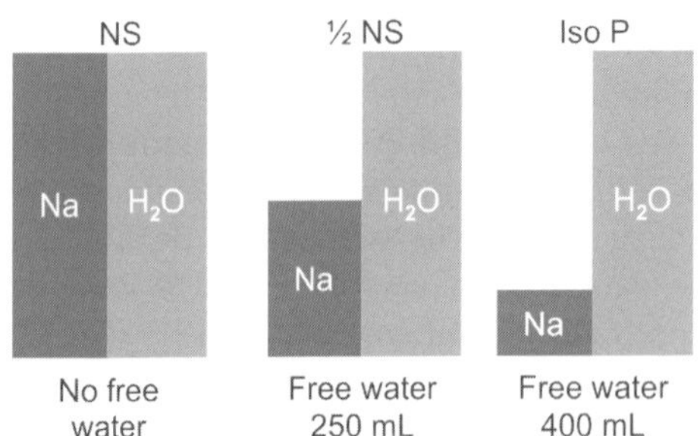

Fig. 2.2.1 Electrolyte free water concept
Abbreviations: NS, normal saline; ½ NS, half normal saline; Iso P, Isolyte P, pediatric maintenance fluid containing 0.18% saline.

WHAT IS THE DIFFERENCE BETWEEN OSMOLARITY AND TONICITY? WHY SHOULD A MAINTENANCE FLUID BE ISOTONIC?

Every clinician should be familiar with these terminologies as well as the composition of commonly used intravenous fluids to understand the concept of transcellular fluid shift **(Table 2.2.3)**. This means pathological shift of fluid from extracellular fluid (ECF) to intracellular fluid (ICF) whenever ECF is hypotonic, resulting in serious complications like cerebral edema.

Osmolarity: Number of osmotically active particles present in one liter of solution.

Osmolality: Number of osmotically active particles present in one kg of solution.

Tonicity: This is the effective osmolarity of a solution, which exerts osmotic force across the cell membrane *in vivo*. Isotonic fluid does not cause fluid shift, whereas hypotonic solution which has excess free water freely moves across cell membrane to cause cerebral edema. For example, a 0.18% NS with 5% dextrose and potassium 20 mmol/L of solution may be considered as isosmolar with respect to plasma but it becomes hypotonic once dextrose is metabolized in few minutes, because tonicity is decided by nonpermeant (which cannot move across cell membrane) osmole like sodium.

Table 2.2.3: Electrolyte composition and tonicity in different types of intravenous fluids

Solution	*Osmolality (mOsmol/L)*	*Sodium content (mEq/L)*	*Osmolality (compared to plasma)*	*Tonicity (with reference to cell membrane)*
Sodium chloride 0.9%	308	154	Isosmolar	Isotonic
Sodium chloride 0.45%	154	77	Hyposmolar	Hypotonic
Sodium chloride 0.45% and glucose 5%	432	75	Hyperosmolar	Hypotonic
Glucose 5%	278	–	Isosmolar	Hypotonic
Glucose 10%	555	–	Hyperosmolar	Hypotonic
Sodium chloride 0.9% and glucose 5%	586	150	Hyperosmolar	Isotonic
Sodium chloride 0.18% and glucose 5%	284	31	Isosmolar	Hypotonic
Ringer lactate	278	131	Isosmolar	Isotonic
Plasmalyte 148	294	140	Isosmolar	Isotonic
4.5% human albumin solution	275	100–160	Isosmolar	Isotonic

What are all the Mechanisms that Lead to Hospitalization Associated Hyponatremia?

Hospitalization associated hyponatremia is explained by the following mechanisms:

- Electrolyte free water added by the hypotonic fluid given as IVMF as per the old protocol
- Inappropriate nonosmotic stimulation of ADH retaining free water
- Few recent studies identified hyponatremia even in children receiving isotonic fluid in full maintenance volume. This is explained by the concept called desalination where high concentrations of sodium is excreted in the urine to cause hyponatremia. So, the current recommendation is to use only isotonic fluid (NS or RL instead of 1/5 isotonic fluid) in reduced volume 60% of the maintenance calculated as per Holliday Segar formula.

WHAT ARE THE CONCLUSIONS OF VARIOUS STUDIES DONE IN THIS SUBJECT?

Despite many studies performed in search of ideal fluid, so far no consensus has been reached. But many favor "more salt less water" concept. This means isotonic fluids at less than 100% maintenance volume should be used somewhere between 60 and 100%.

- A randomized controlled trial done by Kannan et al compared three regimes of fluids, isotonic fluid at standard maintenance rate, 0.18% at standard maintenance rate and third fluid as 0.18% saline at reduced (60%) rate. Their conclusion was least incidence of hyponatremia (1.72%) occurred in 0.9% saline group and worst incidence of (14.3%) noticed in 0.18% at standard rate. Group following 0.18% saline at lower rate fared in the middle (3.8%).
- Meta-analysis performed by Jingjing et al. with 10 published RCTs including 855 subjects showed higher risk of hyponatremia (fall of 3.5 mmol/L) in hypotonic IV fluid group than in the isotonic fluid group. This study concludes that isotonic fluids may be better choice compared to traditional recommendation of 0.18% saline.
- Kristen AN in their prospective, randomized, nonblinded study, studied the risk of hyponatremia in the postoperative period at 8 and 24 hours in 124 children. They compared 0.9% (NS) or 0.45% (N/2) saline solution at 100% or 50% maintenance rates. Plasma sodium concentrations fell in both N/2 groups at 8 hours (T8) with

hyponatremia more common in N2 group than in the NS groups at T8 (30% vs 10%; p = 0.02) but not T24.

Multiple linear regression analysis, showed that fluid type, not rate determined risk of hyponatremia. Their final conclusion was that the risk of hyponatremia was decreased by isotonic fluid administration but not by fluid restriction.

- Steele A et al in their study on post-operative hyponatremia in 22 women who had undergone gynecological procedures observed a curious finding explaining a concept of desalination. 21 out of 22 women developed hyponatremia despite receiving isotonic fluid with a mean fall of 4.2 +/- 0.4 mmol/L and had high sodium content in the urine (284 mmol/L). Free water was generated here during the process of excretion of hypertonic urine which is called desalination process. Further this free water was retained by ADH secretion.
- Other mechanisms considered for postoperative hyponatremia with isotonic fluids are the intracellular shift and redistribution of sodium due to increased membrane permeability known as translocational hyponatremia or sick cell hyponatremia.
- Micheal Yung performed a RCT comparing 4 regimes of maintenance fluid normal saline, 4% dextrose and 0.18% saline, at either the traditional maintenance fluid rate or 2/3 of that rate. Hypotonic fluid 0.18% NS produced significant fall in sodium than NS. Greater fall was observed in full maintenance rate than in restricted volume of maintenance.

Concepts of desalination leading to free water generation and translocation hyponatremia indicate that more salt and less water concept may be the major objective but not the final conclusion. More studies and evidence are needed to arrive at an agreement on an ideal maintenance fluid. But a tailor made customized fluid may not be a solution and in the absence of it, repeated clinical and laboratory monitoring is the only way to fine tune and decide the ideal fluid and ideal rate. Famous words of Buddha "Change is the only thing which is constant in life" is applicable for the science too particularly fluid electrolyte physiology.

WHAT IS THE MOST ACCEPTABLE FLUID OF CHOICE FOR IVMF?

Intravenous fluids are to be considered as drugs and all guidelines for a drug have to be strictly adhered to with reference to dosage particularly sodium content, tonicity, volume and duration. Fluid therapy has to be individualized and these patients' fluid balance and serum sodium levels need to be monitored regularly. Though there is a strong voice for using NS or RL as maintenance fluid, many like to use 5% dextrose ½ normal saline (1/2 GNS) with appropriate potassium (20 mEq/L) for the fear of high sodium load if NS is used in young kids. Rate of infusion is 60–100% of the maintenance volume calculated as per Holliday Segar formula. All the guidelines for IVMF is only for initiation and further titration of type of fluid and rate should be decided by the clinical, biochemical status and monitoring. Hence, one of the following models may be the initial choice of IVMF (1) NS/RL at standard maintenance rate (2) NS/RL at reduced 2/3 maintenance rate (3) Half isotonic fluid (1/2 NS) at standard rate (4) Half isotonic fluid (1/2 NS) at reduced 2/3 maintenance rate. Recommendations given below is only for initial decision. Careful clinical and laboratory monitoring will decide the further modification of the fluid plan.

- *NS/RL at reduced 2/3 maintenance rate:* (Normal salt and reduced water)
  This fluid is indicated in
  - Neurological diseases including CNS infection, traumatic brain injury or following neurosurgical problems. Normal saline with appropriate potassium is given at the rate of 2/3 maintenance. Dextrose is added only in young infants or when there is hypoglycemia. Capillary blood glucose needs to be monitored periodically

to recognize hypo or hyperglycemia, because stress hyperglycemia is a common occurrence in these situations.
- Respiratory problems like bronchiolitis, pneumonia or asthma: Normal saline with appropriate potassium is used at the rate 2/3 maintenance. Additional potassium may be needed because of frequent bronchodilator usage which can promote transcellular shift of potassium. For the same reason potassium has to be estimated frequently.
- *Pre- and perioperative states:* One should ensure euvolemia and hypovolemia should not be missed. Ongoing fluid losses should be monitored and replaced.
- Critically ill children on mechanical ventilation.

• *NS/RL at standard maintenance rate (Normal salt and normal water):*

This is used in situations where nonosmotic stimulation of ADH does not occur.
- Acute diarrheal disorders after correction of dehydration or shock
- Acute febrile illness with vomiting after correction of dehydration

• *Half NS at standard 2/3 maintenance rate (Low salt and low water):*
- *Cardiac failure:* Reduced water and salt is used in cardiac failure. Potassium needs are to be calculated on individual basis and after monitoring serum potassium levels.

• *Half NS at standard at standard maintenance rate (Low salt and normal water):*

This is used in other situations not specified earlier.

Special Situations

Two clinical situations require special mention:

1. *Renal problems:* Insensible water loss plus previous day urine output is the initial choice of fluid. Potassium is not routinely added and decided after the serum potassium status.
2. *Polyuric states:* Apart from specific treatment of underlying disease fluid management is also important till polyuria resolves. Two IV lines should be established. First-line should infuse isotonic fluid equivalent to insensible loss and appropriate dextrose and potassium based on the primary condition and serum levels of electrolytes and glucose. In the second line, the excess volume of urine output, i.e. any output > 4 mL/kg/hr should be replaced with ¼ or ½ isotonic fluid (1/4 or ½ NS) with appropriate potassium. After bladder catheterization, urine output should be measured hourly.

HOW TO MONITOR THE CHILD ON IVMF?

Major difference between oral and intravenous fluid replacement is that IV fluid bypasses the control mechanisms of normal physiology. Oral fluid intake is normally titrated by thirst. Hence, careful monitoring of volume status is mandatory when IF fluids are administered. This includes clinical assessment for signs of dehydration or fluid overload (edema, respiratory distress), daily body weight estimation, measuring urine output, charting fluid intake and output, monitoring pulse rate, volume, respiratory rate and blood pressure. In addition, wherever possible serum electrolyte estimation should be done daily or at a frequency affordable or conforming to local hospital practice.

GENERAL GUIDELINES IN ORDERING THE IV MAINTENANCE FLUID IN PRACTICE?

- IV fluids have saved many lives by correcting shock and dehydration. At the same time it is not without risks. Improper composition and rate of infusion can lead to many iatrogenic issues and some of them may end fatally.
- Preferably fluid orders should be for 12 hours rather than 24 hours. Hydration, pulse volume, respiratory rate, liver span, presence or absence of edema, signs of

increased work of breathing or increase in oxygen requirement, urine output should be monitored and documented at frequent intervals—12 hourly or even more frequently. This will guide further fluid advice.
- Electrolyte estimation at 24–48 hours interval and based on clinical status will be useful.

Points to Remember

- Previous concept of using hypotonic fluid at full maintenance volume is redundant now.
- In most of the children, isotonic fluids like normal saline or Ringer lactate is used with appropriate potassium, usually 20 mEq/L and dextrose usually 5% (D5 NS with 20 mEq/L of potassium).
- In selected situations like CNS disorders isotonic fluid NS is used without dextrose at 2/3 maintenance rates and in pre or perioperative states DNS is used at 2/3 maintenance with appropriate potassium.
- There is no ideal choice or universal acceptance regarding the right composition of fluid, or rate and duration of fluid. But isotonic fluid in 2/3 maintenance may be a favored fluid for many. Whatever be the choice, accurate clinical and laboratory monitoring is essential in any child on IV maintenance fluid to detect complications early. Oral fluid administration is superior and should be used if clinical condition permits.

BIBLIOGRAPHY

1. Bluemle LW, Potter HP, Elkington JR. Changes in body composition in acute renal failure. J Clin Invest. 1956;10:1094-108.
2. Campbell C. Fluid prescription in children. Where are we now? Current Anaesthesia and Critical Care (2008), doi:10.1016/j.cacc.2008.09.001
3. Guglielminotti J, Tao S, Maury E, Fierobe L, Mantz J, Desmonts JM. Hyponatremia after hip arthroplasty may be related to a translocational rather than to a dilutional mechanism. Crit Care Med. 2003;31:442-8.
4. Holliday MA, Segar WE. The maintenance need for water in parenteral fluid therapy. Pediatrics. 1957;19:823-32.
5. Kannan L, Lodha R, Vivekanandhan S, Bagga A, Kabra SK, Kabra M. Intravenous fluid regimen and hyponatraemia among children: a randomized controlled trial. Pediatr Nephrol. 2010;25(11):2303-9. Epub 2010 Jul 29.
6. Lamke LO, Nilson Ge, Reithner L. Insensible perspiration from the skin under standard environmental conditions. Scan J Clin Lab. 1977;37:325-31.
7. Neville KA, Sandeman DJ, Rubinstein, et al. (Prevention of hyponatremia during maintenance intravenous fluid administration: a prospective randomized study of fluid type versus fluid rate. J Pediatr. 2010;156(2):313-9.
8. NHS UK Patient safety alert 22: Reducing the risk of hyponatraemia when administering intravenous infusions to children. National Patient Safety Agency no. 22,28; 2007.
9. Pickering DE, Winters RW. Fluid and electrolyte management in children. Pediatr Clin North Am. 1954. pp. 873-99.
10. Steele A, Gowrishankar M, Abrahamson S, Mazer CD, Feldman RD, Halperin ML. Postoperative hyponatremia despite near-isotonic saline infusion: a phenomenon of desalination. Ann Intern Med. 1997;126(1):20-5.
11. Wang J, Xu E, Xiad Y. Isotonic versus hypotonic maintenance IV fluids in hospitalized children: a meta-analysis. Pediatrics. 2014;133:105-13.
12. Yung M, Keeley S. Randomised controlled trial of intravenous maintenance fluids. J Paediatr and Child Health. 2009;45(1-2):9-14.

Allergy and Immunology

Reviewers: *K Nedunchelian, Jaydeep Choudhury, RV Dhakshayani, P Ramachandran, NC Gowrishankar, Hemchand K Prasad, MKC Nair, S Thangavelu, S Narmada*

3.1 Pediatric Allergy Testing: What, When and How to Do?

S Narmada

Reviewers: *K Nedunchelian, Jaydeep Choudhury, RV Dhakshayani*

Approximately, 20–30% of total population suffer from at least one of the allergic diseases in India. Indian Study on Epidemiology of Asthma, Respiratory Symptoms and Chronic Bronchitis (INSEARCH) showed increased asthma prevalence in children. About 7.2% of our children are affected by allergic disorders.[1]

India has an estimated 15–20 million asthmatics. Proportion of Indian school children suffering from bronchial asthma has increased to more than double in the last 10 years and has reached its highest level ever. The incidence of allergic rhinitis is about 26.1%. Such a high burden of asthma and allergic rhinitis poses a significant financial burden for the family. Burden of asthma affects the patients, their families and society in terms of lost work and school, lessened quality of life and avoidable cause of hospitalizations. **Figure 3.1.1** shows the rise in prevalence of wheezing in different countries over the past 40 years.[2]

ENVIRONMENTAL CHANGES CONTRIBUTING TO INCREASED PREVALENCE

Increased exposure to perennial indoor allergens due to increased time spent indoors, increased conditions for mite and mold growth, decreased ventilation and increased reservoirs (carpets, sofa) for allergens are common. The other reasons have been changes in hygiene such as clean water, eradication of helminthes, introduction of broad-spectrum antibiotics and immunization. There has also been a decline in the play time and dietary changes from the traditional family life that has led to the increased prevalence of allergic disorders.

In short, developing countries are having now all the risk factors suggested for increased prevalence of allergic disorders.[2]

There are various types of allergic disorders in children—allergic asthma, rhinitis, atopic dermatitis, food allergy, medication, venom

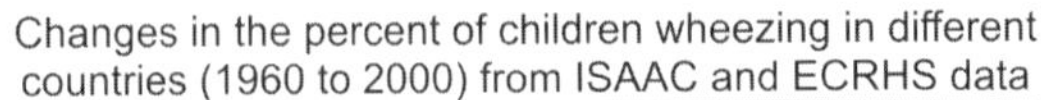

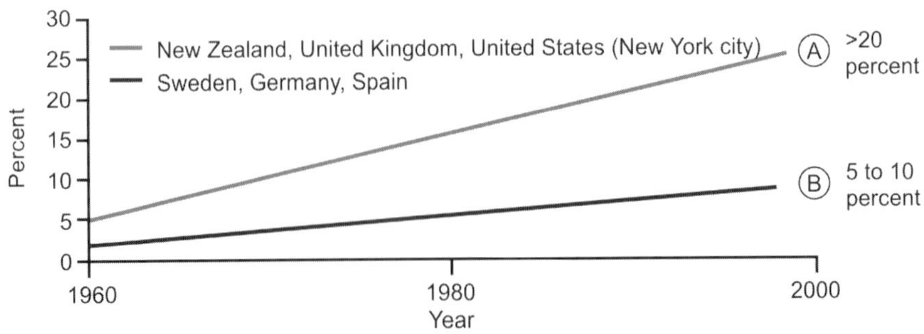

Fig. 3.1.1: Prevalence of wheezing in different countries over decades

and latex allergies. When each of the individual disorders is looked into there are various allergens that are triggering the symptoms.

In atopic dermatitis, food allergies and environmental allergens are playing a major role. About 10–20% of children have food-induced urticaria. Earlier onset and severe atopic dermatitis has been associated with egg, milk or peanut specific IgE. Elimination diet has lead to significant clinical improvement in such children. Similarly in allergic conjunctivitis which affects almost 20% of our population is affected environmental allergens such as pollens, moulds and dust mites have known to trigger the symptoms. When a child has been found to have positive skin prick test to egg or house dust mite in the 1st year of life. They are found to rapidly progress in the path of allergic march from atopic dermatitis to adult onset asthma. Lifestyle avoidance measures of allergens have known to contribute to a reduction in their symptoms.[3]

FACTORS TO PREDICT CHRONIC ASTHMA IN CHILDREN

Several early childhood wheezing phenotypes have been described based upon the natural history and associated risk factors. Accurate classification of young children at high risk to develop persistent asthma may help predict long-term outcomes and identify children who may benefit from secondary prevention interventions. The most important of these epidemiological phenotypes are the episodic (viral) wheezer and multitrigger wheezers. There is a higher association of persistent wheezing and atopic nature with multitrigger phenotypes. In addition, it was found that predisposition to allergy and sensitization with common mold alternaria was associated with higher rate of chronic asthma at age 22.

PREDICTIVE TOOLS IN CHILDREN WITH WHEEZING

Asthma predictive index followed in USA which has been validated in population-based cohort has a high negative predictive value in predicting children having low probability of asthma. The predictive index has major criteria-clinician diagnosed eczema and parental asthma, minor criteria-clinician diagnosed allergic rhinitis, wheezing apart from colds and eosinophilia. Any child having 1 major or 2 minor criteria have 7 times more likely to have asthma.[4] In an attempt to increase the sensitivity of the index in order to provide a better knowledge of predicting future asthma probability allergy skin testing has replaced clinician diagnostic criteria. Allergic sensitization to at least one aero allergen has been predicted as major criteria and sensitization to egg, milk and peanut is one of the minor criteria in the predictive index.[5] In the Prevention of Early Asthma in Kids (PEAK) study, allergic sensitizations has been predicted as afore-mentioned major risk factor.[3] Hence, it is apparent from the above studies that knowledge of sensitizations to various allergic disorders will aid in predicting asthma in later life and help in instituting preventive measures.

TESTS THAT HELP IN FINDING THE OFFENDING ALLERGEN TO REDUCE THE BURDEN

There are three components to the diagnosis of IgE mediated allergic disorder—careful clinical history, demonstration of specific IgE by skin or *in vitro* testing and determination that exposure to the allergen results in symptoms either by history or with challenge procedures.

TESTS FOR IgE-MEDIATED ALLERGIES[6,7]

Prick/Puncture Tests

First described in 1867 by Dr Charles Blackley, skin tests (prick/puncture and intracutaneous test) have evolved as reliable, cost-effective techniques for IgE-mediated hypersensitivity. They are relatively nontraumatic and elicit reproducible results when placed on specific areas of the body (i.e. arms or back). They are used to confirm clinical sensitivity induced by aeroallergens, foods, some drugs and few chemicals.

Skin test allergens used for prick/puncture tests should be potent and stable. To ensure proper interpretation, positive (histamine) and negative (saline or 50% glycerinated HSA–saline) should be performed at the same time as allergen test. In performing the prick test, a sharp instrument (lancet) is passed through a drop of extract or control solutions (histamine, saline) at 45° to 60° angle to the skin. The skin is then gently lifted, creating a small break in the epidermis through which the suspected allergen solution penetrates. Alternatively, the skin device may be passed through a drop at a 90°angle to the skin. This is called puncture test.

Methodology of Prick Test

Procedure

Prick/puncture tests can be performed on the upper back or volar surface of the forearm. Not only is the back more reactive than the forearm, specific locations on the back and forearms vary in reactive intensity. Regardless of location, it is recommended that there should be sufficient space (e.g. Approximately 2–2.5 cm) between each applied allergen, and tests not be placed in areas 5 cm from the wrist or 3 cm from the antecubital fossae. Skin tests should not be performed in skin sites with active dermatitis or severe dermatographism (**Figs 3.1.2A and B**).

Age at which skin tests can be performed: Skin tests may be performed in infants as young as 1 month. Though the reactions tend to be smaller in infants and younger children, they exhibit a high degree of reliability (**Figs 3.1.3A and B**).

Concurrent drugs may affect the validity of prick tests:

- *Antihistamines:* Use of first and second generation antihistamines should be discontinued 2–3 days before skin tests. But variation exists between different antihistamines
- Oral prostaglandin D2 inhibitors—may increase the wheal area
- Leukotriene antagonists—negligible effects
- Short-term oral steroids—do not suppress skin tests, if given in the dosage of 1 mg/kg daily for 2 weeks.

Allergenic extracts used: A limited number of standardized extracts are commercially available, most inhalant and food extracts are not standardized. However, now with recent attempts many standardized extracts are available in the market which have increased the reliability of the reports. Stability and potency of allergenic test extracts are also important issues. They need to be preserved with 50% glycerin and stored in cold conditions (4°C) to ensure stability.

Reading the test results: The peak reactivity of the prick tests is 15–20 minutes at which time both wheal and erythema diameters should be recorded in millimeters and compared with positive and negative controls. Qualitative scoring of 0 to 4+ positive or negative is no longer used. Histamine control should be read 15 minutes after application at the peak of activity. The peak of allergen prick/puncture tests is 15–20 minutes after application. Although some investigators have advocated the importance of wheal diameter, both erythema and wheal should be measured and recorded in millimeters for

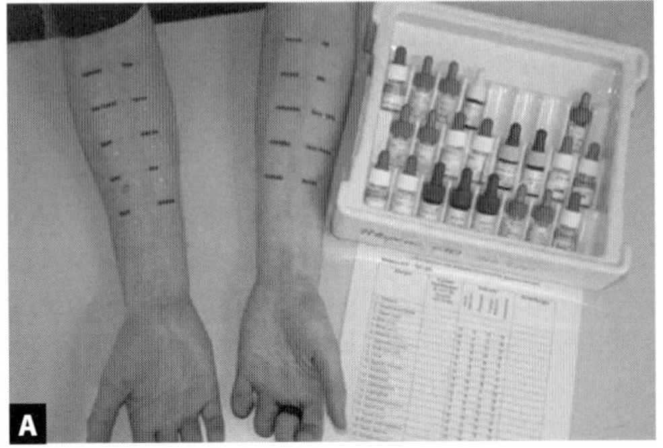

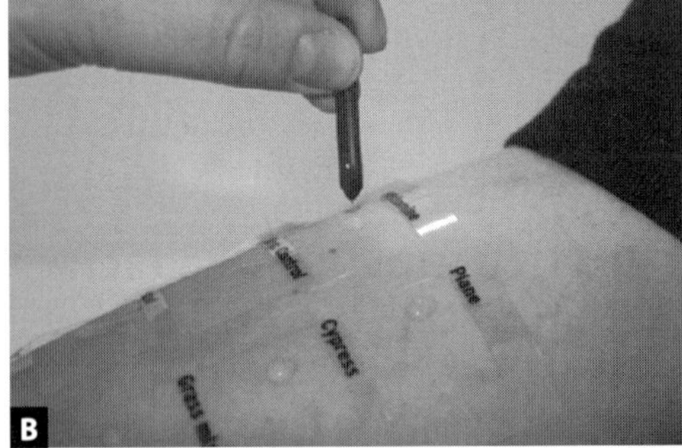

Figs 3.1.2A and B: Methodology of skin testing (*For color version, see Plate 1*)

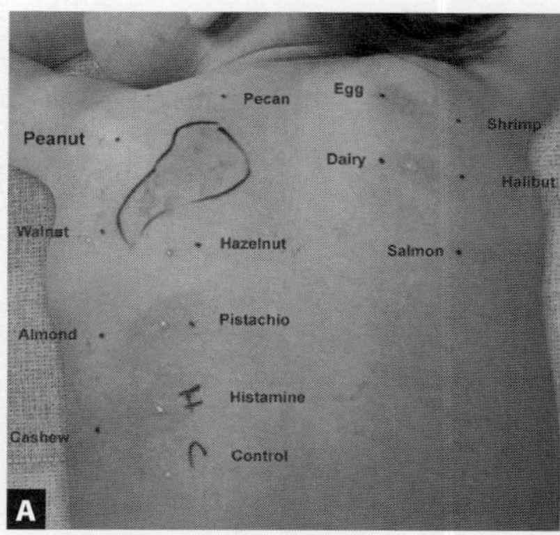

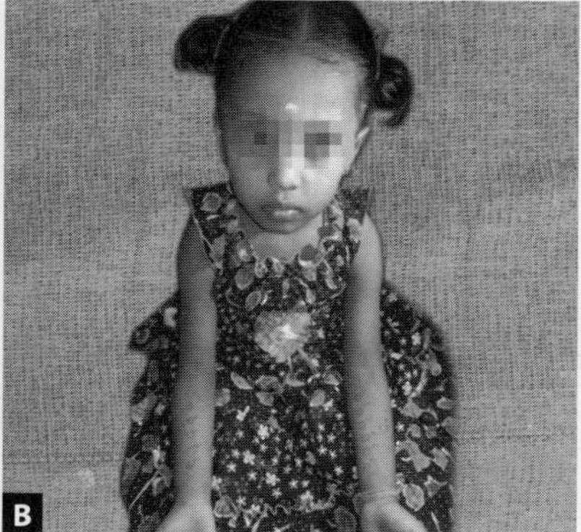

Figs 3.1.3A and B: Allergy skin testing in children (*For color version, see Plate 1*)

appropriate comparison. Since trauma may affect wheal size, an allergen response less than 3 mm generally should not be regarded as positive.

Clinical relevance of skin tests: The diagnostic value of prick/puncture tests has been confirmed as a correlate of clinical sensitivity in double blind randomized control studies under outdoor and indoor conditions. However, compared with clinical history alone, the diagnostic accuracy of prick/puncture tests showed more limited capacity to predict clinical sensitivity for both inhalant and food allergens. However, when it was compared with nasal challenge tests as a standard, the sensitivity of prick/puncture tests range from 85–87% whereas specificity of the tests is between 79–86%.

Limitations: The reliability of prick/puncture tests depends on the skill of the tester, the test instrument, color of the skin, skin reactivity on the day of the test, potency and stability of the test reagents. False positive results can occur due to cross reactive determinants present in another allergen extract.

Safety: Life-threatening generalized systemic reactions are rarely caused by prick/puncture tests. The concurrent use of beta blockers and angiotensin-converting enzyme inhibitors may be a relative contraindication to skin testing as they may mask anaphylactic symptoms.

Number of skin tests: The number of skin tests and the allergens selected for skin testing should be determined based on the patient's age, history, environment and living conditions, occupation and activities. Routine use of large numbers of skin tests or routine annual tests without a definite clinical indication are clearly not justified. Generally, fewer prick/puncture tests need to be performed in infants and very young children because these children are not likely to be sensitized to as many allergens as older children and adults.

Allergen panel to be tested: In toddlers, sensitization is more apt to reflect intense and prolonged exposure to allergens encountered earliest in life such as foods, house dust mites, indoor molds and animal danders rather than pollen. In older children, if inhalation allergy is narrowly confined to single season, then limited number of pollen skin tests would suffice. By contrast, perennial symptoms would require a more extended skin test panel of both indigenous outdoor and indoor inhalant and food allergens but not foods unless a history of food allergy has happened. The general agreement is significant indoor allergens such as house dust mite, prevailing indoor fungal allergens (penicillium, aspergillus and alternaria alternate), cockroach and epidermals (cats, dog, feathers) should be tested in children with perennial respiratory symptoms. The most common pollens reported in Bengaluru which almost have similar vegetation like our region are Parthenium, Casuarinas, Ricinus, Prosopis, Mimosa (touch me not) and Amaranath. The trees are Babhul and shishir. The most common allergenic trees, shrubs and grasses are depicted in **Figures 3.1.4** to **3.1.6**.

COMMON ALLERGENIC TREES (Figs 3.1.4A to D)

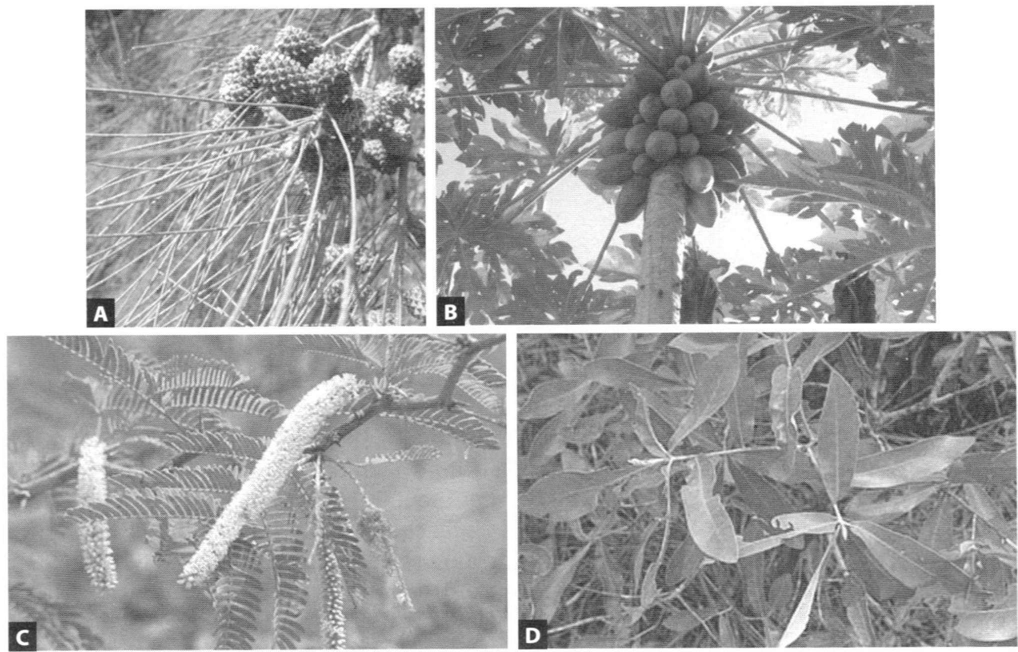

Figs 3.1.4A to D: (A) Casuarina; (B) Carica papaya; (C) Prosopis; (D) Quercus incana (Blue jack oak) *(For color version, see Plate 1)*

COMMON ALLERGENIC SHRUBS AND WEEDS (Figs 3.1.5A to E)

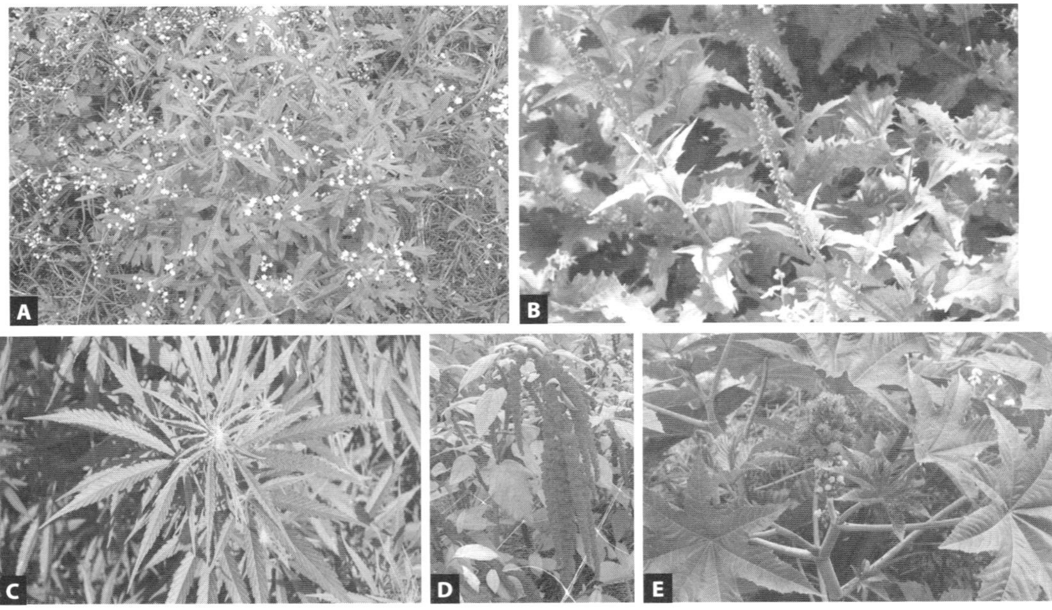

Figs 3.1.5A to E: (A) Parthenium; (B) Chenopodium; (C) Cannabis sativa; (D) Amaranthus; (E) Ricinus communis *(For color version, see Plate 2)*

COMMON ALLERGENIC GRASSES (Figs 3.1.6A to D)

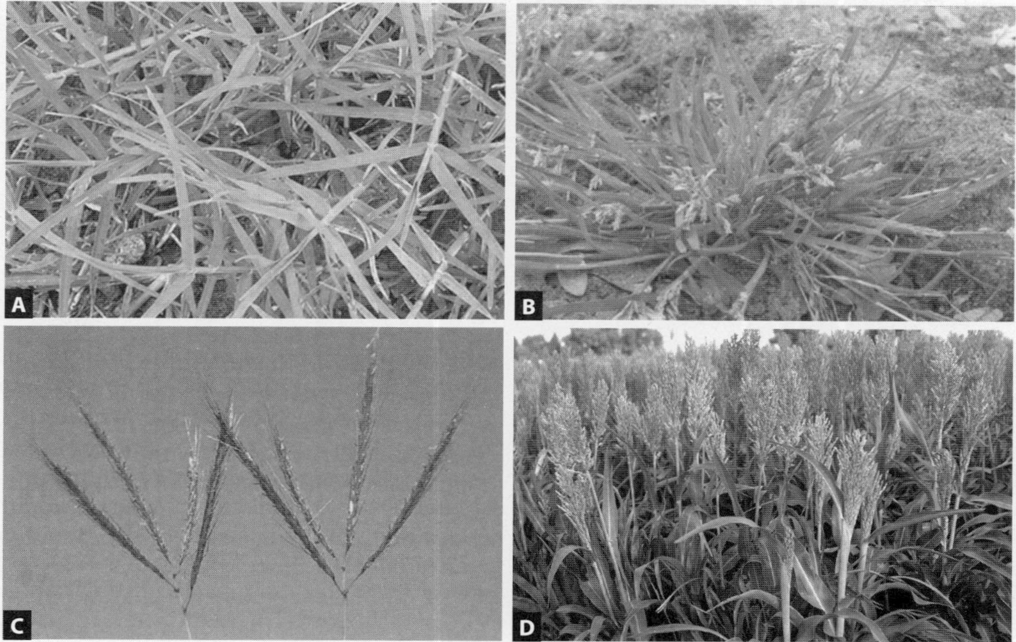

Figs 3.1.6A to D: (A) Cynodon; (B) Poa annum; (C) *Dicanthium annulatum*; (D) *Sorghum*
(*For color version, see Plate 2*)

Food Prick and Puncture Skin Tests

These are excellent diagnostic modalities for the diagnosis of IgE-mediated clinical entities, which include anaphylaxis, food-dependent exercise-induced anaphylaxis, acute urticaria, atopic dermatitis and oral allergy syndrome. Relatively few foods account for most IgE mediated allergic reactions in both children and adults. The more common food allergens in infants and young children are cow's milk, hen's egg, peanuts, tree nuts, soybeans and wheat. Food tests are inappropriate for investigation of chronic idiopathic urticaria.

The scope and number of skin tests for allergy diagnosis reflect the clinician's scientific knowledge and clinical experience.

Type of Allergen Kits Available in India

Two companies are presently supplying allergen kits (**Figs 3.1.7A and B**). One is the indigenously manufactured Credisol company based at Mumbai. The major advantage is the cost and the availability of huge panel of allergens. The major drawback and limitation of using this kit is that the allergens are not standardized. A randomized controlled trial is being done at Christian Medical College, Vellore, Tamil Nadu, comparing the extract with American standard extract and results are yet to be published which will throw a better light on the efficacy of the allergens. The other company is Allergopharma which is an international company. The main advantage is the standardization of the extracts but the major disadvantage is the cost and the restricted number of panels that is available.

IN VITRO DIAGNOSTIC TESTS FOR IMMEDIATE HYPERSENSITIVITY

Total IgE

Measurement of total IgE is an important component of allergic disorders, however, the

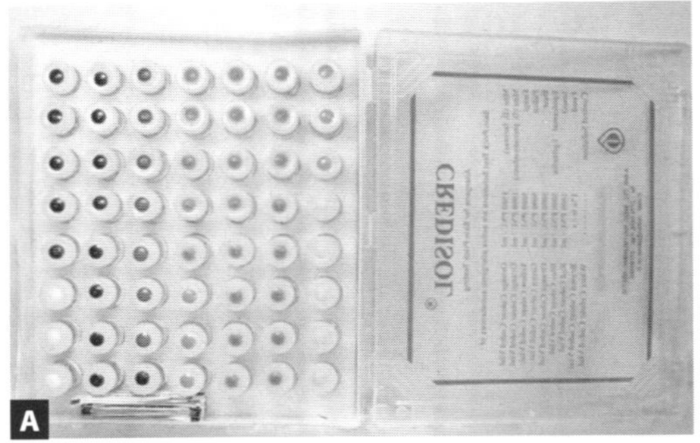

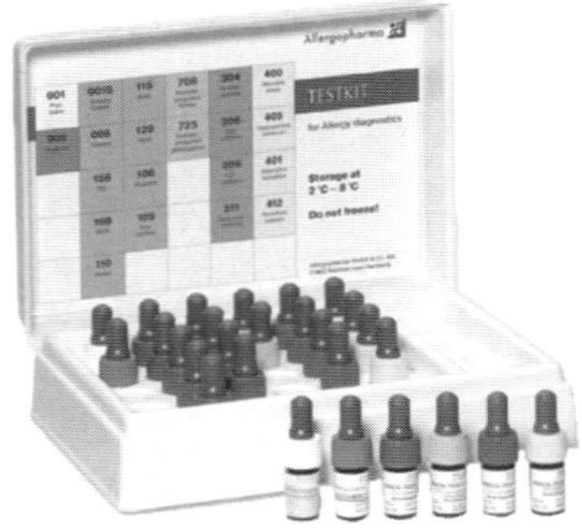

Figs 3.1.7A and B: Allergen skin testing kits available in India (*For color version, see Plate 3*)

clinical significance is doubtful. Total serum IgE levels are age related. Levels are greater and found in asthma, atopic disorders and bronchopulmonary aspergillosis. It may also be increased in parasitic infections, lymphomas, liver diseases and vasculitis. Measurement of total serum IgE concentration are of modest clinical value when used as a screen for allergic disease or for predicting the risk of allergic disease.[6]

It is particularly useful in two clinical situations:

1. When patient has specific symptoms and specific panels are negative an elevated high total IgE count points out a cause of less known inhalant.
2. Doing a total IgE in patients with non-specific symptoms, if it shows a low counts it is an indication not to do a specific panel as it will confuse the clinical picture and indicates a need to look out for other causes of the symptoms.

With the licensing of omalizumab for the treatment of allergic asthma, another application of total serum IgE is verification that the patient is a suitable candidate for anti-IgE therapy with total serum IgE levels between 70 and 800 IU/mL.

Specific IgE Panel

Immunoassay for allergen specific IgE have been used as an alternative to biologic skin tests. The precise sensitivity of these immunoassays compared with prick/puncture skin tests has been reported to range from less than 50% to greater than 90%, with the average being approximately 70–75% for most studies. As with skin tests, the interpretation of specific IgE results requires correlation with the history, physical examination and in some cases symptoms directly observed after natural or laboratory exposure to allergens. A multiallergen upto 15 allergens can screen for atopic status, following which allergen specific tests are required for more definitive evaluation. Commercially, available assays for allergen specific IgE are based on the principle of immunoadsorption. The allergen specific IgE of interest binds to the allergen, which has either been previously bound to a solid phase or becomes bound to a solid phase after the IgE has been bound. The amount of the IgE bound to the allergen is quantified using a labeled anti-human IgE (monoclonal or mixture of monoclonal) antibodies. The label can be a radioactive isotope enzyme or a ligand to which an enzyme or antiligand conjugate is bound. Originally, Radioallergosorbent Test (RAST) immunoassay was used but now improved matrix binding combined with fluroenzymatic or chemiluminescence detection systems which are either semiautomatic or completely automatic are being used **(Figs 3.1.8A to C)**.

Recent advances in lasers, computational power, DNA technology, component miniaturization and other technological advances have allowed for the development of allergen specific IgE multiplexing which is a major improvement over monoplex methods. These arrays use smaller sample sizes and are

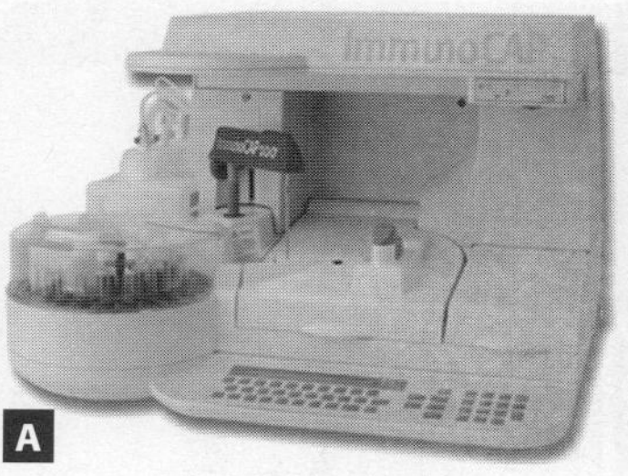

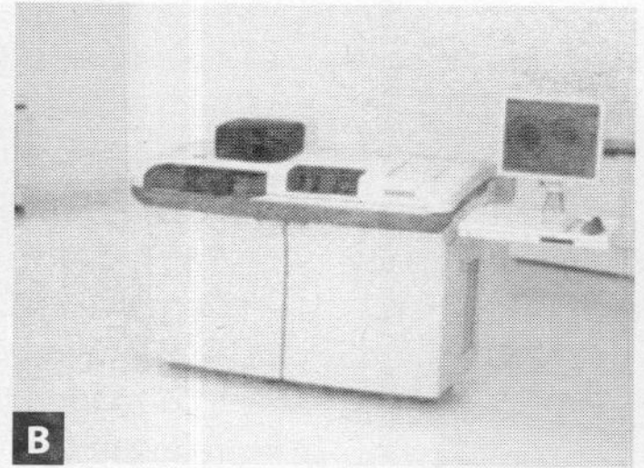
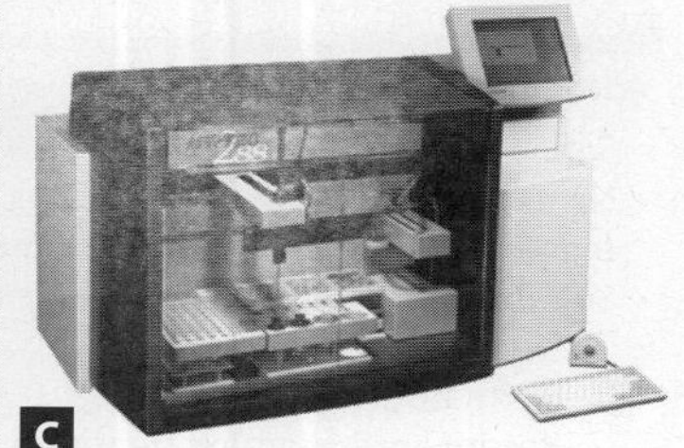

Figs 3.1.8A to C: Various systems with different techniques for doing allergen panel (*For color version, see Plate 3*)

potentially cheaper, faster, more sensitive and more accurate than present day technology.

There are some situations in which immunoassays may be preferable to skin testing for the diagnostic evaluation of patients.

- If the patient has had a near fatal reaction to an allergen, the immunoassay offers the advantage of testing the patient for allergen specific IgE without the risk of inducing a severe reaction from a skin test.
- If patient does not have a sufficient large area of normal skin to allow skin testing, immunoassays for specific IgE are useful for confirming clinical impression, e.g. individuals with dermographism, icthyosis or atopic dermatitis.
- If there is a necessity to determine the patient's sensitivity after a severe reaction during the refractory period immunoassay may be preferable.
- If the patient is on antihistamines and drugs such as tricyclic antidepressants that block the skin test reactivity, it is inadvisable to stop the medications
- When the patient is unable to cooperate with skin testing because of mental or physical impairment, measurement of specific IgE would be preferable.

Quantitative results from clinical IgE antibody assays have allowed investigators to study the quantity of serum IgE antibody has clinical relevance and have found the quantity of serum IgE antibody in serum to peanut, egg white, cow's milk and fish may define clinical sensitivity in many patients. Such correlation has not been consistently observed for respiratory allergens but can give a basic knowledge of sensitivity in situations when allergy skin tests cannot be used.

The types of allergen panel done in the laboratories in our region are either by RAST or by recent advances using cellulose sponge matrix (immunocap) or biotinylated allergens (Siemens immulite). However, cost is a prohibitive factor with these advance technologies.

Test Results

The results of the specific IgE tests are reported as separate classes based on the ranges:

- *Class 0:* Less than 0.35KU/L
- *Class 1:* 0.35 – 0.7 KU/L
- *Class 2:* 0.7 – 3.5KU/L
- *Class 3:* 3.51 – 17.5 KU/L
- *Class 4:* 17.51 – 50 KU/L
- *Class 5:* 50.01 – 100 KU/L
- *Class 6:* Greater than 100 KU/L

Generally, Class 0 has no allergy and class 6 has high significance for allergy.

Relative advantages and disadvantage of *in vitro* diagnostic test over allergy skin test are shown in **Table 3.1.1**.

OTHER LESS DONE TESTS

Basophil Activation Test

A basophil activation test measured by expression of CD 63 and CD 203c and detected by flow cytometry is being evaluated for many IgE-mediated disorders. It has been evaluated in IgE mediated pollen, food, drug, hymenoptera venom and latex reactions. Sera of the

Table 3.1.1: Relative advantages and disadvantages of *in vitro* diagnostic test over allergy skin test

Advantages	*Disadvantages (compared to skin testing)*
• Safe • No experience/expertise/reagents required by the medical practitioner for the performance of the test • Suitable for patients with: – Skin disease – Dermatographism – Recent antihistamine treatment – Infancy/cord blood sampling – Severe anaphylaxis in whom there is a concern that skin testing may provoke an anaphylactic reaction (foods, latex, stinging insects, antibiotics)	• Expensive • Less sensitive than skin tests • RAST tests to "mixes" of allergen may give falsely negative results • Delay before results are available • Information is more abstract, i.e. less immediately relevant to the patient • Stability of allergen a problem for some allergens (particularly food allergens)

patients with chronic idiopathic urticaria also demonstrate basophil-activating antibodies.

Cellular Antigen Stimulation Test

Histamine and leukotriene release measurements from human basophils after incubation with allergen are valuable research tools for *in vitro* investigations of allergy. The recent availability of several sensitive immunoassays for histamine and leukotriene C4 is a significant technological advance for measuring these mediators in various biologic fluids or release from whole blood, basophils, mast cells or other cultured cells. Basophils are the only cells in human peripheral blood that contain histamine. The interaction of specific allergen with the IgE antibody fixed to high affinity Fc epsilon receptors on the basophil membrane initiates release of preformed histamine and other inflammatory mediators associated with immediate hypersensitivity **(Fig. 3.1.9)**. This test detects sensitivity to substances including antibiotics, analgesics, food additives, food colorants, both local and general anesthetics, as well as latex and carboxymethyl cellulose. Tests for bee and wasp venoms, foods, pollens and other aeroallergens are also available.

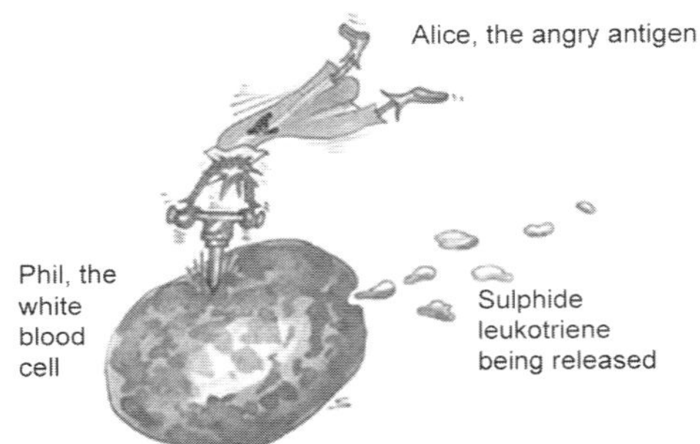

Fig. 3.1.9: Pictorial representation of CAST
(*For color version, see Plate 3*)

Plasma Tryptase Test

Plasma tryptase especially beta-tryptase should be obtained within 4 hours after an anaphylactic episode. Mast cells that have been activated during an IgE-mediated hypersensitivity reaction release proteases and prestored histamine and newly generated vasoactive mediators into surrounding soft tissue. Tryptase is a neutral serine esterase with trypsin like substrate specificity that is found in relatively large quantities in mast cells. Since modest amounts are found in basophils (less than 1% than found in tissue mast cells), tryptase is considered to be a good clinical marker of mast cell activation. Immunoreactive tryptase levels in serum of healthy adults are less than 5μ/L.

Elevated tryptase levels can be detected in serum from 1 to 4 hours after the onset of systemic anaphylaxis with hypotension. Recommended serum collection times for a serum tryptase are 30 minutes to 4 hours after the onset of an acute event.

REFERENCES

1. Allergy situation in India: What is being done? Editorial Indian J Chest Dis Allied Sci. 2013;55:7-8.

2. Platts T, Commins SP. Increasing prevalence of asthma and allergic rhinitis and the role of environmental factors. Wolters Kluwer, 2015.
3. Allergen avoidance in the treatment of asthma and allergic rhinitis. Thomas AE plats-Mills. Wolters Kluwer, 2015.
4. Jose A Castro-Rodriguez. The asthma predictive index: A very useful tool for predicting asthma in young children. J Allergy Clin Immunol. 2010;126(2):212-6. *doi:10.1016/j.jaci.201006.032.*
5. Chang TS, Lemanske Jr R, Gilbert TW, Gern JE, Coen MH, Eans MD, et al. Evaluation of the modified asthma predictive index in preschool children. J Allergy Clin Immunol Pract. 2013; 1(2):*doi:10.1016/j.jaip.2012.10.008.*
6. Bernstein L, Hamilton R, David BK Golden, Blessing J, Randolph CC, Levetin E. Allergy diagnostic testing: An updated practice parameter. Ann Allergy Asthma Immunol. 2008; 100(3):S2-S148.
7. Emanuel S, Di Hawarden. ABC of allergy. Curr Allergy Clin Immunol. 2010;23(1): 28-30.

3.2 Urticaria: Relieving the Itch

S Narmada

Reviewers: *P Ramachandran, NC Gowrishankar, Hemchand K Prasad*

Urticaria is a common heterogeneous group of disorders with a large variety of problems causing marked impairment in school, work or home functioning.

DEFINITION

Urticaria is characterized by the sudden appearance of wheals and/or angioedema.

A wheal is characterized by three typical features:

1. A central swelling of variable size, invariably surrounded by reflex erythema.
2. Associated itching or sometimes burning sensation
3. Transient nature, with skin returning to its normal appearance, usually within 1-24 hours.

Angioedema is associated with sudden, pronounced swelling of lower dermis and sub-cutis, sometimes pain rather than itching, with frequent involvement of mucous membranes, resolution that is slower than for wheals which can take up to 72 hours.

EPIDEMIOLOGY

Life-time incidence of urticaria is 15–20% affecting both genders in adults. However incidence is less in children compared to adults. According to studies, the incidence of urticaria is 0.1–3% per year of age. The cumulative prevalence of urticaria up to the age of 10 years was 14.5% for boys and 16.2% for girls. Variations in incidence of chronic urticaria is noted in different countries. The incidence of angioedema was 6.6% and angioedema associated with urticaria was observed in 15% of children with chronic urticaria. Most cases of chronic urticaria occur in children between 6–11 years.

Incidence in India is not known. In 500 cases of urticaria in India, 37% are physical urticaria.

Admissions for urticaria were 3 times higher in children aged 0–4 years. The greatest increase in hospitalizations was present in those aged 5-34 years (7.8% per year) and for angioedema it was higher in older adults.

CLASSIFICATION

Urticaria can be classified on the basis of its duration and the presence or absence of inducing factors (induced or spontaneous).

Depending on the duration and frequency urticaria is classified as acute when the hives and/or angioedema occur for <6 weeks, whereas episodes lasting longer than 6 weeks are chronic.

The timeline of 6 weeks of daily or near daily symptoms has been chosen as arbitrary dividing point. Acute urticaria is most common in children and chronic urticaria is rare.

Types of Urticaria

Spontaneous urticaria:

- Acute and chronic

Physical urticaria:

- Cold contact urticaria
- Delayed pressure urticaria
- Solar urticaria
- Dermographic urticaria
- Vibratory urticaria

Other inducible urticaria:

- Aquagenic urticaria
- Cholinergic urticaria
- Exercise-induced urticaria

PATHOGENESIS

Though symptomatically urticaria may be seen as an allergic reaction, the disease is often autoimmune or idiopathic in nature. Degranulation of mast cell is the final step and reason for hive formation and on biopsy, a non-necrotizing perivascular infiltration of cells is seen, there is infiltration with granulocytes (neutrophils, eosinophils and basophils) although the magnitude can vary considerably.

T-cells are very prominent and most are CD 4+ with a mixture of *TH1* and *TH2* subtypes. The reason for the spontaneous degranulation has led to the consideration of autoimmune etiology as 30% of patients showed autoreactivity with their serum.

About 5–10% of patients were found to have circulating IgG anti-IgE, which is functional and subsequently 30–40% of patients were found

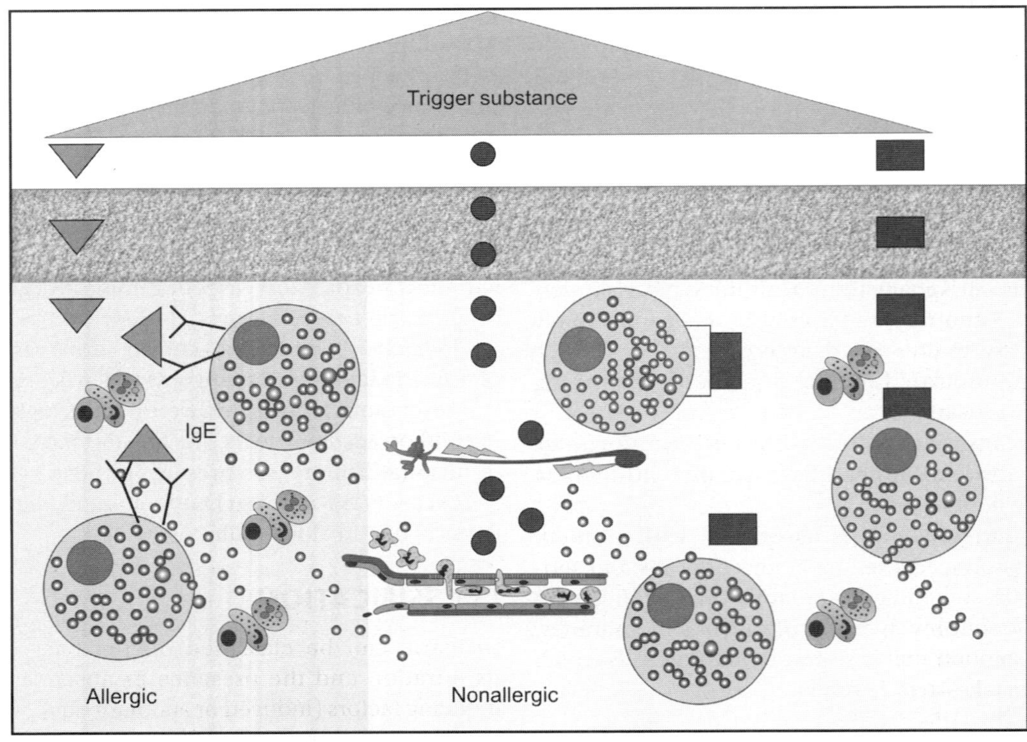

Fig. 3.2.1: Pathogenesis of allergic and non-allergic urticaria
(For color version, see Plate 4)

to have IgG antibody to the alpha subunit of IgE receptor. The thesis is that crosslinking IgE receptors or occasionally IgE itself could activate mast cells. *In vitro* studies support the concept of antireceptor antibody binding which activates complement pathway with release of C5a which further activates basophils and mast cells. Altered basophil subgroups have also been implicated.

In those cases of non-allergic urticaria physical stimuli, infections, and scombroid fish poisoning have known to trigger mast cells directly without IgE mediation **(Fig. 3.2.1)**.

ETIOLOGY

Acute

The most common causes of acute urticaria with or without angioedema are medications, foods, viral infections, parasitic infections, insect venom and contact allergens, particularly, latex hypersensitivity. Medicines commonly implicated are penicillins, sulphonamides, NSAIDs, acetylsalicylic acid, opiates and narcotics. Predominant foods that cause urticaria are milk, eggs, peanuts, trees, nuts, fish and shellfish. In 50% of cases, cause is not known.

Chronic

There are 2 types: chronic autoimmune and chronic spontaneous urticaria

Chronic autoimmune which is associated with thyroid antibodies (27%), vitiligo, rheumatoid arthritis. *Helicobacter pylori* has also been implicated. In the chronic spontaneous type, there seems to be persistent activation of mast cells but cause is not known.

Assessment of Disease Activity in Urticaria Patients

Score	*Wheals*	*Pruritus*
0	None	None
1	Mild (<20 wheals/24 hours)	Mild (present but not annoying or troublesome)
2	Moderate (20–50 wheals/24 hours)	Moderate (troublesome but does not interfere with sleep or activity)
3	Intense (>50 wheals/24 hours or large confluent wheals)	Intense (severe pruritus which interferes with activity or sleep)

DIAGNOSIS

History and Physical Examination

The history and physical examination should include detailed information regarding:

Suggested questions to children with urticaria:
- Time of onset of disease
- Frequency and duration of wheals
- Diurnal variation
- Occurrence in relation to weekends, holidays, and travel
- Shape, size and distribution of wheals
- Associated angioedema
- Associated subjective symptoms of lesions, e.g. itch and pain
- Family and personal history regarding urticaria and angioedema
- Previous or current allergies, infections, internal disease or other possible causes
- Psychosomatic and psychiatric diseases
- Gastric/intestinal problems (stool, flatulence)
- Surgical implantations and events during surgery
- Use of medications
- Induction by physical agents or exercise
- Observed correlation to food
- Relationship to menstrual cycle in adolescence
- Smoking habits in adolescence
- Type of work
- Hobbies
- Stress
- Quality of life related to urticaria and emotional impact
- Previous therapy and response.

Goal of Diagnosis

The goal of diagnostic measures is to:
- Identify urticaria and subtypes

- Identify underlying causes in long-standing or severe chronic spontaneous urticaria

Acute urticaria is associated with speedy recovery, but the identification helps to prevent recurrence, especially when allergy is suspected to be the cause. Although chronic spontaneous urticaria has various etiologies, routine patient evaluation with careful history, physical examination and ruling out systemic disease should be carried out. Extensive investigations should be considered only on an individual basis.

INVESTIGATIONS

- Complete blood count
- Liver function tests
- Determination of ESR and CRP
- Role of *Helicobacter pylori* in causation is controversial
- Screening for thyroid autoimmunity
- IgE-mediated tests in certain cases
- Autologous serum skin test—test to screen for autoantibodies
- Provocation tests—ice cube, cold water test, exercise challenge test
- Skin biopsy in syndromic cases and vasculitis

Urticarial Mimics

- Arthropod bites
- Atopic dermatitis
- Contact dermatitis
- Erythema multiforme
- Henoch-Schönlein purpura
- Pityriasis rosea
- Viral exanthem
- Morbiliform drug reactions

TREATMENT

Interventions before giving medicines:

- Avoidance of physical and other stimuli
- Avoidance of offending drugs
- Treatment of infectious agents
- Dietary modifications
- Nonspecific aggravating factors—overheating, stress and codeine should be minimized
- Cooling antipruritic lotions—calamine or 1% menthol aqueous cream
- Cold compresses

Antihistamines

Second-generation Antihistamines

(Azelastine, bilastine, cetirizine, desloratidine, ebastine, fexofenadine, levocetirizine)

Non-sedating antihistamines have a very good evidence for efficacy, a very good safety profile and low cost. Increasing the dose of second generation antihistamines is recommended because of good safety profile, good evidence of efficacy and low cost.

Antihistamines are most effective, if taken daily, rather on as needed basis. If symptoms are controlled with standard antihistamine doses, it is reasonable to continue treatment for several months, occasionally stopping for brief periods to determine whether urticaria has spontaneously resolved. In patients who do not achieve control with standard doses, it is common practice to increase the antihistamine doses beyond usual recommended doses. Guidelines recommend upto 4 times the usual recommended doses.

First-generation Antihistamines

Double-blind placebo-controlled studies have demonstrated efficacy for several first generation antihistamines with overall similar efficacy to second generation antihistamines. First generation antihistamines have been recommended as add on therapy to patients who have had inadequate control on second generation antihistamines. It is also used in patients who have more nocturnal symptoms. Sedation and cognitive/psychomotor function impairment are side effects of first generation antihistamines, but the degree of these side effects varies between individuals. Therefore, sedating antihistamines are typically recommended as a single nocturnal dose to reduce daytime impairment. First generation antihistamines do not provide additional benefits to those obtained with non-sedating antihistamines.

H_2 Antihistamines

Since 15% of histamine receptors in the skin are H_2 type receptors, H_2 receptor antihistamines, such as cimetidine, ranitidine and nizatidine may also be helpful in some patients with urticaria. However, these agents should not be used as monotherapy as they have limited effects on pruritus. There are experts who consider that the use of H_2 receptor antagonists in association with H_1 antihistamine efficacy is low and such association does not seem to produce any advantage over the use of anti-H_1 antihistamines alone. However, other experts consider the combination to be safe and affordable, sometimes effective and preferable in its risk benefit profile to other second-line treatment options.

Doses of Antihistamines

	Usual adult doses	*Usual pediatric doses*
Second-generation H_1 receptor antihistamines		
Cetrizine	10–40 mg daily	5–10 mL
Desloratidine	5–20 mg daily	2.5–5 mL
Fexofenadine	120–480 mg daily	Not currently indicated for children under 12 years of age
Loratidine	10–40 mg daily	5–10 mL
First-generation H_1 receptor antihistamines		
Hydroxyzine	25–50 mg, 3–4 times daily	30–100 mg daily divided doses
Diphenhydramine	25–50 mg every 6 hours	2.5–20 mL every 4–6 hours
Cyproheptadine	4–20 mg daily	2–4 mg 2 to 3 times daily
Chlorpheniramine	4 mg every 4–6 hours	1 mg every 4–6 hours

Leukotriene Receptor Antagonists

The effectiveness of these drugs has been relatively small. Results from randomized, double-blind studies have been inconsistent. They may be effective in a small subset of patients with urticaria. Altogether, existing evidence of their effectiveness is limited and the grade of recommendation for their use is low. Nonetheless, these drugs may be tried in patients unresponsive to antihistamines in view of their excellent safety profile.

Corticosteroids

Although it is clinically recognized that oral steroids are effective for H_1 antihistamine resistant CU, controlled studies are lacking. In view of the potentially severe side effects associated with long-term treatment, oral steroids should be used for short periods and at the minimally effective dose necessary to achieve control when all other therapies have failed.

Other Treatment Modalities

Dapsone: Isolated case reports have shown efficacy in comparison with desloratidine.

Sulphasalazine: Isolated case reports have suggested its effectiveness but large trials are lacking.

Other immunosuppressive agents: Methotrexate, cyclophosphamide, azathioprine, sirolimus and mycophenolate mofetil have been used to treat in individual case reports.

Omalizumab: Recently, growing number of studies evaluating the effectiveness of omalizumab in different subsets of antihistamine unresponsive CU/angioedema patients have been reported. Efficacy and side effect profile potentially make omalizumab, the future drug of choice for refractory chronic spontaneous urticaria. The main limitations of omalizumab treatment include limited availability, high cost and indefinite long-term clinical benefits.

Intravenous immunoglobulin: Isolated case studies have proved its efficacy. However, large trials are needed for supporting its use and the appropriate dosage. It should be reserved for patients refractory to other therapies.

MANAGEMENT ALGORITHM

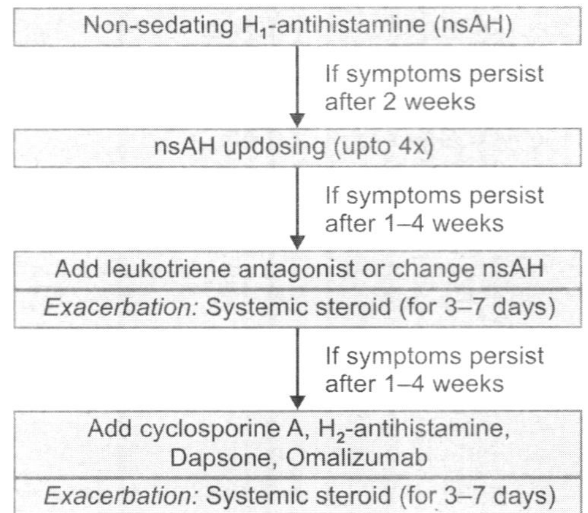

PROGNOSIS

Few studies are available on the prognosis of acute urticaria in children. Two studies indicate that 20–30% of young children with acute urticaria are at risk of chronic or recurrent urticaria. More concerning than repeated episodes of acute urticaria, is the progression of the disease to chronic urticaria.

BIBLIOGRAPHY

1. Bruise I, Standl M, Weidinger S, et al. Epidemiology of urticaria in infants and young children in Germany: Results from the German LISAplus and GINIplus birth cohort studies. Pediatr Allergy Immunol. 2014;25(1):36-42.
2. Consensus statement on the management of urticaria. Indian J Pediatr. 2011;56(5):485-9.
3. Ghaffari J, Hossaini R, Rafatpanah H, et al. Chronic urticaria in children: Etiologies, clinical manifestations, diagnosis and treatment. J Pediatr Rev. 2013;1(2):55-68.
4. Giminez-Arnaeu A, Maurer M, De La Cuadra J, Maibach H. Immediate contact skin reactions, an update of contact urticaria syndrome and protein contact dermatitis—"A never ending story". European Journal of Dermatology. 2010;20:5.
5. Kanani A, Schellenberg R, Warrington R. Urticaria and angioedema. Allergy, Asthma and Clinical Immunology. 2011;7(Suppl 1):59.
6. Sanchez-Borges M, Asero R, et al. Diagnosis and treatment of urticaria and angioedema: A worldwide perspective. WAO Position paper. WAO Journal. 2012;5:125-47.
7. Zuberbier T. A summary of the new international EAACI/GALEN/EDF/WAO guidelines in urticaria. WAO Journal, 2012.

3.3 Investigating a Rheumatologic Disorder: A Pediatrician's Nightmare

Mahesh Janarthanan

Reviewers: *MKC Nair, S Thangavelu, S Narmada*

INTRODUCTION

Investigating a child with rheumatologic disorder can be challenging for a general pediatrician. Baseline knowledge about the most appropriate tests in specific situations is useful.

It is important to bear in mind that in many rheumatologic conditions, the diagnosis is clinical. Placing undue reliance entirely on investigations to make a diagnosis may result in confusion and lead to unnecessary expenditure for the patient. In conditions such as Kawasaki disease, for example, there are criteria which too can help make a diagnosis. Some of these criteria were originally validated for classification purposes from research point of view.

The topic of investigations in rheumatology is vast, and it is not possible to discuss investigations in all rheumatologic conditions. However, an attempt has been made to cover the most common conditions that a general pediatrician can come across in his practice.

BASELINE INVESTIGATIONS IN RHEUMATOLOGY

- Low hemoglobin may signify anemia of chronic disease, hemolysis, bleeding or co-existing iron deficiency.
- Increased white cell count (WCC) may be seen in juvenile idiopathic arthritis (JIA) and vasculitis. A low white cell count in macrophage activation syndrome, low WCC and lymphopenia may be seen in SLE.
- Thrombocytosis may be seen in vasculitis and JIA. Thrombocytopenia may be seen in macrophage activation syndrome and SLE.
- A peripheral smear is always useful to look for abnormal cells.
- Renal function tests may be abnormal in SLE or vasculitis such as Wegener's granulomatosis.
- Liver function tests maybe abnormal in systemic onset juvenile idiopathic arthritis (SOJIA), SLE, juvenile dermatomyositis (JDM) or vasculitis. A low serum albumin may be found in SOJIA, SLE or vasculitis.
- Inflammatory markers CRP and ESR may be generally high in inflammatory disorders, but a rapidly dropping ESR with an elevated ferritin level in an unwell child should raise the suspicion of macrophage activation syndrome (MAS), a potentially fatal condition. MAS may arise as a complication of SOJIA, SLE, vasculitis or JDM. When the CRP is very high infection must be ruled out. A high CRP in a child with SLE may indicate serositis.

SCENARIO 1

A 9-year-old female child presents with swelling of the right knee since 6 months **(Fig. 3.3.1)**. There is no history of trauma or fever. The pain is worse in the mornings. What are the investigations that may be necessary?

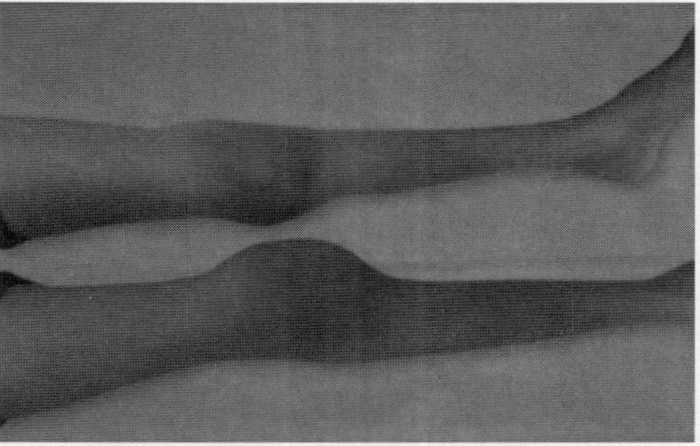

Fig. 3.3.1: Oligoarthritis right knee. The diagnosis in this scenario is most likely oligoarticular JIA (*For color version, see Plate 4*)

- The CBC may be completely normal in Oligo JIA or may show modest elevation in counts and ESR.
- Rheumatoid factor (RF) and anti-nuclear antibody (ANA) testing may be useful in this scenario. RF should not be used to diagnose JIA, as >90% of childhood JIA is RF negative. It has more of prognostic value indicating that the course of the disease may be protracted and severe. RF is likely to be positive in an adolescent child with polyarticular onset, with small and symmetrical joint involvement similar to adult onset Rheumatoid arthritis.
- The presence of ANA positivity in a child with arthritis signifies risk of uveitis. All children with JIA irrespective of their ANA status should have their eyes screened for uveitis at the time of diagnosis and annually. In addition young children, particularly, those with Oligo-JIA and ANA positivity should have their eyes checked at 3 monthly intervals.
- It may be necessary to rule out TB before making a diagnosis of Oligo-JIA.
- When the diagnosis is in doubt a joint aspiration +/− a synovial biopsy may be needed.
- A bone marrow may be needed in children with features of systemic onset arthritis when diagnosis is in doubt or when leukaemia is suspected. Excruciating bone or joint pain, night pain and lymphocyte predominance

in the differential count, leukopenia, and low normal platelet count should alert the possibility of leukemia.
- HLAB27 should be checked when the patient is a boy > 6 years with arthritis of joints predominantly of lower segment of body, enthesitis, sacroiliitis, acute anterior uveitis or has family history of HLAB27 related disease like inflammatory bowel disease, ankylosing spondylitis, etc.
- Anticyclic citrullinated peptide (Anti-CCP) antibodies are positive in a proportion of patients with RF positivity and erosive joint disease. However, this is less when compared to adult RA patients. Many centres do not do this test as a routine in children with arthritis.

SCENARIO 2

A 6-year-old female presents with 3 month history of rash on her knuckles **(Fig. 3.3.2)**. She was diagnosed as contact allergy by her family physician, but has no improvement with topical steroid. She has difficulty in climbing stairs and parents have noticed change in her voice. On examination, she has a red macular rash on cheeks and eyelids, red papules on all her metacarpophalangeal joints (MCPs) and proximal interphalangeal joints (PIPs).
- In this scenario, CBC may be normal, differential count may show lymphopenia and inflammatory markers ESR and CRP may be elevated.
- Serum CPK levels may be grossly elevated, but rarely can be normal.
- Other enzymes such as LDH, aldolase and ALT may also be increased with disease activity. ANA positivity is variable between 10–85%. Anti-Jo-1 antibodies may be positive in JDM with interstitial lung disease.
- Though EMG has been traditionally used to make a diagnosis of JDM, currently it is seldom used as a diagnostic tool in tertiary pediatric rheumatology centres.
- An MRI of the thighs in early stages shows increased soft tissue density caused by edema of the muscle and subcutaneous tissue and in chronic cases may show areas of calcification.
- A muscle biopsy needs interpretation by a pathologist with expertise in this field and therefore may not be always feasible. When done it may show evidence of inflammatory change and perifascicular atrophy.

SCENARIO 3

A 13-year-old girl presents with history of low grade fever for 3 months, recurrent oral ulcers and multiple joint pain. On examination, she has alopecia and a rash on her cheeks which gets worse with exposure to sunlight **(Fig. 3.3.3)**.
- A CBC is likely to show mild-to-moderate anemia, leukopenia, lymphocytopenia and thrombocytopenia.
- ESR may be high and CRP maybe normal. A high CRP in a child with SLE should lead to suspicion of infection or serositis.
- Coagulation abnormalities maybe present due to lupus anticoagulant

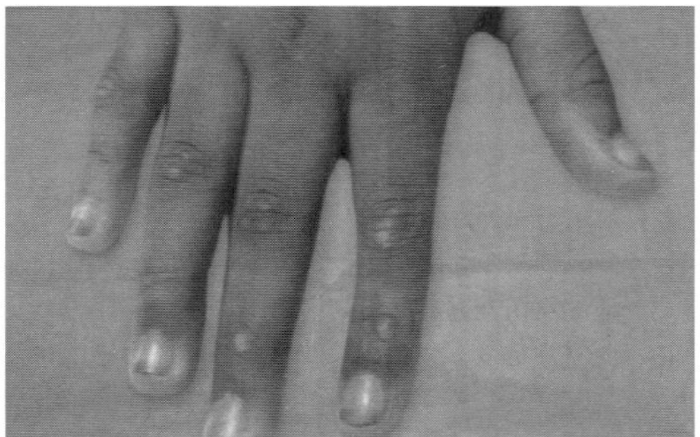

Fig. 3.3.2: Gottron's papules. The diagnosis is juvenile dermatomyositis (*For color version, see Plate 4*)

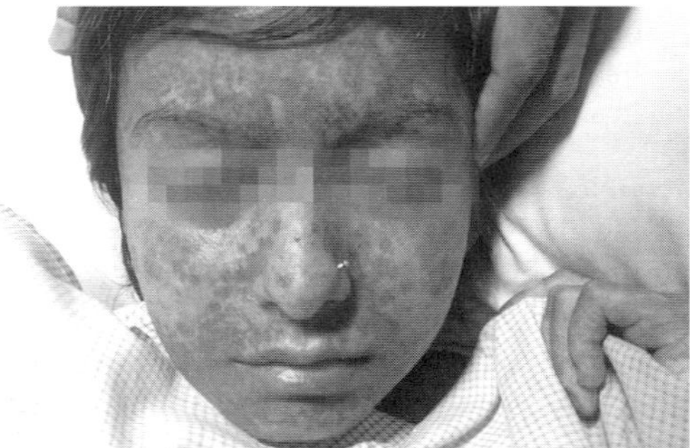

Fig. 3.3.3: SLE-malar rash. The diagnosis in this case is SLE (*For color version, see Plate 5*)

and antiphospholipid antibodies (anticardiolipin antibodies and anti beta-2-glycoprotein antibodies) may be positive.

- Urine routine examination should be done to look for presence of protein, blood and casts. If urine routine examination is abnormal, urine protein estimation either urine protein creatinine ratio or 24-hour estimation is necessary.
- Direct Coomb's test is likely to be positive.
- Complements C3 and C4 may be low.
- ANA by immunofluorescence technique should be requested and is positive in almost all children with SLE.
- In SLE, ds DNA is pathognomonic and high titres are present in active disease and in nephritis. Anti-Sm antibodies maybe present in CNS lupus and are one of the diagnostic criteria **(Table 3.3.1)**.

What to Do when ANA is Positive?

The flow chart for further evaluation based on ANA is given in **Flow chart 3.3.1**.

Flow chart 3.3.1: ANA testing

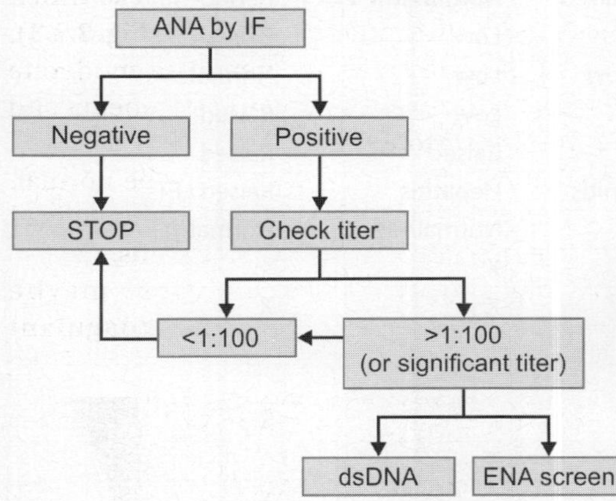

ANA is likely to be positive in significant titres in SLE, mixed connective tissue disorder, overlap syndromes, Sjögren's syndrome, scleroderma and to a lesser degree in juvenile arthritis. It is important to check with the local immunology lab regarding the significance of titers. ANA maybe positive in normal individuals in lower titers. It could also be positive in infections such as TB, EBV, infective endocarditis, etc.

Table 3.3.1: Common extractable nuclear antigen (ENA) disease associations in pediatric rheumatology

Antibody	*Disease association*
Anti-Ro/Anti SS-A	SLE /Sjögren's/Neonatal lupus/congenital heart block (CHB)
Anti-La/Anti SS-B	Neonatal lupus/ Congenital heart block
Anti-histone	Drug-induced lupus
Anti-RNP	Mixed connective-tissue disease (MCTD)
Anti-SCL-70/Anti-centromere	Systemic sclerosis
Anti-LKM/Smooth muscle antibodies	Autoimmune hepatitis
Anti-Sm	SLE /CNS lupus

Systemic Lupus International Collaborating Clinics (SLICC) Classification Criteria for SLE 2012

These criteria were introduced for classification purposes from a research basis. Increasingly clinicians are utilizing this to make a diagnosis. The SLICC criteria requires 4 or more of these criteria to be present with at least 1 clinical and 1 immunological criteria or biopsy proven nephritis with the presence of ANA or dsDNA **(Table 3.3.2)**.

Table 3.3.2: Systemic Lupus International Collaborating Clinics (SLICC) classification criteria

Clinical criteria	*Immunological criteria*
Acute cutaneous lupus	ANA
Chronic cutaneous lupus	Anti-DNA
Oral or nasal ulcers	Anti-Sm
Non-scarring alopecia	Antiphospholipid Antibody
Arthritis	Low complements
Serositis	Direct Coomb's test (DCT)
Renal involvement	
Neurological involvement	
Hemolytic anemia	
Leukopenia	
Thrombocytopenia	

SCENARIO 4

A 12-year-old boy presents with history of fever for 3 months, abdominal pain and a discolored toe **(Fig. 3.3.4)**.

- The diagnosis in this scenario could be medium vessel vasculitis such as polyarteritis nodosa or small vessel vasculitis, e.g. Granulomatosis with polyangitis (Wegener's) or SLE +/- Antiphospholipid syndrome. The CBC could show raised WCC with neutrophilia and thrombocytosis in vasculitis.
- Urine routine examination may show hematuria, proteinuria or casts. Renal functions maybe deranged.
- Apart from the investigations mentioned for SLE, testing for anti-neutrophil cytoplasmic antibody (ANCA) may be useful in this situation. Wegener's granulomatosis (granulomatosis with polyangitis) is associated with cytoplasmic C-ANCA with specificity against PR3 (Proteinase 3). Microscopic polyangitis and Churg-Strauss syndrome (eosinophilic granulomatosis with polyangitis) is associated with perinuclear p-ANCA with specificity against

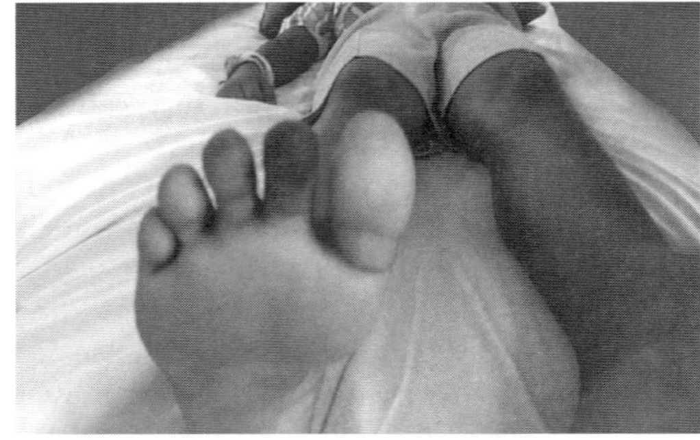

Fig. 3.3.4: Gangrene of right second toe in a child with suspected vasculitis (Discolored toe) *(For color version, see Plate 5)*

Table 3.3.3: Summary of investigations

Investigations	*JIA*	*JDM*	*SLE*	*Vasculitis*
Hb	Low	Normal/low	Low	Low
WCC	Normal/raised	Normal/raised	Normal/low	Raised
Neutrophils	High	Normal	Low	Raised
Lymphocytes	Normal	Normal/low	Low	Normal
Platelets	Raised	Normal	Low	Raised
ESR	Raised	Raised	Raised	Raised
LFT	abnormal SOJIA	Transaminitis	Hepatitis	Raised LFTs
RFT	Normal	Normal	Normal/raised	Normal/raised
CPK/LDH		X	X	
ANA	X	X	X	X
RF	X			
HLAB27	X			
dsDNA			X	X
ENA			X	
ANCA				X
DCT			X	
C3C4			X	X
Lupus anticoagulant APL antibodies			X	X
Urine routine	X	X	X	X
Echo	X	X	X	X
US abdomen	SOJIA		X	X
Imaging	MRI joint	MRI thighs		Angiogram
Tissue biopsy	Synovial	Muscle	Skin/kidney	Organ involved

myeloperoxidase (MPO). Tissue biopsy of the skin (cutaneous polyarteritis nodosa) or involved organ (e.g. kidney or nasal mucosa in Wegener's disease) may show features consistent with vasculitis.

- A digital subtraction angiography or CT angiogram maybe useful in diagnosis when systemic polyarteritis nodosa or Takayasu's arteritis is suspected.
- A CT chest may be required in Wegener's disease in those with lung lesions.

Table 3.3.3 shows the summary of tests that maybe necessary in investigating a child with suspected rheumatologic disorder. An X mark indicates that the investigation is possibly needed for the condition suspected. Extensive investigations maybe needed in the context of SOJIA or vasculitis to rule out infection and malignancy. Not all investigations mentioned under each column may be needed and the diagnosis in most cases is clinical. The investigations should help confirm clinical diagnosis rather than being used as a screening method. Some of these tests such as complements, quantitative dsDNA and ANCA may be used to monitor disease activity.

CONCLUSION

No investigation can substitute a thorough clinical examination and investigations should only be used as corroborative evidence. Basic maneuvers such as BP check including 4 limb BP measurement, urine dipstick and palpation of peripheral pulses must be done as part of routine examination as they may provide valuable clinical information. It is important to bear in mind that many rheumatologic conditions can present atypically and children maybe very ill during their first presentation of illness. Therefore a high degree of suspicion and prompt appropriate investigations followed by aggressive management is needed to avoid long-term morbidity and possible mortality.

BIBLIOGRAPHY

1. Foster H, Brogan PA. Handbook in Paediatric Rheumatology. Oxford University Press, 2016.
2. Lee, et al. A clinical overview of autoantibodies in general practice rheumatology. Br J Gen Pract. 2014;64(626):e599–e601.
3. Petri, et al. Derivation and Validation of Systemic Lupus International Collaborating Clinics Classification Criteria for Systemic Lupus Erythematosus. Arthritis Rheum. 2012; 64(8):2677-86.
4. Petty, Laxer, Lindsley, Wedderburn. Textbook of Paediatric Rheumatology, 7th edn. Saunders Elsevier, 2015.
5. Phan, et al. Autoantibodies to extractable nuclear antigens: making detection and interpretation more meaningful. Clin Diagn Lab Immunol. 2002;9(1):1-7.

CHAPTER 4

Infections

Reviewers: *MKC Nair, S Thangavelu, S Narmada, P Ramachandran, NC Gowrishankar, Hemchand K Prasad*

4.1 Investigating Malaria and Typhoid
(Old Wine in a New Bottle)

U Umadevi
***Reviewers:** MKC Nair, S Thangavelu, S Narmada*

MALARIA

Malaria is a life-threatening disease caused by *Plasmodium* species of parasites that are transmitted to people through bites of infected female anopheles mosquitoes. About 3.2 billion people—almost half of the world's population are at risk of malaria. Infants, children under 5 years, pregnant women, patients with HIV/AIDS and non-immune travelers from malaria-free areas are particularly vulnerable to severe form of malaria. According to the latest WHO estimates, the global disease burden is estimated to be 214 million cases with 438,000 deaths.

Of the 5 species of malarial parasites known to infect humans (including the recently added species *Plasmodium knowlesi*), *Plasmodium vivax* causing benign tertian malaria, and *Plasmodium falciparum* causing malignant tertian malaria, cause majority of the malarial infections. As there is enormous burden of illness and substantial mortality due to falciparum malaria, especially in a tropical country like India, specific and rapid laboratory diagnosis of malaria is very critical to initiate early treatment **(Fig. 4.1.1)**.

Laboratory diagnosis involves conventional peripheral blood film microscopy, fluorescence microscopy, Quantitative Buffy Coat (QBC) microhematocrit concentration method, rapid antigen detection tests (RDTs), antibody detection methods and nucleic acid amplification (NAAT) tests. In this article, the wide choice of available malarial diagnostic tests, their utility, advantages and limitations are discussed.

PERIPHERAL BLOOD FILM MICROSCOPY

Parasite morphologic analysis by microscopy is considered to be the 'Gold Standard' for malaria diagnosis. Peripheral blood film should be examined at least twice daily until parasites are detected. Parasites can be visualized on both thick and thin blood smears stained with Giemsa or Wright or Wright Giemsa or Field stain. Giemsa stain is superior to other stains as it allows detection of certain morphologic forms such as Schuffner's dots, Maurer's clefts, etc. that may not be seen with other stains. Ideally thick smears are used to detect presence of parasites (screening) while thin smears are used for parasite identification. Quantification can be done on both thick and thin smears (prognosis monitoring). In addition to species identification, thin smears have the advantage of identification of the stages of the parasite found in blood, e.g. trophozoites, gametocytes etc.

Critical factors in determining sensitivity and specificity of light microscopy are frequency of peripheral blood smear examination, collection of a good specimen—capillary blood which is free flowing and not squeezed from fingers/toes, proper maintenance of microscope, quality control of staining reagents and competency of the microscopist.

FLUORESCENCE MICROSCOPY

Kawamoto technique is used in malaria fluorescence microscopy, in which blood

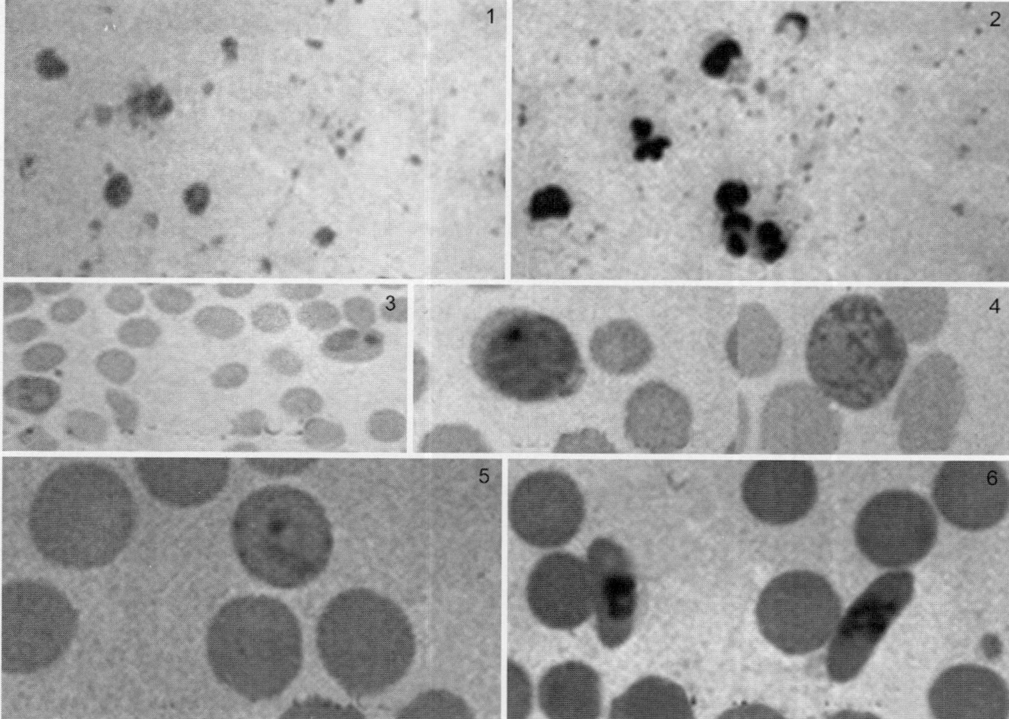

Fig. 4.1.1: Malarial parasites in light microscopy. (1) *P. vivax*—trophozoites and gametocytes, (2) *P. falciparum*—rings and gametocytes, (3) *P. vivax*—trophozoites, (4) *P. vivax*—schizont *P. vivax* gametocytes, (5) *P. falciparum*—trophozoites, (6) *P. falciparum*—gametocytes (*For color version, see Plate 5*)
Source: Approach to Malaria Diagnosis, TAG Archives: Rapid Diagnosis of Malaria. Srinivas/Feb.25.2015/Diagnosis. *www.malariasite.com*

smears on slide are stained with acridine orange and examined with the fluorescent microscope. Parasitic nuclear DNA is stained green and cytoplasm red. This aids in rapid screening of the smear, but availability of fluorescent microscope is restricted as it is expensive.

QUANTITATIVE BUFFY COAT MICROHEMATOCRIT EXAMINATION

Patient's whole blood is collected in special capillary tubes coated with acridine orange and subjected to microhematocrit centrifugation to form buffy coat, where the parasites are concentrated and are visualized as brilliant green-yellow fluorescing bodies against a dark red background under fluorescence microscope.

The quantitative buffy coat (QBC) microscopy is useful for screening large number of samples, as it is quick and saves time. It is reported to have good sensitivity and has an added advantage of possibility to detect other hemoparasites like microfilaria and babesia. The limitations of this method are difficulty in species identification and quantification, high cost of the capillary tubes and equipment.

RAPID DIAGNOSTIC TESTS (RDTs)

- Immunochromatographic assay for target malaria antigen/s detection **(Table 4.1.1)**
- Dipstick or cassette format
- Results are available within 30 minutes
- RDTs for malaria are available in India. Cost ranges from ₹ 50 to ₹ 150/test.

Table 4.1.1: Target antigens and their significance

Target antigens	*Significance*
HRP-2	Specific for *Plasmodium falciparum*, but other species cannot be detected, hence mixed infections may be missed. Persists after parasite death. Hence therapeutic monitoring cannot be done
Aldolase	Found in all *Plasmodium* species, hence can be utilized as 'Pan Malarial' antigen. Closely reflects parasite viability and hence a prognostic indicator
LDH (Lactate dehydrogenase of *Plasmodium* species)	Can be genus specific and species specific if monoclonal antibodies are used against each species. Closely reflects parasite viability. Potential for monitoring treatment efficacy
Combination of antigens Various formats are available	HRP2 and aldolase/pLDH pf and Pan /pLDH pf and pV/HRP2, pLDHPan/ HRP2 pLDH Pan and pLDHpV

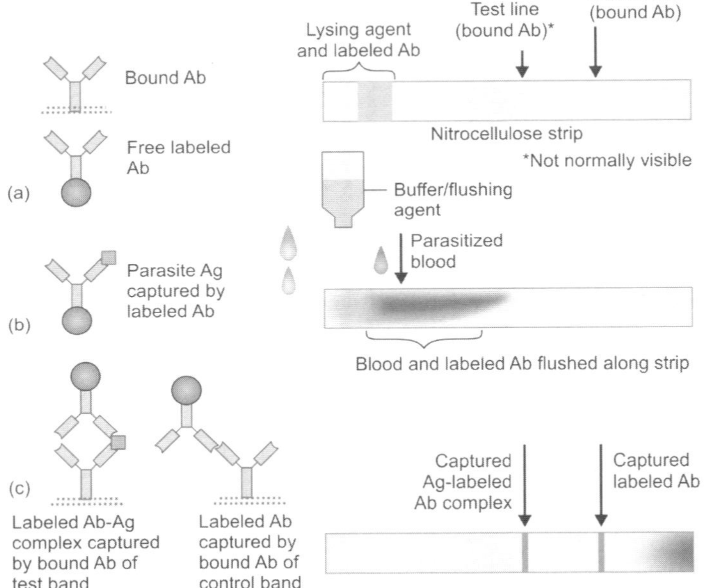

Mode of action of common malaria RDT format.

(a) Dye-labeled antibody (Ab), specific for the target antigen, is present on the lower end of the nitrocellulose strip or well-provided with the strip. Antibody, also specific for the target antigen, is bound to the strip in a thin (test) line, and either antibody specific for the labeled antibody, or antigen (Ag), is bound at the control line.

(b) Blood and buffer, which have been placed on the strip or in the well, are mixed with the labeled antibody and are drawn up the strip across the lines of bound antibody.

(c) If antigen is present, some labeled antibody will be trapped on the test line. Other labeled antibody is trapped on the control line.

Fig. 4.1.2: Mode of action of antigen detecting malaria RDTs
Source: Bell D, Wongsrichanalai C, Barnwell JW. Ensuring quality and access for malaria diagnosis: how can it be achieved? Nature Reviews Microbiology 2006;4:682-95. doi:10.1038/nrmicro1474.

RDTs have several advantages such as they do not require sophisticated equipment or expertise, and the tests are fairly sensitive and specific (Sensitivity of most kits >95% for *Plasmodium falciparum* and 75% to 90% for non-*falciparum*). With targeted antigens, the diagnosis can be made at species level. But they have limitations like low sensitivity in patients with lesser parasite density. Also no gold standard is available for antigen titration by RDTs **(Fig. 4.1.2)**.

The potential applications for RDTs are diagnosis of malaria in remote areas and confirmation of dubious microscopy diagnosis, rapid outbreak investigation and laboratory-based screening/diagnosis.

Wide array of RDTs are available for malarial parasitic antigens. The following critical points should be considered in order to achieve accuracy from RDTs:

- Use of standard kits should be strictly adhered to

- Validation of performance—both of performance and individual test performance are mandatory
- Technical competence of personnel should be regularly monitored and evaluated

POLYMERASE CHAIN REACTION (PCR)

Threshold of detection by PCR is 5 parasites/µL. Species-specific diagnosis is possible. Major application of PCR is in the area of anti-malarial drug resistance by identifying genetic mutations in the parasite. May have use in epidemiologic studies. But PCR is cost-ineffective and requires specialized equipment, reagents, and training. PCR is not done as a routine diagnostic testing, and only used for research purpose and for epidemiological studies, in referral centers like National Center for Disease Control (NCDC) in India. It is also useful to identify drug resistance.

SUMMARY

The WHO recommends that all cases of suspected malaria be confirmed using parasitebased diagnostic testing (either microscopy or RDTs) before administering treatment. Results of parasitological confirmation can be available in 30 minutes or less. Treatment, solely based on symptoms, should only be considered when parasitological diagnosis is not possible **(Table 4.1.2)**.

TYPHOID FEVER

The term "enteric fever" is a collective term that refers to typhoid fever caused by *Salmonella enterica serovar typhi* and paratyphoid fever caused by *Salmonella paratyphi A, B and C.* Worldwide an estimated 22 million cases of typhoid fever with 6 lakh deaths and 6 million cases of paratyphoid fever occur annually. Highest incidence is seen in south central and southeast Asia, especially in young children and adolescents. Though *S. typhi* infection is more common, enteric fever caused by *S. paratyphi* A is shown to be increasing in incidence especially in India in recent years.

LABORATORY DIAGNOSIS OF ENTERIC FEVER

The definitive diagnosis of typhoid fever depends on isolation of *S. typhi* from blood, bone marrow or a specific anatomic lesion. Detection of specific antibody response is suggestive of typhoid fever but not definitive.

CULTURE ISOLATION OF *SALMONELLA* SPECIES

Specimens: Blood, bone marrow, rose spots (punch biopsy), stool, urine, duodenal aspirate (especially in children) and pus from any suppurative lesion.

Table 4.1.2: Comparison of methods for diagnosing *Plasmodium* infection

Parameter	*Microscopy*	*PCR*	*Fluorescence*	*Dipstick HRP-2*	*Dipstick pLDH, ICT-Pf/Pv*
Sensitivity (parasites/microl)	50	5	50	>100	>100
Specificity	All species	All species	*P. falciparum* good, others difficult	*P. falciparum*	*P. falciparum* and *P. vivax* good
Parasite density measurement	Yes	No	No	Crude estimation	Crude estimation
Time for result	30–60 min	24 hr	30–60 min	20 min	20 min
Skill level	High	High	Moderate	Low	Low
Equipment	Microscope	PCR thermal cycler	QBC apparatus or fluorescence microscope	Kit only	Kit only
Cost /test	Low	High	Moderate/low but equipment cost is high	Moderate	Moderate

BLOOD CULTURE

Blood culture is the mainstay in specific diagnosis of typhoid fever. Volume of blood is one of the most important factors in the isolation of *S. typhi* from typhoid patients. 10–15 mL of blood should be collected from young children and adults, and 2–4 mL from children less than 5 years, in order to achieve the optimal isolation rates.

Critical Factors Responsible for Optimum Isolation

- Appropriate volume of blood broth ratio 1 in 10 (older children and adults), 1 in 6 (children less than 5 years)
- Number and timing of cultures—blood drawn during febrile spike, more than one culture—better yield
- Use of standard selective and non-selective media
- Laboratory competence in isolation techniques.

In manual blood culture method, blood collected is inoculated into brain heart infusion broth and after 24–72 hours of incubation subcultured onto selective and non-selective media and observed for growth after further 24 hours incubation. Limitation of conventional culture method is long turnaround time, i.e. the time taken from sample collection to release of report. This can be overcome by automated radiometric-based blood culture system, where the equipment detects the presence of growth in the bottles by a continuously monitoring sensor. So when the growth is detected, subcultures are made immediately thereby reducing the turnaround time.

CLOT CULTURE

Clot cultures yield better isolation. After clotting, the blood clot is lysed with streptokinase or manually, which will release the bacilli trapped inside the cells. But streptokinase is expensive.

STOOL OR RECTAL SWAB CULTURES

These cultures are useful especially in carriers and patients during the 3rd or 4th week of illness. Stool sample is collected in Selenite F. Broth and processed further. It is useful in outbreak investigations.

BONE MARROW CULTURE

Though bone marrow culture is the most ideal specimen, it is only opted in patients with strong clinical suspicion of enteric fever, in whom multiple blood cultures with recommended volume of blood are negative, especially in patients treated with antibiotics. Duodenal aspirate culture is also a very good specimen for culture isolation especially in children.

Advantages of Culture Isolation

- Gold standard, as it identifies the pathogen up to species level
- Antibiotic susceptibility testing guides in specific therapy
- Emergence of drug resistance can be studied
- Used in prognosis assessment.

Limitations of Culture Isolation

- Facility for culture isolation is not available in primary and many secondary health care centers
- As the sensitivity of blood culture is volume dependent, it is not feasible in patients in whom large volume of blood cannot be drawn
- Prolonged turnaround time, i.e. results are available earliest by 72 hours after blood culture
- Variable sensitivity during different phases of disease
- Sensitivity is also dependent on competency of the laboratory in isolation methods.

Antibiotic Susceptibility Testing Guidelines

- CLSI standard—Clinical Laboratory Standards Institute (USA)
- EUCAST—European Committee on Antimicrobial Susceptibility Testing
- Testing methods
  - Kirby Bauer Disk Diffusion
  - Minimum inhibitory concentration (MIC) measured by micro/macro broth dilution tests, and e-tests
- Report
  - For susceptible strains of *Salmonella typhi*
    - Susceptibility to first-line drugs like ampicillin, sulphamethoxazole-trimethoprim and chloramphenicol would be reported
  - For resistant strains
    - Susceptibility to second-line drugs like fluoroquinolones (e.g. Ciprofloxacin), 3rd generation cephalosporins (e.g. Ceftrioxone, cefotaxime), monobactum (e.g. aztreonam) and a macrolide (e.g. azithromycin) would be reported with a mention about resistant status.

MDR strains are now prevalent globally. CLSI reviews and modifies guidelines every year. As per CLSI 2013, nalidixic acid was used as the surrogate marker for in vitro susceptibility testing of all quinolones. But as with CLSI 2014 and 2015, nalidixic acid is not the marker for quinolones resistance, and zone of inhibition of each drug in the quinolone group tested, should be reported individually.

SEROLOGICAL DIAGNOSIS OF TYPHOID FEVER

Felix Widal Test

Popularly known as Widal test, this test measures agglutinating antibody levels against O and H antigens of *S. typhi* and H antigens of *Paratyphi A and B*. Usually O antibodies appear on days 6 to 8 and H antibodies appear on days 10 to 12 after the onset of the disease. O agglutinins appear early and disappear early and indicate recent infection. H agglutinins appear late and disappear late. O antibodies are serotype non-specific. They are raised in all infections, i.e. *S. typhi, S. paratyphi A* and *B*. But H antibodies are more specific. It is performed by tube agglutination method which, if positive, is reported in titers. Slide agglutination method with colored antigens is rapid but can only be qualitative or semiquantitative **(Table 4.1.3)**.

Both acute and convalescent sera are required to observe rise in titers (4-fold rise). To arrive at the significant titers, the baseline titres of that geographic region should be studied periodically by population studies, which varies with different regions based on the endemicity of the disease. In a comparative analysis of baseline titer of O and H agglutinins in different regions of India and Nepal, the baseline titers of *S. typhi* "O" was found to be 1:40, *S. typhi* "H" was 1 in 80 in southern India by studies done by Patil et al., Sneha et al. and Peshattiwar et al. Base line titers of *S. paratyphi* are AH 1:40, BH 1:40 according to various studies from South India.

Significant titers are at least one titer higher than baseline titer.

Table 4.1.3: Interpretation of Widal test

Widal test result	*Suggestive of*
Rise of TO and TH antibody	Enteric fever due to *S. typhi*
Rise of TO and AH antibody	Enteric fever due to *S. paratyphi A*
Rise of TO and AH antibody	Enteric fever due to *S. paratyphi B*
Rise of only TO antibody	Recent infection: Due to any serotype—*S. typhi* or *S. paratyphi A or B*
Rise of only TH antibody	? Convalescent stage/Anamnestic response
Rise of all TH, AH, BH antibodies	Post-TAB vaccination

Source: Essentials of Medical Microbiology, Edn. 1. Apurba Sankar Sastry, Sandhya Bhat K. ISBM:978-93-5152-987-3.

Limitations of Widal Test

- Both acute and convalescent sera are required to demonstrate fourfold rise in titer in patients with low acute phase titers, which is difficult to obtain
- False positive results are seen in unrelated infection like malaria, dengue in persons who have had enteric fever (Anamnestic response) and in persons with prior immunization (with TAB vaccine)
- False negative results are seen in first week of illness, patients on antibiotics and due to prozone effect (antibody excess)

Other Antibody Detection Tests

Various commercial methods available are shown in **Table 4.1.4**.

KEY POINTS

Diagnosis of enteric fever should be considered depending upon duration of illness **(Table 4.1.5)**.

Table 4.1.4: Other antibody detection tests (RDTs)

Name of test	*Principle*	*Antigens used*	*Utility*	*Limitations*
IDL Tubex test	Chromogenic test	• LPS • O9 (specific antigen for *S. typhi*	• Very specific test as it detects IgM antibodies against *S. typhi* only • Invaluable test for rapid diagnosis of current infection	• Kits are very temperature sensitive, hence need stringent storage conditions • Sensitivity of the test varies between 65–80%
Typhidot	Dot EIA	50 KD OMP antigen	• Detects both IgM and IgG antibodies • Useful in diagnosis of typhoid fever in early (1st week) and middle phases (2nd and 3rd week)	• Cannot differentiate between current infection and re-infection in carriers, as IgG response would mask IgM antibodies
Typhidot-M (modification of Typhidot)	Dot EIA	OMP antigen	• Detects only IgM, by blocking IgG response • Hence useful in diagnosis of current infection as well as re-infection in carriers • Sensitivity 100%; Specificity 98%; Very good positive and negative predictive values	• Kits are very temperature sensitive, hence need stringent storage conditions
IgM dipstick test	Immuno chro-matography	LPS antigen	• Detects IgM anti-LPS antibodies • Results are available after 3 hours	Sensitivity of the test varies between 65% and 77%

Source: Adapted from Background document: The Diagnosis, treatment and prevention of typhoid fever: Communicable disease surveillance and response: Vaccines and Biologicals, WHO/W&B/03.07. May 2003

Table 4.1.5: Diagnosis of enteric fever depending upon duration of illness

Duration of illness	*Specimen used and test(s) done*
First week	Culture of blood, bone marrow aspirate, duodenal aspirate
Second week and Third week	Serum for antibody detection by Widal test/RDTs Stool and urine culture, blood culture can be tried in second week, if the patient had not received antibiotics
Fourth week	Stool and urine culture
Carriers	Stool and urine culture, serum for detection of antibodies to Vi antigen Sewage culture—indirect way

Source: Essentials of Medical Microbiology, Edn. 1. Apurba Sankar Sastry, Sandhya Bhat K. ISBM:978-93-5152-987-3.

As RDTs are simple, rapid, easy-to-perform and fairly economical, they are likely to replace conventional Widal test in future in the developing world. When used in conjunction with culture method these rapid tests provide an invaluable tool in accurate diagnosis of typhoid fever.

BIBLIOGRAPHY

1. Background document: The Diagnosis, Treatment and Prevention of Typhoid Fever; Communicable diseases, surveillance and response, vaccines and biologicals WHO/V&B/03.07 May 2003
2. Cumitech 1C Blood cultures IV—edition 1st American Society for Microbiology; ASM Press, 2005.
3. Document on malaria diagnosis - Laboratory identification of parasitic diseases of public health concern-CDC's division of parasitic diseases and malaria (DPDx) http//www.cdc.gov/malaria/diagnosis_treatment/rdt.html
4. WHO publications:
   - Information note on recommended selection criteria for procurement of malaria RDTs (2016)WHO/HTM/GMP/2015.12.rev1
   - Summary results of WHO product testing of malaria RDTs: Rounds 1- 6 (2008-2015) ISBN 978924150042
   - Malaria Microscopy quality assurance manual-version 2 (2016)

4.2 Diagnostic Armamentarium in Dengue, Leptospirosis and Scrub Typhus

Somu Sivabalan, MVN Malleswari

Reviewers: *MKC Nair, S Thangavelu, S Narmada*

DENGUE ILLNESS

Dengue is caused by a single-stranded RNA virus belonging Flaviviridae with 4 serotypes which are genetically and antigenically different. The severity of disease ranges from asymptomatic infection to mild undifferentiated fever, to fatal shock; dengue illnesses exhibit an extensive array of clinical presentations with unpredictable evolution.

CLINICAL DIAGNOSIS

Clinically dengue is a dynamic disease which may have three stages—febrile, critical and recovery. Presently, according to the revised WHO guidelines, it is being classified based on its severity as: (a) Dengue without warning signs, (b) Dengue with warning signs, (c) Severe dengue **(Fig. 4.2.1)**. This classification is highly likely to be of practical use.

LABORATORY DIAGNOSIS

The objectives of laboratory investigations in Dengue are (i) to confirm the clinical diagnosis, and (ii) to provide information for epidemiological surveillance. Laboratory diagnosis is not necessary for clinical management except in atypical cases or when carrying out differential diagnosis with other infectious diseases.

The diagnostic method to confirm an acute infection depends on the time of clinical illness. The febrile phase is coincident with the presence of viremia, some viral components and replication products in blood; the critical and convalescent phases coincide with the development of antibodies **(Fig. 4.2.2)**.

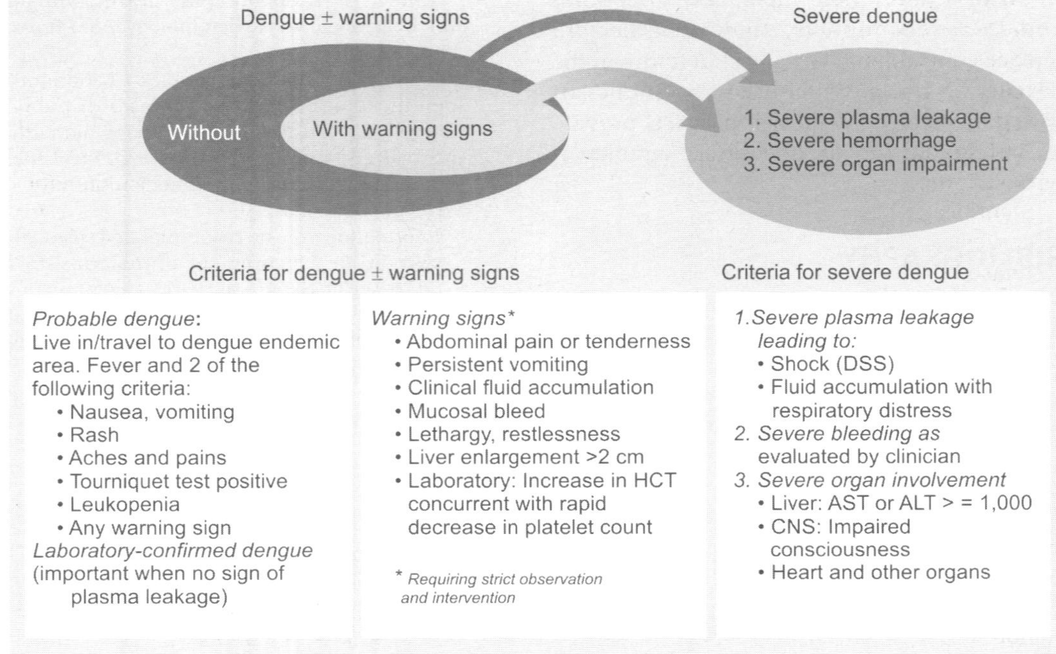

Fig. 4.2.1: Severity-based clinical classification of dengue

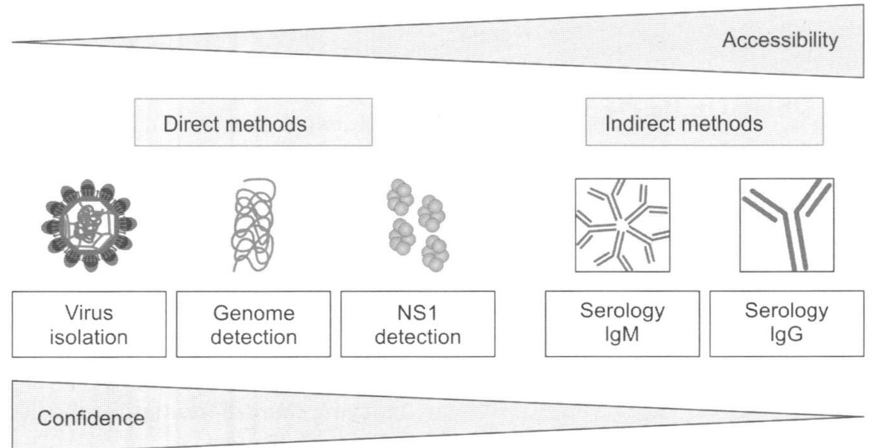

Fig. 4.2.2: Diagnostic test for dengue

FEBRILE PHASE (DAY 1 TO DAYS 4–5 OF FEVER)

1. *Viral isolation:* The infective virus can be isolated in serum by inoculation in tissue culture (mosquito cell cultures) and mosquitoes. This method allows for identification of the viral serotype. Results are available within 1–2 weeks time.

2. *Viral nucleic acid detection (Genome detection):* Virus genome detection using reverse transcriptase polymerase chain reaction (RT-PCR) and real-time RT-PCR confirms an acute dengue infection. Turnaround time is 1–2 days. Both methods have a high sensitivity and allow serotype identification and quantification of genome copies. The test may be negative in acute phase specimen, i.e. within first 5 days of symptom due to undetectable levels of viruses.

   Both viral isolation and nucleic acid detection are expensive, require expertise, and cannot distinguish between primary and secondary dengue infection. The virus is extremely heat sensitive and hence the sample needs to be rapidly transported at 4°C to the laboratory and be processed as soon as possible. If specimen delivery cannot be performed in the first 24–48 hours, freezing at –70°C is recommended. These tests can be performed in necropsy tissue specimens also. Presently *both these methods are reserved for research purpose.*
3. *Viral antigen detection:* NS1 antigen test, i.e. nonstructural protein 1 is produced by all flaviviruses. This glycoprotein antigen can be detected in all patients with both primary and secondary dengue from first day of symptom up to nine days and even, at times, up to 18 days post-onset of symptoms. This test can be done by ELISA or by other rapid methods like immune chromatography, where results are obtained in minutes. ELISA test due to its specificity may be useful for differential diagnostics between flaviviruses but other rapid tests have the drawback of gross reactivity across the flavivirus group. Currently, these assays are not type-specific, are expensive and under evaluation for diagnostic accuracy and cost-effectiveness.

CRITICAL AND CONVALESCENT PHASES (AFTER DAYS 4–5 OF ILLNESS)

Serology

Primary infections are characterized by high levels of IgM and low levels of IgG, while low levels of IgM with high levels of IgG characterize secondary infections. Specific IgM by MAC-ELISA is the best marker of a recent dengue infection. It has good sensitivity and specificity only when done on five or more days after the onset of illness. A single serum sample collected after day 5 of fever onset is useful for IgM determination. Low or undetectable levels of dengue IgM response in some secondary infection reduces the diagnostic accuracy of IgM ELISA test. Moreover, IgM antibodies to dengue may remain elevated for 2–3 months after illness.

A diagnosis of dengue infection is confirmed by the detection of the virus, the viral genome

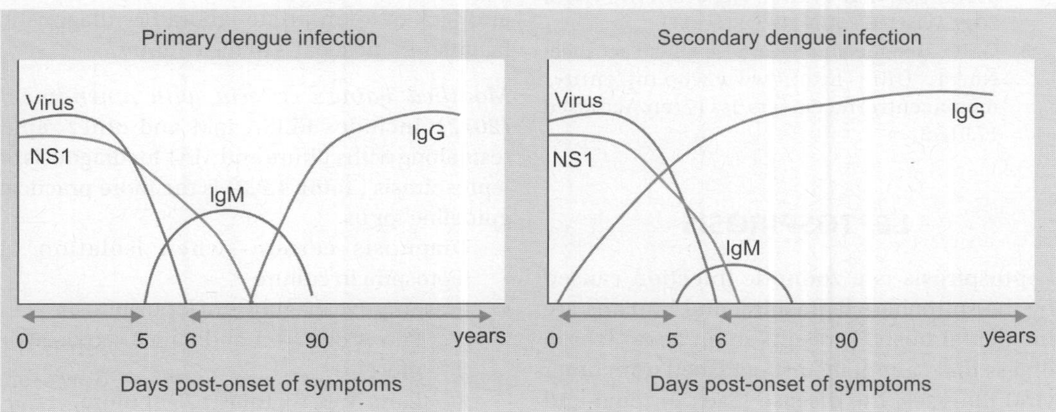

Fig. 4.2.3: Relationship in the presence of NS1, IgM and IgG in dengue

Table 4.2.1: Summary of test and their interpretation for dengue

	Method	*Interpretation*	*Sample characteristics*
Confirmed dengue infection	Viral isolation	Virus isolated	Serum (collected at 1–5 days of fever) Necropsy tissues
	Genome detection	Positive RT-PCR or positive real-time RT-PCR	
	Antigen detection	Positive NS1 Ag	
		Positive immunohistochemical	Necropsy tissues
	IgM seroconversion	From negative IgM to positive IgM in paired sera	
	IgG seroconversion	From negative IgG to positive IgG in paired sera or 4-fold increase; IgG levels among paired sera	Acute serum (days 1–5) and convalescent serum (15–21 after first serum)
Probable dengue infection	Positive IgM	Positive IgM	Single serum collected after day 5
	High IgG levels	High IgG levels by ELISA or HI (≥ 1280)	

Abbreviations: ELISA, enzyme-linked immunosorbent assay; IgG, immunoglobulin G; IgM, immunoglobulin M; NS1 Ag, non-structural protein 1 antigen; RT-PCR, reverse transcriptase polymerase chain reaction.

or NS1 Ag, or seroconversion of IgM or IgG (from negative to positive IgM/IgG or four-fold increase in the specific antibody titer) in paired sera. The relationship of NS1, IgM and IgG is depicted in **Figure 4.2.3** and an overall summary in **Table 4.2.1.** A low platelet, NS1 and serology does not indicate severity or complication and need to be correlated clinically.

BIBLIOGRAPHY

1. Dar L, Broor S, Sengupta S, Xess I, Seth P. The first major outbreak of dengue hemorrhagic fever in Delhi, India. Emerg Infect Dis. 1999;5:589-590.
2. Dengue. Guidelines for diagnosis, treatment prevention and control. Geneva, TDR/WHO, 2009. WHO/HTM/NTD/DEN/2009.
3. WHO. Dengue and Severe Dengue. Fact sheet No. 1. URL: http://www.who.int/entity/mediacentre/factsheets/fs117/en.Accessed 17.01.12.

LEPTOSPIROSIS

Leptospirosis is a zoonotic infection caused by the spirochete leptospira, and humans are incidental hosts. It results in an acute febrile illness that cannot be distinguished from other viral illnesses, the disease leads to renal and hepatic dysfunction with hemorrhage also known as Weil's disease or icteric leptospirosis which may be associated with multisystem organ dysfunction in form of pulmonary, cardiac, and central nervous system affection.

According to Indian leptospirosis society's criteria, leptospirosis should be suspected in a child presenting with history of abrupt onset of high fever >39°C and bodyache/headache with any one or more of the following features (i) jaundice (ii) oliguria (iii) cough and breathlessness (iv) hemorrhagic tendency (v) signs of meningeal irritation or altered sensorium or convulsions. Leptospirosis has been under-reported and underdiagnosed from India due to a lack of awareness of the disease and lack of appropriate laboratory diagnostic facilities in most parts of the country.

Modified Faine's criteria with amendment (2012): Includes ELISA IgM and other rapid tests along with culture and MAT for diagnosis of leptospirosis **(Table 4.2.2)** is the more practical guideline for us.

- Diagnosis certain—when isolation of leptospira in culture
- Presumptive diagnosis of leptospirosis
  - Part A or Part A and Part B score: 26 or more
  - Parts A, B, C (Total) : 25 or more
- Possible diagnosis -20 to 25

These criteria designed for adults also can be applied to older children.

LABORATORY DIAGNOSIS

Specific Investigations

1. *Demonstration of leptospira from body fluids:* Leptospires may be isolated from blood (first 7 days), cerebrospinal fluid, and most tissues during the septicemic phase which lasts for about 5–7 days. However, since this phase usually presents with non-specific symptoms, it is usually missed. The immune stage is characterized by circulating antibodies and disappearance of leptospires from the circulation. However, leptospires may still be isolated from urine for several weeks up to 2 months post-infection. The leptospires can be identified by:
   - *Dark-field microscopy or direct fluorescent-antibody assay.*
   - *Culture:* Isolation of leptospira organism by culture of blood, CSF and urine are the most definite way of confirming leptospirosis. Culture does not contribute to an early diagnosis as results come late, weeks or even months after inoculation of culture medium.
   - *Detection of DNA by PCR* is the only available diagnostic test available in the first week of leptospirosis. It is a complicated and expensive test.
2. *Serology:* Seroconversion usually occurs after 5–7 days after the onset of disease but may sometimes occur only after 10 days or longer. IgM class antibodies usually appear somewhat earlier and may be present for up to 2 months after the infection and at lower titers for years. IgG antibody is usually erratic and often may not be detected or may be detectable for only relatively short periods of time. Thus, the presence of antibodies is by itself no proof of current infection, as some antibodies may persist for long periods after an infection.
   - *Microscopic agglutination test (MAT):* The MAT is considered to be the gold standard for diagnosis and can identify specific serotypes. The MAT uses a battery of antigens from common endemic leptospire serovars, is complicated and requires dark field microscopy. Test accuracy is affected by selection of antigens for the test. This test is important from the epidemiologic point of view to identify the serovar. Repeat samples are required for confirming diagnosis and the cut-off titers are controversial. Interpretation of MAT:
     - *Single titer:*
       - Significant criteria—1:100
       - Diagnostic criteria
         (a) Endemic area—1:400 (1:800, 1:1,600)
         (b) Nonendemic area—1:100, 1:200
         (c) Sero-survey—1:50
     - *Repeat titer:* Four-fold rise or seroconversion
3. *ELISA:* The presence of IgM antibodies may indicate current or recent leptospirosis. A patient's serum may be positive 5–10 days after onset of symptoms and may remain detectable for several years. If the initial sample was taken at an early stage in the infection, the ELISA test may be positive but MAT negative. Therefore, a follow-up sample is required. Test may be negative if the serogroup of the infecting strain does not react with the serovar strain used as the antigen. If antibiotics are given from the beginning of the illness, the immune and antibody response may be delayed.

- *Macroscopic slide agglutination test (MSAT)*
- *Other rapid serological tests include*—Latex agglutination test, Lepto dipstick, Leptotek lateral flow Leptotek Dri-Dot test.

Diagnostic tests cannot identify the serogroup but have the following advantages:

- A single positive sample adequate for diagnosis,
- Simple, sensitive and specific
- Becomes positive earlier than MAT
- Can be done also in small rural hospitals

Table 4.2.2: Modified Faine's criteria 2012

Clinical data (Part A)		*Epidemiological factors (Part B)*		*Bacteriological and laboratory findings (Part C)*	
Headache	2	Rainfall	5	Isolation of leptospira in culture—Diagnosis certain	
Fever	2	Contact with contaminated environment	4	PCR	25
Temperature >39°C	2	Animal contact	1	Positive serology	
Conjunctival suffusion	4			ELISA IgM positive*	15
Meningism	4				
Myalgia	4	Total	10	SAT-Positive*	15
Conjunctival suffusion + Meningism + Myalgia	10			Other rapid tests**	15
				MAT- Single positive in high titer*	15
Jaundice	1			MAT (paired sera): Rising titer/Seroconversion	25
Albuminuria/ Nitrogen retention	2				
Hemoptysis/Dyspnea	2				

* Any one of the tests only should be scored
** Latex agglutination test/Lepto dipstick/Lepto Tek lateral flow/Lepto Tek Dri-Dot test
Abbreviations: SAT, slide agglutination test; PCR, polymerase chain reaction; MAT, microscopic agglutination test.

- Can be easily done for a large number of patients during epidemics

Confirmed case of leptospirosis is a suspect or probable case with any one of the following:
- Isolation of leptospires from clinical specimens
- Positive PCR result
- Seroconversion from a negative to positive or four-fold rise in titer by MAT
- Titer by MAT of 400 and greater in a single sample.

Where laboratory capacity not well established: Positive by two different rapid diagnostic tests could be considered as laboratory confirmed case.

BIBLIOGRAPHY

1. Human Leptospirosis: Guidance for diagnosis, surveillance and control. World Health Organization and International Leptospirosis Society 2003. ISBN 92 4 154589 5 (http://www.who.int/csr/don/en/WHO_CDS_CSR_EPH_2002.23.pdf)). Accessed on 15 April 2016.
2. Shiva Kumar S. Indian Guidelines for the Diagnosis and Management of Human Leptospirosis. In: Muruganathan A, editor. Medicine Update. 23rd edn. pp.23-9 (http://www.apiindia.org/medicine_update_2013/chap07.pdf). Accessed on 15 April 2016.

SCRUB TYPHUS

Rickettsial diseases are considered some of the most covert emerging and re-emerging diseases and are being increasingly recognized in India. It occurs more frequently during the rainy season. However, outbreaks have been reported during the cooler season in southern India. They are difficult to diagnose due to low index of suspicion, nonspecific signs and symptoms, and absence of widely available sensitive and specific diagnostic tests but are extraordinarily easy and inexpensive to treat if diagnosed early.

SPECIFIC LABORATORY INVESTIGATIONS

Rickettsiae are not evident on blood smear findings and do not stain with most conventional stains. No rapid laboratory tests are available to diagnose rickettsial diseases early in the course of illness.

Serology

Serologic assays that demonstrate antibodies to rickettsiae are:

1. *Weil-Felix OX-K Agglutination test* is based on the cross-reactive antigens of *Proteus*

vulgaris strains. Serologic findings usually take 10–12 days to become positive. The value of testing 2 sequential serum or plasma samples together to show a rising antibody level is considerably more important in confirming acute infection because antibody titers may persist in some patients for years after the original exposure. Titer of 1:80 is to be considered possible infection. However, baseline titers need to be standardized for each region. An IgM titer >1:32 and/or a four-fold increase of titers between two sera confirm a recent infection. Fifty percent of patients have a positive test result during the second week. This test should be carried out only after 5–7 days of onset of fever. This test is now being replaced by a complement-fixation test. However, due to cross-reactions among serotypes, it is difficult to identify accurately a specific serotype.

2. *Immunofluoroscence Assay (IFA):* This is a reference serological method for diagnosis of rickettsial diseases and is considered serological 'gold standard'; however, cost and requirement of technical expertise limit its wide use. Therefore, it is recommended only for research and in areas where sero-prevalence of rickettsial diseases has been established and a reference facility is already available.
3. *Indirect Immuno-peroxidase (IIP)* is a modification of the standard IFA method that can be used with a light microscope, and the results of these tests are comparable to those from IFA.
4. *IgM and IgG ELISA:* ELISA techniques, particularly immunoglobulin M (IgM) capture assays for serum, are probably the most of sensitive tests available for rickettsial diagnosis and the presence of IgM antibodies, indicate comparatively recent infection. A significant IgM antibody titer is observed at the end of 1st week, whereas IgG antibodies appear at the end of 2nd week. The cut-off value is Optical Density of 0.5. Baseline titers need to be established keeping in view the regional variations.
5. *Commercial Rapid Diagnostic Kits* provide reliable and well-accepted preliminary results within one hour, but the availability of these tests is severely limited by their cost. However, other serological tests must be used in order to obtain confirmation of *O. tsutsugamushi* infection. ELISA provides more sensitivity and equal specificity when compared to commercial test kits.

Non-serological

1. *Culture:* The organism can be grown from the blood of patients with scrub typhus but results are not available in time to guide clinical management.
2. *Polymerase Chain Reaction (PCR)* is possible from skin rash biopsies, lymph node biopsies or ethylene-diamine-tetra-acetic acid (EDTA) blood. Real-time PCR assays are as sensitive as standard PCR but are more rapid and can give quantitative results.
3. *Eschar:* Mite bites are painless; patients are unaware even with eschar and/or fever. The infection begins as a red induration, within 48 hrs enlarges to 8–12 mm in diameter that eventually vesiculates and ruptures to form an eschar. It is seen in around 50% to up to 95% of cases, and is usually painless and single, though occasionally pruritic. Tender lymphadenopathy may be seen in the draining basin. The eschar resolves in 3–4 weeks with no sequelae, but may occasionally cause scarring or hyperpigmentation. Eschar **(Fig. 4.2.4)** at the bite site is the single most useful diagnostic clue, all febrile patients without localizing signs of infection should be examined.
4. *Therapuetic Trial:* Antibiotic therapy brings about prompt disappearance of the fever and dramatic clinical improvement by 24–48 hrs. Rapid defervescence after antibiotic treatment is so characteristic that it is used as a diagnostic test. Antibiotics are recommended, treatment duration is 7–14 days. If the antibiotic treatment is discontinued too quickly, relapses may occur. No significant morbidity or mortality

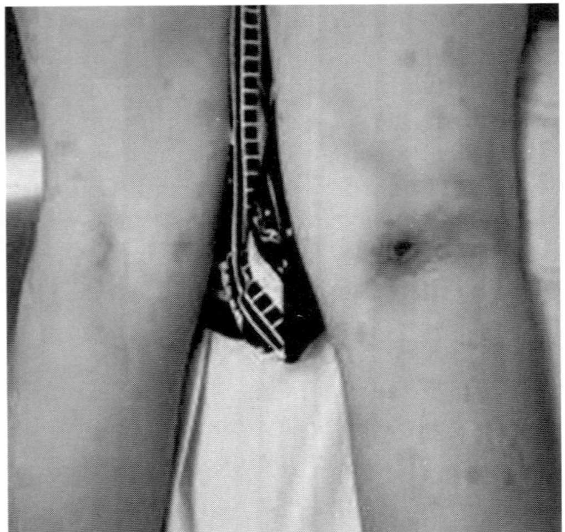

Fig. 4.2.4: Eschar in scrub typhus
(For color version, see Plate 6)

occurs in patients who receive appropriate treatment. There are no obvious differences between tetracycline, doxycycline, telithromycin or azithromycin. Rifampicin may be better than tetracycline in areas where scrub typhus appears to respond poorly to standard anti-rickettsial drugs.

CASE DEFINITION

For the purpose of management, the following definitions have been provided by guidelines on the basis of clinical and various laboratory parameters.

Suspected/Clinical Case

Acute undifferentiated febrile illness of 5 days or more with or without eschar (If eschar is present, fever of less than 5 days duration should be considered as scrub typhus). Other presenting features may be headache and rash (rash more often seen in fair persons), lymphadenopathy, multi-organ involvement like liver, lung and kidney involvement.

Probable Case

A suspected clinical case showing titers of 1:80 or above in OX2, OX19 and OXK antigens by Weil Felix test and an optical density (OD) > 0.5 for IgM by ELISA are considered positive for typhus and spotted fever groups of Rickettsiae.

Confirmed Case

- Rickettsial DNA is detected in eschar samples or whole blood by PCR (or)
- Rising antibody titers on acute and convalescent sera detected by Indirect Immune Fluorescence Assay (IFA) or Indirect Immunoperoxidase Assay (IPA).

BIBLIOGRAPHY

1. Bozeman FM, Elisberg BL. Serological diagnosis of scrub typhus by indirect immuno-fluorescence. Proc Soc Exp Biol Med. 1963;112: 568-73.
2. Janani S. Rickettsial infections. IAP-IJ PP CME 2011. Indian Journal of Practical Pediatrics. 2012;14:11-4.
3. Kelly DJ, Wong PW, Gan E, Lewis GE Jr. Comparative evaluation of the indirect immunoperoxidase test for the serodiagnosis of rickettsial disease. Am J Trop Med Hyg. 1988;38(2):400-6.
4. Mahajan SK, Kashyap R, Kanga A, Sharma V, Prasher BS, Pal LS. Relevance of Weil-Felix test in diagnosis of scrub typhus in India. J Assoc Physicians India. 2006;54:619-21.
5. Panpamich R, Garner P. Antibiotics for treating scrub typhus. Cochrane Database Syst Rev. 2002;3:CD 002150.
6. Rahi M, Gupte MD, Bhargava A, Varghese GM, Arora R. DHR-ICMR Guidelines for diagnosis and management of Rickettsial diseases in India. Indian J Med Res. 2015;1414:417-22.
7. Shivbalan S, Sendil KD. The Eschar of Scrub Typhus. Indian J Pediatr. 2010;77:918.
8. Singhsilarak T, Leowattana W, Looareesuwan S, et al. Detection of *O. tsutsugamushi* in clinical samples by quantitative real-time polymerase chain reaction. Am J Trop Med Hyg. 2005;72:640-1.

4.3 Insight into the Tests for Intrauterine Infections

Palani Gunasekaran

Reviewers: *MKC Nair, S Thangavelu, S Narmada*

INTRODUCTION

Infections during pregnancy carry a risk of intrauterine transmission resulting in fetal or neonatal damage. Microorganisms may gain access to the fetus before delivery and the magnitude of intrauterine infections depends on the type of pathogenic agents, which cause fetal or neonatal diseases ranging in severity from mild and transient symptoms to a fatal disease. About 25% of preterm births are associated with intrauterine infection and the clinical assessment process essentially comprises laboratory diagnostic tests that facilitate clinical intervention during pregnancy and at the neonatal stage. Fetuses are uniquely susceptible to pathogens because of the immature functions of physiologic and immunologic systems. This necessitates clinical and diagnostic laboratories to adopt distinct methods for rapid and accurate diagnosis for intrauterine infections with high sensitivity and specificity. The chapter discusses overview of these infections and the insights into the diagnostic methods for effective clinical intervention.

INTRAUTERINE INFECTIONS

Intrauterine infection is defined as the invasion of the amniotic cavity by pathogenic microbes causing both clinical as well as asymptomatic features. They are the major cause of premature labor involving the intact or ruptured membranes, and increase the fetal morbidity and mortality rates. Risk factors such as prolonged rupture of membranes, prolonged labor, multiple vaginal examinations, meconium-stained amniotic fluid, smoking, etc. are identified as risk factors for intrauterine infections.

Several microorganisms are known to gain access to the fetus before delivery and the establishment of these intrauterine infections occurs through the following routes:

- Ascending infection from the vagina or cervix;
- Transplacental hematogenous dissemination (transplacental infection);
- Retrograde seeding from the peritoneal cavity via fallopian tubes; and
- Accidental introduction by invasive procedures such as chorionic villous sampling (CVS), amniocentesis, shunting, etc.

Among these four routes, incidence by ascending infection from the vagina or cervix is more common and this infection induces inflammation in each placental compartment and subsequent intra-amniotic, maternal, and fetal inflammatory responses. The microbial products elicit a fetal inflammatory response which may result in premature labor with multi-system organ involvement in the human fetus and a higher rate of perinatal morbidity. It is to be noted that the earlier the gestational age at delivery, the higher the frequency of intra-amniotic infection.

Ascending infection, a significant problem in patients of premature rupture of the membranes (PROM), is proposed to follow a four-stage process leading to intrauterine infection:

Stage I: The process starts in Stage I that consists of a change in the vaginal or cervical microflora or the presence of pathogenic agents in the cervix. Bacterial vaginosis is an example for a manifestation of Stage I.

Stage II is characterized by the access of microorganism to the intrauterine cavity followed by colonization of the placenta deciduas causing the localized inflammatory reaction (deciduitis) and subsequent colonization of the chorion and amnion.

Stage III is characterized by the invasion of microorganisms through the fetal vessels, amnion and the amniotic cavity. Without rupturing the membranes, microorganisms can cross them for producing an intra-amniotic infection.

From amniotic cavity, they gain entry to the fetus by various means (Stage IV) such as aspiration of the infected fluid by the fetus (e.g. congenital pneumonia), direct spreading of pathogenic microbes from infected amniotic fluid (e.g. otitis, conjunctivitis, omphalitis, etc.) and dissemination from any of these sites to the fetal circulation (e.g. bacteremia and sepsis). The fetal infection (Stage IV) is the most advanced and critical stage of ascending intrauterine infection. The mortality rate of neonates due to congenital sepsis is in the range of 25% to 90%.

MICROBIOLOGY OF INTRAUTERINE INFECTIONS

Intrauterine infections are caused by a range of viral, bacterial and protozoan agents and consequently may lead to preterm birth. The infection or the products of infecting agents evoke an inflammatory response by means of the placental release of proinflammatory cytokines. Fetal infection is associated with infections involving the amnion and chorion rather than the amnion alone. This is likely secondary to invasion and inflammation being closer in proximity to the fetus. Infection of the umbilical cord, funisitis, has a higher rate of clinical chorioamnionitis and neonatal sepsis than those without infection.

Commonest bacterial isolates: The most common bacterial isolates associated with spontaneous preterm labor with intact membranes are *Ureaplasma urealyticum*, *Fusobacterium* species, *Gardnerella vaginalis*, *Mycoplasma hominis*, *Staphylococcus aureus* and Bacteroides species. Rarely, *Escherichia coli*, *Neisseria gonorrhoea*, *Lactobacillus* spp., *Enterococcus faecalis*, and *Peptococcus* spp. **(Table 4.3.1)**. Group B *Streptococcus* (GBS), the bacteria colonizing the vaginal canal, is having the maternal to fetus transmission risk of about 20%. *Chlamydia trachomatis* is capable of causing congenital pneumonia through ascending intra-amniotic infection. Diagnosis of bacterial infection from amniotic cavity may reveal that >50% of the patients exhibiting infection by more than one microorganism.

Commonest viral isolates—Rubella virus (RV), cytomegalovirus (CMV), varicella-zoster virus (VZV), herpes simplex virus (HSV), parvovirus B19 and human immunodeficiency virus (HIV) are the six most significant intrauterine viral infections. Fetus is infected with virus probably through maternal viremia and viral replication in the placenta. The ability of viruses to cross the placenta, infect the fetus and cause damage depends on the mother's immune status against the specific virus.

Table 4.3.1: Location of intrauterine infection and the bacteria implicated in the infection

Location	*Bacteria*
Between maternal and fetal membranes	Group B streptococci, *Escherichia coli*, *Chlamydia trachomatis*, *Neisseria gonorrhoea*, *Mycoplasma hominis*, *Trichomonas vaginalis*
Within the fetal membranes (chorioamnionitis)	Group B streptococci, *Escherichia coli*, *Chlamydia trachomatis*, *Neisseria gonorrhoea*, *Mycoplasma hominis*, *Trichomonas vaginalis*
Within the placenta	*Klebsiella pneumoniae* and *Staphylococcus sp*
Within the amniotic fluid (intra-amniotic infection, amnionitis)	*Ureaplasma urealyticum*, *Fusobacterium* species, *Mycoplasma hominis*
Within the umbilical cord (funisitis)	*Klebsiella pneumoniae* and *Staphylococcus sp*
Within the fetus	Group B streptococci, *Escherichia coli*, *Chlamydia trachomatis*, *Neisseria gonorrhoea*, *Mycoplasma hominis*, *Trichomonas vaginalis*

Exposure to maternal virus often is a result of chronic infection caused by cytomegalovirus (CMV), HIV, HSV, hepatitis B, or hepatitis C. For these viruses, the prevalence of infection in women of childbearing age and the incidence of new infections during pregnancy contribute to the overall prevalence of fetal or neonatal infection.

In contrast, viruses such as rubella, varicella-zoster virus (VZV), enteroviruses, and parvovirus B19 that produce acute infections in the mother are transmitted to the fetus to produce disease and this depends on the timing of maternal infection in relation to gestation. The risk of transmission to the fetus in primary CMV infection is 30–40%.

Vector-borne viruses such as West Nile virus, Chikungunya virus and Zika virus also infect fetus through maternal infection with varying degree. Certain maternal viral infections such as dengue and adenovirus can affect only the placenta without causing fetal infection and thereby affect the outcome for the infant. The proportion of morbidities such as preterm birth or poor fetal growth can be attributed to viral infection of the mother of fetus.

Diagnosis of Intrauterine Infections, Challenges and Prospects

Diagnosis of intrauterine infection is primarily based on the:

- Observation of fever >37.8°C;
- Rupture of placental membranes; and
- Two or more of the following conditions: maternal or fetal tachycardia, uterine tenderness, malodorous amniotic fluid, or peripheral leukocytosis with no other site of infection.

Low glucose level in amniotic-fluid is a rapid, simple, and inexpensive indicator of microbial invasion of the amniotic cavity; however, the method lacks sensitivity and specificity. Syphilis, toxoplasmosis, rubella, CMV and herpes simplex virus (HSV) are the pathogens frequently implicated in intrauterine infections and these pathogens are grouped under the acronym STORCH. More number of viral pathogens such as chicken pox, hepatitis (B, C and E), enterovirus, AIDS and parvovirus are included in CHEAP TORCHES, an expansion of STORCH.

DIAGNOSIS OF BACTERIAL INFECTIONS

The diagnosis of bacterial infections is generally performed through isolating the microorganisms from amniotic fluid with standard *culture techniques*. Though the differential culture methods are helpful in diagnosing much of the intrauterine bacterial infections, these methods are not useful in detecting *Chlamydia trachomatis* as these microbes cannot be isolated by standard culture techniques.

The use of molecular methods such as *polymerase chain reaction* (PCR) can help to detect specific sequences for such viable non-cultivable microorganisms. PCR for nucleic acid amplification methods are not only sensitive and specific but also rapid and less expensive than the culture methods. These methods require scrupulous handling of specimens to avoid contamination and false-positive results. Strategies of PCR to detect bacterial infections in the amniotic fluid cover the detection of highly conserved 16S ribosomal DNA and the detection of specific gene sequences of an infecting agent.

Multiplex PCR approach can be used to detect multiple intrauterine infections of bacterial and viral origins. Multiplex PCR methods are currently available as diagnostic panel of intrauterine infection that helps in diagnosing single and multiple bacterial infections such as *Ureaplasma urealyticum, Gardnerella vaginalis, Fusobacterium* spp., *Mycoplasma hominis, Escherichia coli, Peptostreptococcus anaerobius, Chlamydia trachomatis, Bacteroides fragilis, Neisseria gonorrheae, Haemophilus influenzae, and Streptococcus* spp. using amniotic fluid in preterm labor.

Since amniotic fluids during intrauterine infections show elevated levels of *proinflammatory cytokines* such as IL-1, IL-6 and TNF-α, their expression levels and the extent of inflammation can be assessed by immunological and reverse transcriptase PCR methods.

DIAGNOSIS OF VIRAL INFECTIONS

Prenatal diagnosis is performed primarily for viral detection.

Nucleic acids of adenovirus, cytomegalovirus, and enterovirus are commonly detected in the amniotic fluid of low- or high-risk pregnancies. Unlike bacterial 16S ribosomal RNA, which is common to many different bacterial species, the absence of a global marker for viral genomes limits current molecular methods to screening for specific, known viruses.

Invasive procedures are used to obtain samples representing the fetus such as amniotic fluid, chorionic villi and cord blood. The conventional virus detection relies on *isolation of virus in cell culture* which is regarded as "gold standard" assay for virus detection. This assay uses viral susceptible cell lines for infection and culturing of virus from the specimens (**Table 4.3.2**). Upon infection, the cells are periodically observed for viral-induced changes such as *cytopathic effect (CPE)* or *the ability to haemadsorb*. The identity of the isolated virus may be confirmed, or if necessarily typed by methods such as neutralization, fluorescent antibody, hemadsorption-inhibition tests. Cell cultures vary greatly in their susceptibility to different viruses and it is important to use the most sensitive cell cultures available for the isolation of suspected viruses in the clinical specimen. The method suffers the following limitations: (1) the duration required for appearance of CPE usually takes a few days to a few weeks except few viruses of intrauterine infections such as herpes simplex viruses and enteroviruses, where CPE may appear within one day of inoculation; (2) cell cultures are very susceptible to bacterial contamination and requires experienced personnel to perform; (3) sensitivity is often low and depends on the quality of the clinical specimen received; (4) cell culture is not applicable to viruses which grow poorly or not in cell culture (e.g. hepatitis and parvoviruses).

More rapid and sensitive diagnostic methods have been developed in recent years. Among them, direct antigen detection by specific antibodies or antibody detection by viral antigens by serological techniques and amplification and detection of viral nucleic acids by molecular methods are the two categories of laboratory methods used for assessment of viral infections. Though serological methods are sensitive, these methods often cannot indicate the time of infection, which is needed for risk assessment. Conventional serological tests measure antibody levels without distinguishing the levels of IgM and IgG, and usually require two samples for determination of seroconversion or a substantial increase in titer. However, a range of modern ELISA methods can distinguish between IgG and IgM and may allow diagnosis in one serum sample. However, biological and technical difficulties including reduced sensitivity and specificity due to cross-reactions, false-positive and false-negative results are the major concerns.

Antibody avidity test is also used for diagnosing intrauterine viral infections and this depends on the strength of interaction of an antibody with a multivalent antigen. Antibody avidity is low after primary antigenic challenge, becomes

Table 4.3.2: Cell lines useful for propagation of viruses causing intrauterine infections

Virus	*Cell lines used to propagate the virus*	*Duration for CPE observation*
Rubella	Vero and Vero/SLAM	3 to 5 days
CMV	Human diploid fibroblast cells either primary, such as human embryonic cells and human foreskin cells, or continuous cultures such as MRC-5 and WI-38 cells	3 days to 5 weeks
VZV	MRC-5 cells, and A-549 cells	2 to 3 weeks
HSV	Vero cells	1 to 4 days

Table 4.3.3: Diagnosis of common intrauterine viral infection from clinical specimens

Virus	*Diagnosis*	
	Maternal Infection	*Fetal Infection*
Rubella	IgM and IgG ELISA; Confirmation by IgG avidity assay	IgM ELISA using fetal blood; RT PCR using clinical samples of chorionic villous and amniotic fluid
CMV	Primary or recurrent infection is assessed by serology using IgM, IgG and IgG-avidity assays	Detection of CMV in amniotic fluid is done by virus culturing and/or PCR
VZV	IgG and IgM	IgM ELISA and PCR using amniotic fluid; for virus culture, amniotic fluid should be sampled after 18 weeks of pregnancy; immunofluorescent staining using monoclonal anti-VZV antibody
HSV	Type-specific IgG assays	Virus culture or PCR
HIV	IgG enzyme immunoassay; confirmation by western blot or immunofluorescence assay	Prenatal laboratory assessment of congenital HIV infection is not recommended as it increases the risk of infecting the fetus
Parvovirus B19	IgG and IgM assays based on recombinant conformational epitopes of VP1 and VP2	Cannot be grown in cell lines; ELISA IgM and IgG assays; PCR

higher with time and it usually involves IgG antibodies. **Table 4.3.3** describes the diagnosis of common intrauterine viral infections from clinical samples.

There are challenges in diagnosing these IU infections as there is no single diagnostic method or standard procedure or panel of tests available to identify the agent and interpreting the condition. Often, both serological and molecular diagnostic tests need to be performed to confirm the infection as well as to determine the extent of infection based on the load of the infective agents. The duration between exposure to an infectious agent and diagnostics is very critical for the interpretation of the test result. The findings of pathogen-specific antibodies or sonographic abnormalities do not accurately predict the severity or outcome of fetal infection. There is a need for precise diagnosis to guide appropriate counseling, clinical intervention by adopting therapeutic strategies and individual fetal risk assessment.

BIBLIOGRAPHY

1. Agrawal V, Hirsch E. Intrauterine infection and preterm labor. In: Seminars in Fetal and Neonatal Medicine. 2012;17(1):12-9.
2. Calvet G, Aguiar RS, Melo AS, Sampaio SA, de Filippis I, Fabri A, Tschoeke DA. Detection and sequencing of Zika virus from amniotic fluid of fetuses with microcephaly in Brazil: a case study. The Lancet Infectious diseases. 2016:16(6):653-60.
3. Delorme-Axford E, Sadovsky Y, Coyne CB. The placenta as a barrier to viral infections. Annual Review of Virology, 1,2014; pp. 133-46.
4. Fritel X, Rollot O, Gérardin P, Gauzere BA, Bideault J, Lagarde L, Sampériz S. Chikungunya virus infection during pregnancy, Reunion, France, 2006. Emerg Infect Dis. 2010;16(3): 418-25.
5. Gonçalves LF, Chaiworapongsa T, Romero R. Intrauterine infection and prematurity. Mental retardation and developmental disabilities research reviews. 2002;8(1):3-13.
6. Lamont RF. The role of infection in preterm labour and birth. Hospital Medicine, 2003; 64(11);644-7.
7. Long SS, Pickering LK, Prober CG. Principles and practice of pediatric infectious disease. Elsevier Health Sciences. 2012.
8. Mendelson E, Aboudy Y, Smetana Z, Tepperberg M, Grossman Z. Laboratory assessment and diagnosis of congenital viral infections: Rubella, cytomegalovirus (CMV), varicella-zoster virus (VZV), herpes simplex virus (HSV), parvovirus B19 and human immunodeficiency virus (HIV). Reproductive Toxicology. 2006;21(4):350-82.
9. Overall JC. Viral infections of the fetus and neonate. In: Feigin RD, Cherry JD (Eds). Textbook of Pediatric Infectious Diseases, 1981;(1):924-59.
10. Widome MD. Principles and Practice of Pediatric Infectious Diseases. JAMA. 2009; 302(11):1232-5.

4.4 Malaria: Treatment Guidelines

P Ramachandran

Reviewers: *MKC Nair, S Thangavelu, S Narmada*

The near elimination of malaria seemed possible in the mid-1960s; thanks to the concerted action of various agencies. But this effort received a setback with gradual resurgence of the disease with malaria cases peaking by the year 1976. Though the overall incidence started coming down since then, the incidence of *Plasmodium falciparum* remains unchanged. Drug resistance in *P. falciparum* is one of the important contributory factors for this status. This resulted in formulation of national guidelines for the treatment of malaria which was revised periodically **(Fig. 4.4.1)**.

TREATMENT IN MALARIA

The aims of the malaria case management are:

- To provide prompt and complete treatment to all suspected/confirmed cases of malaria
- To prevent progression of mild cases of malaria into severe or complicated form of malaria
- To prevent deaths from severe and complicated malaria
- To prevent transmission of malaria
- To minimize risk of spread of drug resistant parasites by use of effective drugs in appropriate dosage by everyone.

All fever cases diagnosed as malaria by either rapid diagnostic test (RDT) or microscopy should be promptly given effective treatment.

Three main factors are to be taken into consideration before initiating treatment:

1. Infecting *Plasmodium* species
2. Clinical status of the patient
3. Drug susceptibility determined by the geographic area of infection.

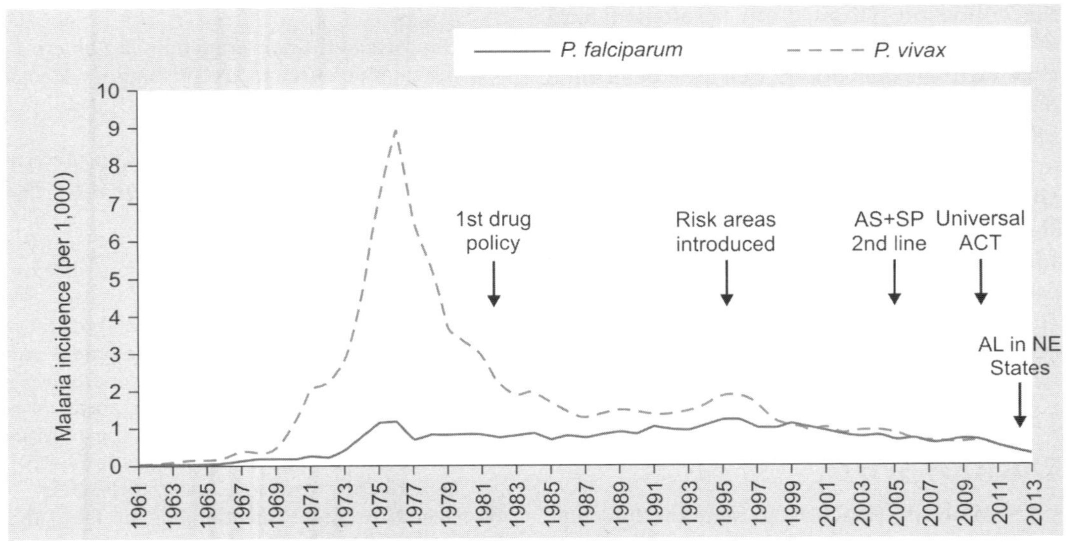

Fig. 4.4.1: Reported malaria incidence and the evolution of the National Drug Policy for malaria in India, 1961-2013.

Abbreviations: AS, artesunate; SP, sulphadoxine-pyrimethamine; ACT, artemisinin-based combination therapy; AL, artemether lumefantrine; NE, North-East.

Source: National Vector-borne Disease Control Programme, New Delhi.

UNCOMPLICATED MALARIA

Smear Positive for *P. vivax*

- Treat with: Chloroquine (CQ) 3 days + Primaquine (PQ) 0.25 mg per kg body weight daily for 14 days
- Primaquine is contraindicated in infants, pregnant women and individuals with G6PD deficiency

Chloroquine is administered in a dose of 25 mg/kg over 3 days; an initial dose of 10 mg/kg followed by 5 mg/kg after 6 hours and 5 mg/kg once daily on day 2 and 3 is found to be the most optimal regimen.

Chloroquine is available as 250 mg tablet containing 150 mg base. Starting treatment on empty stomach is to be avoided. Dose should be repeated if vomiting occurs within 30 minutes.

Though there have been some reports of chloroquine resistance, presently drug resistance is not a major concern in *P. vivax*. Presumptive treatment of malaria with a single dose of chloroquine has been stopped.

The relapse rate in *P. vivax* infection is up to 40%. Primaquine is given to prevent relapse in a dose of 0.25/kg/day for 14 days from day one. Primaquine is usually available as 2.5 mg tablet. A complete course of 14 days is important for maximal effectiveness. Recent articles suggest that a dose of 0.5 mg/kg/day may be more effective.

Smear Positive for *P. falciparum* (Pf)

For Pf malaria, the treatment is initiated with artemisinin based combination therapy (ACT) in the form of artesunate with sulfadoxine-pyrimethamine (SP) for 3 days, followed by primaquine in a single dose on second day.

The treatment recommendation for North Eastern states alone is different. There ACT-AL (Artesunate-Lumifantrine) combination is given for 3 days followed by a single dose of PQ on second day.

Artemisinin

Artemisinin compounds are synthesized from the plant *Artemisia annua*. These compounds are artesunate, artemether and arteether. They act by inhibiting the protein synthesis by the parasite. They have the advantage of very rapid parasite clearance in comparison to quinine. They are potent against all developmental stages of the asexual forms of malaria. It is important that artemisinins should be given in combination to prevent resistance.

Artemisinin Combination Therapy

Artemisinin combination therapy (ACT) refers to an artemisinin derivative combined with a long-acting antimalarial. The possible partner drugs in ACT regimens include amodiaquine, atovaquine, proguanil, clindamycin, doxycycline, lumefantrine, mefloquine, piperaquine, pyronaridine and sulfadoxine-pyrimethamine. The ACT used in the national programme is artesunate + sulfadoxine-pyrimethamine (SP) combination known as ACT-SP except in North Eastern region. *Artemisinin derivatives must never be administered as monotherapy for uncomplicated malaria.*

Dose

1. *ACT-SP:* Artesunate 4 mg/kg body weight daily for 3 days + Sulfadoxine (25 mg/kg body weight) - Pyrimethamine (1.25 mg/kg) on day 1
2. *Primaquine:* 0.75 mg/kg body weight on day 2.

Smear Positive for Mixed Infection (Both *P. falciparum* and *P. vivax*)

All cases of mixed infection are to be treated as for *P. falciparum*. The standard SP-ACT is given for 3 days as per the dose mentioned above. Primaquine is given 0.25/kg body weight for 14 days as for the radical treatment of *P. vivax*.

Severe/Complicated Malaria

The criteria for severe malaria are given in **Box 4.4.1**. If not treated within 24 hours, *P. falciparum* malaria can progress to severe illness often leading to death. Treatment with IV artesunate compounds are associated with greater reduction in mortality and lower risk of hypoglycemia compared to IV quinine in adults. In children with severe malaria, similar

Box 4.4.1: Severe malaria

Asexual forms in peripheral smear PLUS
- Altered consciousness with or without seizures
- Respiratory distress or ARDS
- Circulatory collapse
- Metabolic acidosis
- Renal failure, hemoglobinuria (blackwater fever)
- Hepatic failure
- Coagulopathy with or without DIC
- Severe anemia or massive intravascular hemolysis
- Hypoglycemia

mortality and clinical outcomes with artesunate and quinine were observed.

Still artemisinin is preferred for severe malaria in view of its ease of administration and greater safety compared to quinine.

Artesunate for Severe Malaria

Initial parenteral treatment is given for at least 48 hrs: Artesunate is administered 2.4 mg/kg IV or IM on admission (time = 0), then at 12 hours and 24 hours, then once a day. Artesunate powder is diluted in 5% sodium bicarbonate provided in the drug pack.

The alternative is artemether: 3.2 mg/kg i.m. given on admission, then 1.6 mg/kg per day.

Follow-up treatment: Once the patient can take oral medication oral ACT-SP is started in the same dose as for uncomplicated *Pf* malaria and given for 3 days and a single dose of primaquine 0.75 mg/kg is given on second day of oral therapy.

Quinine

When quinine is chosen to treat severe malaria, it is given as 20 mg quinine salt/kg IV infusion in 5% GDW/5% GNS over a period of 4 hours and followed by maintenance dose of 10 mg/kg 8 hourly. If parenteral quinine therapy needs to be continued beyond 48 hours, dose should be reduced to 7 mg/kg 8 hourly. Infusion rate should not exceed 5 mg/kg per hour.

Never give Bolus Injection of Quinine

Follow-up treatment: Oral quinine is given in a dose of 10 mg/kg TID for total of seven days (including the days when parenteral quinine was administered) plus doxycycline 3 mg/kg OD or clindamycin 10 mg/kg BD (in pregnant women and children under 8 years of age) for total duration of 7 days.

SEVERE MALARIA DUE TO *P. VIVAX*

Recently there have been some case reports of severe malaria due to *P. vivax*. In such a clinical presentation the treatment is same as given for severe *falciparum* malaria. In addition, a fourteen day course of primaquine is given for radical cure.

Supportive Treatment in Severe Malaria

Optimal maintenance of airway, breathing and circulation along with organ support is important. In cerebral malaria, use of mannitol and corticosteroids is better avoided as the outcome may be adverse. Recent studies from Africa show that aggressive fluid boluses may be associated with poor outcome in resource poor settings.

Treatment of *Plasmodium ovale* and *Plasmodium malariae*

In India, these species are very rarely found. *P. ovale* should be treated as *P. vivax*. *P. malariae* should be treated as *P. falciparum*.

TREATMENT OF UNCOMPLICATED MALARIA IN PREGNANCY

Artemisinin compounds are not recommended in 1st trimester. Quinine salt is advised in a dose of 10 mg/kg three times daily for 7 days. One should watch for hypoglycemia with quinine use. In 2nd and 3rd trimester, ACT as per dosage schedule can be used.

Prophylaxis

Doxycycline: 100 mg once daily for adults and 1.5 mg/kg once daily for children. The drug should be started 2 days before travel and continued for 4 weeks after leaving the malarious area. Doxycycline is contraindicated in children below 8 years.

Mefloquine: This is recommended in adults in a dose of 250 mg weekly. It is started two weeks before reaching the malarious area, continued during the stay and for four weeks after leaving.

Use of personal protection measures including insecticide-treated bed nets (ITN)/ long-lasting insecticidal nets (LLIN) should be encouraged for pregnant women and other vulnerable population including travellers for longer stay.

Malaria guidelines over the last four decades (1982–2013) have been summarized in **Table 4.4.1**.

Table 4.4.1: National treatment guidelines for malaria

		Treatment after confirmation		*Special groups*			
Year	*Presumptive treatment*	*P. falciparum malaria*	*P. vivax malaria*	*Severe malaria*	*Malaria in pregnancy*	*Chemoprophylaxis or MDA*	*Criteria for CQR*
Late 1950s	CQ or AQ (10 mg/kg SD)	PQ (0.25 mg/kg for 5 days)				MDA: Presumptive+ PYR (adult SD 50 mg)	
1982	CQS: CQ (10 mg/kg SD) in ACD, DDCs and FTDs	CQS: CQ (10 mg/kg SD) + PQ (0.75 mg/kg SD)	CQ (10 mg/kg SD) + PQ (0.25 mg/kg for 5 days)	Parenteral CQ or quinine	Contraindications: PQ	MDA in migrants: CQ (10 mg/kg) + PQ (0.75 mg/kg)	Areas with established CQ resistance by in vivo tests
	CQR: AQ (10 mg/kg SD) in ACD DDCs, FTDs and SLP (adult SD 1000/50 mg) in PCD	CQR: SLP (adult SD 1000/50 mg) + PQ (0.75 mg/kg SD)					
1995	Low risk: CQ (10 mg/kg SD)	Low risk: CQ (10 mg/kg SD) + PQ (0.75 mg/kg SD)	Low: CQ (10 mg/kg SD) + PQ (0.25 mg/kg for 5 days)	Parenteral artemisinin derivatives or quinine	" "	CQS: CQ (10 mg/kg LD then 5 mg/kg weekly)	" "
	High risk: CQ (25 mg/kg over 3 days) + PQ (0.75 mg/kg SD)	High risk CQS: no further treatment	High risk: PQ (025 mg/kg for 5 days)			CQR: CQ (5 mg/kg weekly) + proguanil (100 mg daily)	
		High risk CQR: SP (adult dose 1500/75 mg) with PQ (0.75 mg/kg SD)					
2002	" "	" "	" "	" "	Contraindications: PQ: Artemisinins in first trimester	" "	n>30, failure more than 25% in a PHC
2004	" "	Low risk: CQ (25 mg/kg over 3 days) + PQ (0.75 mg/kg SD)	CQ (25 mg/kg over 3 days) + PQ (0.25 mg/kg for 5 days)	" "	" "	" "	" "

Contd...

Contd...

		Treatment after confirmation		*Special groups*			
Year	*Presumptive treatment*	*P. falciparum malaria*	*P. vivax malaria*	*Severe malaria*	*Malaria in pregnancy*	*Chemoprophylaxis or MDA*	*Criteria for CQR*
		High risk CQS and high risk CQR: same					
2005	" "	Low risk and high risk CQS: same CQR: AS (4 mg/kg daily for 3 days) + SP (adult dose 1500/75 mg SD)	" "	" "	" "	" "	" "
2007	No presumptive therapy; CQ (25 mg/kg over 3 days) if lab diagnosis is not available within 24 h	CQS and CQR: same	CQ (25 mg/kg over 3 days) + PQ (0.25 mg/kg for 14 days)	" "	" "	" "	n > 50, failure more than 10% in clusters of a PHC's
		Treatment failure: Oral QN + tetracycline or DOX					
2008	Same but with full treatment for RDT negative cases also	" "	" "	" "	" "	Short term: DOX daily Long-term: MQ weekly	n > 50, failure more than 10% in clusters of blocks
2010	" "	AS (4 mg/kg daily for 3 days) + SP (adult dose 1500/75 mg SD) + PQ (0.75 mg/kg SD)	" "	" "	QN (1st trimester) or AS+SP (2nd and 3rd trimester	" "	" "
2013	" "	Same (AS+SP) for all over India except North Eastern States; artemether lumefantrine (80+480mg adult dose) in North Eastern States	" "	" "	" "	" "	" "

Abbreviations: CQ, chloroquine; AS, artesunate; CQR, chloroquine resistant; CQS, chloroquine sensitive; ACD, active case detection; DDC, Drug distribution centers; ACD: active case detection; AS, artesunate; CQ, chloroquine; DOX, doxycycline; FTD, fever treatment depot; LD, loading dose; MDa, mass drug administration; Mq, mefloquine; PHC, primary health center; QN, quinine; RDT, rapid diagnostic test; SD, single dose; SP, sulfaodoxine pyrimethamine; PYR, pyrimethamine; AQ, amodiaquine; PQ, primaquine; SLP, sulfalene-pyrimethamine; PCD, passive case detection; RDK, rapid diagnostic kit.
Source: Anvikar AR, Arora U, Sonal GS, Mishra N, Shahi B, Savargaonkar D, et al. Antimalarial drug policy in India: Past, present and future. Indian J Med Res. 2014;139(2):205-15.[1]

HIGHLIGHTS OF CURRENT NATIONAL RECOMMENDATION ON MALARIA THERAPY

- Artemisinin monotherapy was banned in India in 2009.
- Antimalarial therapy is to be instituted only after parasitological confirmation of the diagnosis to reduce drug pressure for resistance, prevent side-effects, decrease drug costs, and improve the management of other causes of febrile illness.
- The current first-line therapy for *P. falciparum* is AS+SP, which shows high efficacy across the nation.
- ACT in North Eastern States has been changed to artemether lumefantrine in view of the resistance to partner drug SP.
- Chloroquine continues to be recommended for *P. vivax* malaria. Though there were reports of chloroquine resistance in *P. vivax*, studies showed there was 100% therapeutic efficacy.

New Developments

- *New ACTs in pipeline:* Fixed dose ACTs including artesunate + mefloquine, dihydroartemisinin + piperaquine, arterolane + piperaquine, and pyronaridine + artesunate. Arterolane is a synthetic analogue of artemisinin and has the potential to replace plant-derived artemisinin.
- The bivalent rapid diagnostic kits (RDKs) have recently been introduced all over the nation and will improve the diagnosis.

Future Challenges

- The emergence of chloroquine resistance in *P. vivax* which is responsible for half of the national malaria burden.
- The spread and increase in SP resistance, which is likely to be inevitable, may decrease the present high efficacy of AS+SP in India and necessitate the switch to a different combination therapy.
- Present ACT is not a fixed drug combination (FDC)
- Access to therapy in remote areas is still a problem
- Awareness about national drug policy needs to percolate to all health personnel, both in Government and private sector.
- Wide variation in prescriptions, available formulations should be minimised.
- Compliance especially radical treatment with primaquine is still not good.

BIBLIOGRAPHY

1. Anvikar AR, Arora U, Sonal GS, Mishra N, Shahi B, Savargaonkar D, et al. Antimalarial drug policy in India: Past, present and future. Indian J Med Res. 2014;139(2):205-15.
2. Diagnosis and Treatment of Malaria in India. Directorate of National Vector-borne Disease Control Programme. Ministry of Health and Family Welfare, New Delhi, 2013.
3. Guidelines for Diagnosis and Treatment of Malaria in India. National Institute of Malaria Research and National Vector-borne Disease Control Programme, 2009.
4. Jones KL, et al. Cochrane database of systematic review 2007;4: Art No CD 005967.
5. Mathew JL. Artemisinin derivatives versus quinine for severe malaria in children: A systematic review and meta-analysis. Ind Pediatr. 2010;47:423-8.
6. National Vector-borne Disease Control Programme, Delhi.
7. Sharma RS, Sharma GK, Dhillon GPS. New Delhi: Ministry of Health and Family Welfare, National Malaria Eradication Programme, Directorate General of Health Services, Government of India; 1996. Epidemiology and control of malaria in India 1996.

4.5 Being Rational with Acute Pharyngotonsillitis

A Somasundaram

Reviewers: *P Ramachandran, NC Gowrishankar, Hemchand K Prasad*

INTRODUCTION

Acute pharyngitis is defined as an infection of the pharynx and/or tonsils. It is a common problem in children and adolescents. Although viruses cause most of the acute pharyngitis episodes, group A beta hemolytic *Streptococcus* (GABHS) causes 37% of cases of acute pharyngitis in children older than 5 years. Other bacterial causes of pharyngitis are group C *Streptococcus* (5% of total cases), *Chlamydophila pneumoniae* (1%), *Mycoplasma pneumoniae* (1%) and anaerobic species (1%). Among the viruses—rhinovirus, corona virus and adenovirus account for the 30% of the total cases, Epstein Barr virus for 1%, influenza and parainfluenza virus for about 4%. The absence of pharyngeal inflammation or the presence of rhinorrhea is much more likely to be associated with viral infection. However, no physical findings clearly separate GABHS from viral, other bacterial, or non-infectious causes. The diagnostic facilities for accelerated detection of most common and most dangerous bacterial pathogen, GABHS is often lacking and this has led to widespread injudicious antimicrobial therapy. Tonsillectomy is often recommended with recurrence, although indications may be questionable.

ETIOLOGY

Pharyngitis refers to the inflammation of the pharynx which includes erythema, edema, exudates or an enanthem [ulcer]. It can be of either non-infectious etiologies or due to acute infections.

The following are the non-infectious causes:

- Environmental exposure to tobacco smoke, air pollutants and allergens
- Contact with caustic substances, hot food and liquids
- Periodic fever, aphthous stomatitis, pharyngitis, cervical adenitis (PFAPA) syndrome
- Kawasaki disease, SLE, inflammatory bowel disease
- Steven Johnson syndrome.

Acute infections of the pharynx and tonsils can be caused by numerous etiologic agents. The herculean task is to differentiate important potentially serious treatable causes of acute pharyngitis from those that are self-limited and requires no specific treatment or follow-up. The infections causing acute pharyngitis are given in **Table 4.5.1**.

CLINICAL PRESENTATION

Viruses

Viral upper respiratory infections are usually mild except for infectious mononucleosis and usually spread by contact with oral and respiratory secretions. Certain clues will help in identifying the virus. Vesicles or ulcers in the oropharynx with vesicles on the extremities and palms and soles are found in hand-foot-mouth disease. It is usually caused by Coxsackie A16 and also by Enterovirus 71 and Coxsackie A6.In pharyngoconjuctival fever, pharyngitis occurs with conjunctivitis.

Splenomegaly or hepatomegaly may be the clue to infectious mononucleosis.

Bacteria

GABHS causes pharyngitis in children usually in the age group of 5–15 years. Group C and group G *Streptococcus* cause pharyngitis in adolescents. Gonococcal pharyngitis presents with fever and cervical lymphadenitis in children subjected to sexual abuse. In diphtheritic pharyngitis, sore throat along with fever, dysphagia, hoarseness

Table 4.5.1: Infectious agents that cause pharyngitis

Organisms	*Clinical syndrome(s)*
Bacteria	
Group A *Streptococcus*	Pharyngotonsillitis, scarlet fever
Group C and Group G *Streptococcus*	Pharyngotonsillitis
Arcanobacterium haemolyticum	Scarlatiniform rash, pharyngitis
Neisseria gonorrhoea	Tonsillopharyngitis
Mixed anaerobes	Vincent's angina
Fusobacterium necrophorum	Lemierre's syndrome, peritonsillar abscess
Francisella tularensis	Tularemia (oropharyngeal)
Yersinia pestis	Plague
Yersinia enterocolitica	Enterocolitis, pharyngitis
Viruses	
Adenovirus	Pharyngoconjunctival fever
Herpes simplex virus 1 and 2	Gingivostomatitis
Coxsackievirus	Herpangina
Rhinovirus	Common cold
Corona virus	Common cold
Influenza A and B	Influenza
Parainfluenza	Cold, croup
EBV	Infectious mononucleosis
Cytomegalovirus	CMV mononucleosis
HIV	Primary acute HIV infection
Mycoplasma	
Mycoplasma pneumoniae	Pneumonitis, bronchitis
Chlamydia	
Chlamydophila pneumoniae	Bronchitis, pneumonia
Chlamydophila psittaci	Psittacosis

Table 4.5.2: Clinical features suggestive of group A streptococcal and viral pharyngitis

Group A streptococcal	*Viral*
• Sudden onset of sore throat • Age 5–15 years • Fever • Headache • Nausea, vomiting, abdominal pain • Tonsillopharyngeal inflammation • Patchy tonsillopharyngeal exudates • Palatal petechiae • Anterior cervical adenitis (tender nodes) • Winter and early spring presentation • History of exposure to strep pharyngitis • Scarlatiniform rash	• Conjunctivitis • Coryza • Cough • Diarrhea • Hoarseness • Discrete ulcerative stomatitis • Viral exanthema

and a characteristic membrane are present. The clinically distinguishing features of Group A streptococcal and viral pharyngitis are given in **Table 4.5.2**.

DIAGNOSIS

There is significant overlap between the clinical presentations of streptococcal and viral pharyngitis. Clinically scoring by McIsaac and a judicious use of throat culture and rapid antigen detection tests (RADTs) help in differentiating streptococcal pharyngitis from other infectious agents. The modified Centor score **(Table 4.5.3)** can be used to help physicians decide which patients need no testing, throat culture/rapid antigen detection testing, or empiric antibiotic therapy.

- McIsaac (Modified Centor) score
- Throat swab
- Rapid antigen detection test

Table 4.5.3: McIsaac scoring

	Score
Absence of cough	1
Exudates in the tonsil	1
Tender anterior cervical lymphadenopathy	1
Temperature > 38°C	1
Age	
3–14 years	1
15–44 years	0
45 years or older	–1

Mnemonic for modified Centor Score—"CENTA"

C - Cough
E - Exudates
N - Nodes
T - Temperature
A - Age

The algorithm for the diagnosis and management of acute tonsillitis is given in **Flow chart 4.5.1**.

THROAT CULTURE

Culture of a throat swab on a sheep-blood agar plate has been the standard for the documentation of the presence of group A streptococci (GAS) in the upper respiratory tract and for the confirmation of the clinical diagnosis of acute streptococcal pharyngitis. If performed correctly, culture of a single throat swab on a blood agar plate is 90–95% sensitive for detection of GAS pharyngitis.

Rapid Antigen Detection Tests (RADTs)

A major disadvantage of throat cultures is the delay of minimum 24 hours in obtaining results.

Flow chart 4.5.1: Algorithm for the management of acute tonsillitis

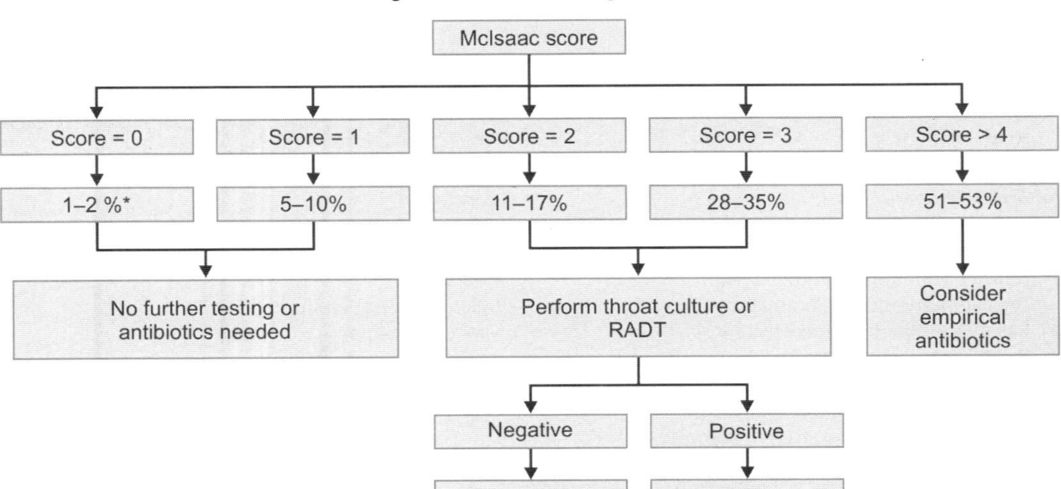

Source: American Family Physician www.aafp.org/afp Volume 79, Number 5. March 1, 2009
* Risk of Group A Streptococcal pharyngitis

RADTs have been developed for the rapid identification of GAS pharyngitis and the results are available in minutes.

RADTs currently available are highly specific (approximately 95%) when compared with blood agar plate cultures.

Anti-streptococcal antibody titers are not recommended in the routine diagnosis of acute pharyngitis as they reflect past but not current events.

TREATMENT

There is no specific therapy for most viral pathogens causing pharyngitis. Nonspecific symptomatic treatment for the relief of fever and throat pain can be given by paracetamol or ibuprofen. Throat lozenges and warm water gargle can provide symptomatic relief in children.

Antibiotic therapy depends on the organism identified. A variety of antimicrobial agents are effective in GABHS. GABHS are universally sensitive to pencillin and other beta lactam antibiotics. The recommended treatment for acute streptococcal pharyngitis is given in **Table 4.5.4**.

Pearls of Treatment

- Total duration of treatment is 10 days except for azithromycin which is 5 days.
- Antibiotics not recommended are tetracyclines, fluoroquinoline and sulphonamides
- A clinical response is usually achieved within 24–48 hours of therapy.
- Antibiotics prevent acute rheumatic fever even when given up to 9 days after the onset of illness.
- Follow-up post-treatment throat cultures or RADTs are not recommended routinely.

Accurate diagnosis of streptococcal pharyngitis followed by appropriate antimicrobial therapy is important for the prevention of complications and to minimize the potential adverse effects of inappropriate antimicrobial therapy.

INDICATIONS FOR TONSILLECTOMY

- Recurrent group A streptococcal tonsillitis [Paradise criteria] **(Table 4.5.5)**
- Recurrent infections with modifying factors: Multiple antibiotic allergy/intolerance Periodic fever/aphthous stomatitis and pharyngitis/adenitis
- History of peritonsillar abscess
- Persistent foul taste or breath due to chronic tonsillitis not responsive to medical therapy
- Chronic or recurrent tonsillitis associated with streptococcal carrier state and not

Table 4.5.4: Recommended treatment for acute streptococcal pharyngitis

Drug	*Dose*	*Route*	*Frequency*	*Days*
Amoxicillin	50 mg/kg	Oral	Od	10 days
Penicillin V	Weight < 27 kg – 250 mg Weight > 27 kg – 500 mg	Oral	bid	10 days
Benzathine penicillin G	Weight < 27 kg – 6,00,000 units Weight > 27 kg – 1.2 million units	IM	–	Once
For penicillin allergic individuals				
Cephalosporin	Variable	Oral		10 days
Erythromycin estolate	20–40 mg/kg/day	Oral	bid	10 days
Clarithromycin	15 mg/kg/day	Oral	bid	10 days
Azithromycin	Day 1:12 mg/kg Day 2–5:6 mg/kg	Oral	od	5 days
Clindamycin	20 mg/kg/day	Oral	tid	10 days

Table 4.5.5: Paradise criteria for tonsillectomy

	Criterion	*Definition*
1.	Frequency criteria: Minimum number of pharyngitis episodes	Past 1 year: 7 episodes Past 2 years: 5 episodes per year for both years Past 3 years: 3 episodes per year for all three years
2.	Episode criteria	Each pharyngitis episode must include at least ONE of the following criteria in addition to sore throat: 1. Temperature >100.9°F (38.3°C) 2. Tender cervical adenopathy or cervical lymph nodes >2 cm in size 3. Tonsillar exudate 4. Group A beta hemolytic *Streptococcus* culture positive
3.	Treatment criteria	Each pharyngitis episode must have been treated with standard protocol Antibiotics at conventional dosing for suspected or proven streptococcal pharyngitis
4.	Documentation criteria	Medical record documents each pharyngitis episode including above criteria or Observation by clinician for at least 2 subsequent episodes that meet above criteria, typically over a 12-month period

responding to beta-lactamase resistant antibiotics

- Sleep-disordered breathing.

COMPLICATIONS AND PROGNOSIS

Purulent bacterial otitis media and sinusitis may occur following a viral pharyngitis. Influenza may be complicated by secondary bacterial pneumonia.The complications of streptococcal pharyngitis include local complications such as cervical adenitis, peritonsillar abscess, retropharyngeal abscess, parapharyngeal abscess, otitis media, mastoiditis, and sinusitis and later nonsuppurative illness such as acute rheumatic fever and acute postinfectious glomerulonephritis.

The prognosis for a patient with viral pharyngitis is excellent. In patients with infectious mononucleosis, fever disappears in approximately 10 days. Lymphadenopathy and splenomegaly disappear in approximately 4 weeks. The prognosis of treated cases of streptococcal pharyngitis with the right antibiotic for the right duration is extremely good.

BIBLIOGRAPHY

1. Clinical Practice Guideline for the Diagnosis and Management of Group A Streptococcal Pharyngitis: 2012 Update by the Infectious Diseases Society of America.
2. Clinical Practice Guideline: Tonsillectomy in Children. American Academy of Otolaryngology—Head and Neck Surgery Foundation 2011.
3. Nelson Textbook of Pediatrics, First south Asia edition.
4. Update on the management of acute pharyngitis in children. Italian Journal of Pediatrics, 2011; 37:10.

Neurology

Reviewers: *P Ramachandran, NC Gowrishankar, Hemchand K Prasad, MKC Nair, S Thangavelu, S Narmada*

5.1 Status Epilepticus: What is New in Therapy?

TS Ekambaranath, S Shanthi

Reviewers: *P Ramachandran, NC Gowrishankar, Hemchand K Prasad*

Status epilepticus (SE) is a medical emergency. It may be the first manifestation of an epilepsy. The mortality may range from 9% to 27%. A protocol based management reduces the mortality and improves neurologically intact survival.

DEFINITION

Status epilepticus is defined as continuous seizures lasting 5 min or more, or two or more discrete seizures with incomplete recovery of consciousness in between the episodes.

The International League Against Epilepsy (ILAE) recently proposed a new definition of SE, as follows:

Status epilepticus is a condition resulting either from the failure of the mechanisms responsible for seizure termination or from the initiation of mechanisms, which lead to abnormally prolonged seizures (after time point t_1). It is a condition, which can have long-term consequences (after time point t_2), including neuronal death, neuronal injury, and alteration of neuronal networks, depending on the type and duration of seizure.

For tonic-clonic seizures, t_1 describes the duration of seizure activity after which it is likely to continue, if not treated, i.e. when it should be considered abnormally prolonged (or continuous) and requiring treatment. The second time point, or t_2, defines the length of continuous seizure activity after which there is a risk of long-term consequences.

For generalized convulsive status epilepticus (CSE), t_1 is estimated to be 5 min, and t_2 is 30 min. For focal SE, t_1 is considered 10 min, and t_2 is 60 min.

Status epilepticus can be classified as convulsive and nonconvulsive SE **(Table 5.1.1)**.

Table 5.1.1: Convulsive and nonconvulsive SE

Convulsive SE	*Nonconvulsive SE*
Generalized 1. Overt 2. Subtle *Focal* 1. Simple 2. Complex	1. Associated with coma or paralysis 2. Following prolonged convulsive seizures

Convulsive SE

It is the most common type. It can progress to nonconvulsive status during or after treatment.

Nonconvulsive SE

Patient will be pain responsive or unresponsive. There will not be any tonic clonic movements. Clinical clues for NCSE are conjugate eye deviation, nystagmus/roving eye movements, eyelid twitch, twitching of angle of mouth. EEG is confirmatory. Consider NCSE, if a status epilepticus patient becomes unresponsive and not regained baseline mental status. In all patients with unexplained coma the eyes should be examined for subtle seizure activity.

Diagnostic Dilemma

All abnormal movements described by the mother are not seizures. Tonic posturing is often interpreted as "fits" by the parents and physicians. Do not mistake posturing as seizure. Posturing can be secondary to hypoxia, hypoperfusion, raised ICP.

Case Scenario

A 1-year-old girl presented with fever of 1 day duration. She was brought to the hospital with abnormal movements of limbs lasting for 5 min. On examination has generalized tonic-clonic seizures.

Box 5.1.1: Complications of SE

- Hypoxia
- Hypercapnia
- Acidosis
- Hypertension followed by hypotension
- Hyperglycemia followed by hypoglycemia
- Raised ICT
- Hyperpyrexia, hyperkalemia

The management goals are to:

- Maintain vital functions and prevent complications
- Terminate seizures rapidly
- Evaluate and treat underlying cause.

Anticipate complications in a child with status epilepticus and manage them accordingly **(Box 5.1.1)**.

MANAGEMENT IN PREHOSPITAL SETTING

Midazolam is the drug of choice in prehospital settings as it is effective when given intramuscularly. The dose is 0.2 mg/kg [Class 1, level A]

- Watch for respiratory depression. Patient has to be monitored till he reaches a hospital setting.
- Recent evidences show that midazolam by buccal/intranasal routes could also be a safe and effective alternative in prehospital setting (Level 1B, Grade A). Rectal diazepam in a dose of 0.5 mg/kg (max 10 mg) can be given as an alternative.
- All benzodiazepines can cause respiratory depression. Hence bag and mask should be available to ventilate the patient, if need arises.

MANAGEMENT: IN-HOSPITAL SETTING

Management starts with care of airway, breathing and circulation

- Stabilize the airway by head tilt/chin lift and by jaw thrust in trauma
- Suction using Yankauer catheter
- Introduce nasogastric tube to decompress the stomach
- Bag valve mask ventilation is often needed in convulsive SE as these patients have inadequate respiratory efforts. *Untreated hypoxia >5 min can cause permanent neurologic sequelae*
- Connect to a cardiorespiratory monitor

Circulation: Correct shock, if present. Anticipate shock, if convulsions are prolonged. SE patients presenting late to ED have myocardial dysfunction most of times secondary to hypoxia. So small volume fluid boluses of 5–10 mL/kg may suffice. If these patients have underlying sepsis or hypovolemia, may need more fluids.

Treat documented hypoglycemia (<60 mg/dL according to PALS) with 2 mL/kg of 25% dextrose.

Consider pyridoxine 100 mg IV push, if patient is less than 18 months old.

ANTICONVULSANT THERAPY

Benzodiazepines (BNZ) are considered the first line anticonvulsant for status epilepticus **(Table 5.1.2)**. *Lorazepam* is the drug of choice. It is less lipid soluble, and hence does not undergo rapid redistribution in tissues. So it has a longer duration of action and less risk of relapse, compared to diazepam or midazolam.

It also causes less respiratory depression (Level 1B, Grade A).

The most commonly employed second line anticonvulsant is phenytoin or fosphenytoin.

Phenytoin is given as an IV infusion in the loading dose of 20 mg/kg (max 1g) @1mg/kg/min. Phenytoin is better avoided if shock, hypotension and myocardial dysfunction are present.

Fosphenytoin: IV/IM—20mg phenytoin equivalent/kg @3 mg/kg/min. Fosphenytoin

Table 5.1.2: Benzodiazepines

Drug	*Dose*
Lorazepam	0.1 mg/kg IV (max-4 mg)
Midazolam	IV 0.15–0.2 mg/kg IM 0.15–0.2 mg/kg Nasal 0.2–0.3 mg/kg Buccal 0.5 mg/kg
Diazepam	0.2–0.3 mg/kg

is preferred because of its favorable side effect profile including less risk of phlebitis and local irritation. It can also be given intramuscularly. Respiratory depression is exceedingly rare with its use and it does not cause sedation.

If seizures persist, an additional 10 mg/kg may be given intravenously.

A recent prospective randomized controlled study states that phenytoin, valproate, and levetiracetam are safe and equally efficacious following lorazepam in CSE. The choice of AEDs should be individualized based on comorbidities. In patients with hypotension, myocardial dysfunction and shock, one of the following drugs can be used as second-line anticonvulsants after benzodiazepines

- Levetiracetam
- Sodium valproate
- Phenobarbitone.

Levetiracetam (LEV) [Class IIb, Level C]

Many centers have started using levitiracetam in pediatric status epilepticus.

Advantages of Levetiracetam

- It is a safe drug with no reports of cardio-respiratory depression, hence, intubation can be avoided.
- It does not produce or aggravate any organ damage and can be used safely in liver failure and in presence of bleeding diathesis.
- It has a different mode of action.
- It has less drug interaction.
- *Dose:* 20–30 mg/kg (max 4 g) as IV infusion in 15 min.
- May be used, if other drugs are contra-indicated and/or the SE is refractory.

Sodium Valproate or Valproic Acid (VPA)

Many recent trials suggest sodium valproate is either equally effective or superior in efficacy compared to phenytoin. Sodium valproate also has the advantage of less sedation and less cardiopulmonary depression.

- Dose 20–40 mg/kg (6 mg/kg/min) followed by an infusion of 1–2 mg/kg/hr.
- Common side effects of sodium valproate are hepatic dysfunction, hyperammonemia, dose-dependent thrombocytopenia,and possibly increased bleeding despite normal platelet count. Try to avoid valproate in patients with intracranial bleeding or those requiring neurosurgical intervention

It is contraindicated in <2 years (hepatotoxicity 1 in 500), liver diseases or suspected metabolic disease, thrombo-cytopenia, possible recent intracranial bleed.

Phenobarbitone

It is a very good drug for status epilepticus particularly in infants. There are randomized trials which state that the incidence of respiratory depression with phenobarbitone is comparable to other drugs. But the risk is still present, if it is used after two or more doses of benzodiazepines. It is preferable to use phenobarbitone in an ED or PICU setting where intubation could be done, if needed. Hypotension, respiratory depression and sedation are the major side-effects. High dose phenobarbitone has also been used for refractory status epilepticus in intensive care setting.

Dose: 20 mg/kg in NS @ 1.5 mg/kg/min.

REFRACTORY SE (RSE)

Refractory SE is defined as seizures which persist despite the administration of two appropriate anticonvulsants at acceptable doses. RSE accounts for 35–40 % of SE cases.

Super-refractory status epilepticus is defined as SE that continues or recurs 24 hour or more after the onset of anesthetic therapy.

Patients who do not return to their pre-convulsive neurologic baseline within 20 minutes should be connected to EEG monitoring to diagnose subclinical electrographic seizures.

MANAGEMENT OF REFRACTORY SE

Midazolam

This is the most preferred anesthetic agent for refractory status epilepticus in children.

Dose: 0.2 mg/kg bolus followed by infusion 1 µg/kg/min, increasing the infusion by 1 µg/kg/min every 5–10 min (max 12 µg/kg/min, may go up to 36 µg/kg/min). Maintain infusion for 48 hrs. Decrease by 1 µg/kg/min q4h. One of the main limitation of this drug is development of tachyphylaxis, particularly, if used for >72 hours.

Several reports have demonstrated its efficacy in RSE.

Advantages of midazolam are its rapid onset, easy titration, greater water solubility, and circumvention of the metabolic acidosis associated with the propylene glycol vehicle of other benzodiazepines and barbiturates.

It is unclear what is the end point of nonconvulsive electrographic seizures and nonconvulsive SE.

Controversy exists regarding the electrographic target of continuous infusions. Some advocate for seizure suppression; others prefer burst suppression or even complete background suppression.

If SE still not controlled with midazolam infusion any of the following drugs can be used

Thiopentone

This is another anesthetic agent which can be used in RSE.

Dose: 2–4 mg/kg bolus followed by infusion of upto 10 mg/kg/hr.

Discontinue midazolam and phenobarbitone once thiopentone is started. Maintainence phenytoin can be continued.

Side effects: Hypotension and heart failure, and sometimes pharmacologic support for maintaining BP and circulation is necessary.

Contraindication: Presence of hypotension, cardiogenic shock, sepsis.

IV Propofol: Propofol is a short-acting IV anesthetic agent used in RSE.

Dose: 1–3 mg/kg bolus followed by an infusion of 2–10 mg/kg/hr.

Side effects: If used at high doses and for prolonged periods, may cause "propofol syndrome" involving metabolic acidosis, rhabdomyolysis, arrhythmias, heart failure, hypertriglyceridemia, kidney failure, hepatomegaly, and possible death. These effects are common in children. If used for more than a few hours monitor ABG, CPK, and triglycerides.

OTHER DRUGS FOR REFRACTORY SE

Repeated bolus doses of phenobarbitone 10 mg/kg every 30 min.

Topiramate

It has multiple mechanisms of action including blockage of voltage sensitive Na^+ channels, L-type Ca^{2+} channels and enhancement of GABA activity. There are case reports of oral topiramate being used in refractory status epilepticus in children (age 4 months to 11 years). It was reported to result in rapid CSE resolution (<24 hour) with no hemodynamic or sedative side effects.

Dose: Topiramate is administered by nasogastric tube at 5–10 mg/kg/day for two days followed, if there is a response, by maintenance at 5 mg/kg/day.

Possible side effects: Metabolic acidosis, decreased sweating, glaucoma.

Ketamine

Ketamine acts as an N-methyl-D-aspartate (NMDA) glutamate receptor antagonist, and can be useful in refractory CSE. It has additional neuroprotective potential.

Dose: Load: 1.5 mg/kg IV every 3–5 min until seizures stop (max 4.5 mg/kg). Infusion, 1.2 mg/kg/h, maintenance 0.3–7.5 mg/kg/h.

Possible side effects: Hypertension, cerebellar toxicity.

It is contraindicated in cases with intracranial hypertension, tachycardia.

Lacosamide

There are only limited case reports of use of lacosamide in pediatric CSE. There are no case control or randomized studies to strongly suggest its use in pediatric CSE.

Dose : 25 mg/kg/day IV

Precautions: May prolong PR interval, so its use should be carefully evaluated in patients with heart concerns.

Alternate therapies available for treatment of refractory SE are:
- Lidocaine
- Paraldehyde, general anesthesia.

Nondrug options include: Resective surgery
- Vagus nerve stimulation.

Ketogenic Diet

Several studies have found success in treating adults and children for RSE in the inpatient setting. Patients had seizure termination within 3 days of starting the diet. The type of SE was not specified. Further research is needed to assess the value of the KD in RCSE; preliminary results are promising.

Hypothermia

Hypothermia activates many anticonvulsant and neuroprotective mechanisms. A recent systematic review found very low-grade evidence to support the use of therapeutic hypothermia in RSE . Underlying seizure type was not described. The well-tolerated level of hypothermia used in humans has minimal effect on the EEG, and deeper levels, which are neuroprotective and strongly anti-seizure in animal models, may be unsafe.

ELECTROCONVULSIVE THERAPY

Immunomodulatory Treatments

New onset refractory status epilepticus (NORSE) accounts for approximately 40% of RSE cases.

Many are of autoimmune or paraneoplastic in nature. About 52% remained cryptogenic after extensive evaluations. Immunomodulatory treatments such as high dose parenteral corticosteroids, intravenous immunoglobulin, and plasmapheresis are increasingly being tried in treatment of these cases, in addition to traditional anti-epileptic agents. No randomized, double-blinded case-control clinical trials currently exist.

CONCLUSION

Lot of progress is being made in determining the best treatment protocol for CSE. Benzodiazepines remain established as first-line treatment. Recent studies proved the utility of IM, nasal and buccal BNZ in cases where IV access is not obtainable, including in the pre-hospital setting. VPA is effective at treating CSE—at least as effective as phenytoin and better tolerated.

LEV has increasing evidence supporting it as an effective treatment option, but further study is needed. In cases of unexplained RSE of any type with no obvious cause after a couple of days, this qualifies as NORSE; evidence is emerging that immunomodulatory treatment may be beneficial in these cases, especially when given early. The ketogenic diet and surgery have roles in selected severe cases.

BIBLIOGRAPHY

1. Alldredge BK, Gelb AM, Isaacs SM, et al. A comparison of lorazepam, diazepam, and placebo for the treatment of out-of-hospital status epilepticus. N Engl J Med. 2001;345(9):631-7.
2. Arya R, et al. Efficacy of nonvenous medications for acute convulsive seizures: a network meta-analysis. Neurology. 2015;85(21):1859-68.
3. Blumkin L, et al. Pediatric refractory partial status epilepticus responsive to topiramate. J Child Neurol. 2005;20(3):239-41.
4. Brigo F, et al. A common reference-based indirect comparison meta-analysis of buccal versus intranasal midazolam for early status epilepticus. CNS Drugs. 2015;29(9):741-57.
5. Brophy GM, et al. Guidelines for the evaluation and management of status epilepticus. Neurocrit Care. 2012;17(1):3-23.
6. Caraballo RH, et al. Ketogenic diet in pediatric patients with refractory focal status epilepticus. Epilepsy Res. 2014;108(10):1912-6.
7. Crawford TO, Mitchell WG, Fishman LS, Snodgrass SR, et al. Very-high-dose phenobarbital for refractory status epilepticus in children. Neurology. 1988;38:1035-40.

8. Epilepsia. 2015;56(2):254-62.
9. Epilepsy Res. 2015;114:52-8.
10. Eric H, et al. Treatment of convulsive status epilepticus. Curr Treat Options Neurol. 2016; 18:11.
11. Fawaz, et al. Crit Care Clin. 2014;30:751-64.
12. Gaspard N, et al. New-onset refractory status epilepticus: etiology, clinical features, and outcome. Neurology. 2015;85(18):1604-13.
13. Igartua J, Silver P, Maytal J, et al. Midazolam coma for refractory status epilepticus in children. Crit Care Med. 1999;27(9):1982-5.
14. Kahriman M, et al. Efficacy of topiramate in children with refractory status epilepticus. Epilepsia. 2003;44(10):1353-6.
15. Kalviainen R. Intranasal therapies for acute seizures. Epilepsy Behav. 2015;49:303-6.
16. Khawaja AM, et al. New-onset refractory status epilepticus (NORSE): The potential role for immunotherapy. Epilepsy Behav. 2015;47:17-23.
17. Koul RL, Raj Aithala G, Chacko A, et al. Continuous midazolam infusion as treatment of status epilepticus. Arch Dis Child. 1997; 76(5):445-8.
18. Lowenstein, et al. Epilepsia. 1999;40(1):120-2.
19. Mishra D, et al. Indian Pediatrics. 2014;51:975.
20. Moseley BD, et al. Refractory status epilepticus treated with trigeminal nerve stimulation. Epilepsy Res. 2014;108(3):600-3.
21. RAMPART, Epilepsia. 2011.
22. Shafer A, et al. Complications of sedation with midazolam in the intensive care unit and comparison with other sedative regimens. Crit Care Med. 1998;26(5):947–56
23. Silbergleit R, et al. N Engl J Med. 2012;366: 591-600.
24. Sreenath TG, et al. Eur J Paediatr Neurol. 2010; 14:162-8.
25. Status epilepticus: A critical review of available therapies and a clinical treatment protocol. Brain. 2011;134(10):2802-18.
26. Treiman DM, et al. A comparison of four treatments for generalized convulsive status epilepticus. Veterans Affairs Status Epilepticus Cooperative Study Group. N Engl J Med. 1998;339:792-8.
27. Trinka E, et al. A definition and classification of status epilepticus—report of the ILAE task force on classification of status epilepticus. Epilepsia. 2015;56(10):1515-23.
28. Wilkes R, et al. Pediatric intensive care treatment of uncontrolled status epilepticus. Crit Care Clin. 2013;29:239-57.
29. Yasiry Z, et al. Seizure. 2014;23(3):167-74.
30. Zeiler FA, et al. Therapeutic hypothermia for refractory status epilepticus. Can J Neurol Sci. 2015;42(4):221-9.

5.2 Approach to Single-enhancing CT Lesions

N Thilothammal

Reviewers: *P Ramachandran, NC Gowrishankar, Hemchand K Prasad*

Single-enhancing CT lesions (SECTL) are the most common radiological abnormality in Indian patients with new onset of seizures. In few cases, the lesion may be tuberculoma especially in presence of evidence of tuberculosis elsewhere. However, histopathological studies have proved that neurocysticercosis (NCC) is the most frequent cause for the lesions.

INCIDENCE

Wadia, et al. observed that 26% of patients with partial seizure showed these lesions and the incidence was higher among children as 40% of his patients were below 15 years. Murthy et al. reported single CT lesions in 23.4% of in patients with all types of epilepsies. Incidence as high as 72–78% of SECTL have been reported after the first seizures especially in children. Poor hygienic conditions of children make them more vulnerable to infection than adults.

It is difficult to estimate community prevalence of SECTL. Neuroimaging was done for patients with partial seizures identified in population-based epilepsy surveys. Estimated community prevalence by this method is 4% but other studies mention it to be responsible for half all partial seizures.

ETIOLOGY

Single-enhancing CT lesions are seen in neurocysticercosis, tuberculoma, metastatic tumors, CNS lymphomas, abscesses, toxoplasmosis, fungal granulomas and rarely with infarction.

CLINICAL PICTURE

Patients with SECTL often present with focal, focal becoming generalized seizures and rarely status epilepticus. Children may present with motor deficits such as monoplegia, hemiplegia or ataxia. Large lesions may manifest with features of increased intracranial pressure.

NEUROIMAGING

SECTL is a clinicoradiological entity. Clinical presentation and neuroimaging remain the mainstay of diagnosis in the developing world.

CT SCAN FEATURES

Lesions due to neurocysticercosis appear as irregular hypodense lesion in plain CT scan and contrast study shows smooth, thin walled ring- enhancing lesion or disc lesion. The scolex may be seen as contrast-enhancing eccentric dot within the cystic lesion **(Figs 5.2.1A and B)**.

There is no specific site predilection but, they are seen often at the gray-white matter junction. Ventricular and meningeal lesion may lead to hydrocephalus.

Tuberculous granulomas appear as large (>20 mm), irregular thick-walled lesions, conglomerulating when they are multiple with significant perilesional edema.

The various stages of NCC with radiologic correlation are shown in **Table 5.2.1.**

In patients with new onset seizures these unenhanced cystic lesions have never been demonstrated. Second and third stages, which represent dying stages of cysticercus larva, are seen in CT scans of Indian patients with epilepsy. Acute development of inflammation and surrounding cerebral oedema is responsible for new onset seizures in these patients. Because of intense inflammation in and around the parasite in acute stage, patients experience cluster of seizures.

In India, 75–85% patients with NCC present with single degenerating (stage 2 and 3) cysticercus. Whereas in Latin America and China substantial proportion of infected individuals present with a few viable (Stage 1) brain cyst. Several studies have shown that 10–20% of symptom-free population with one or

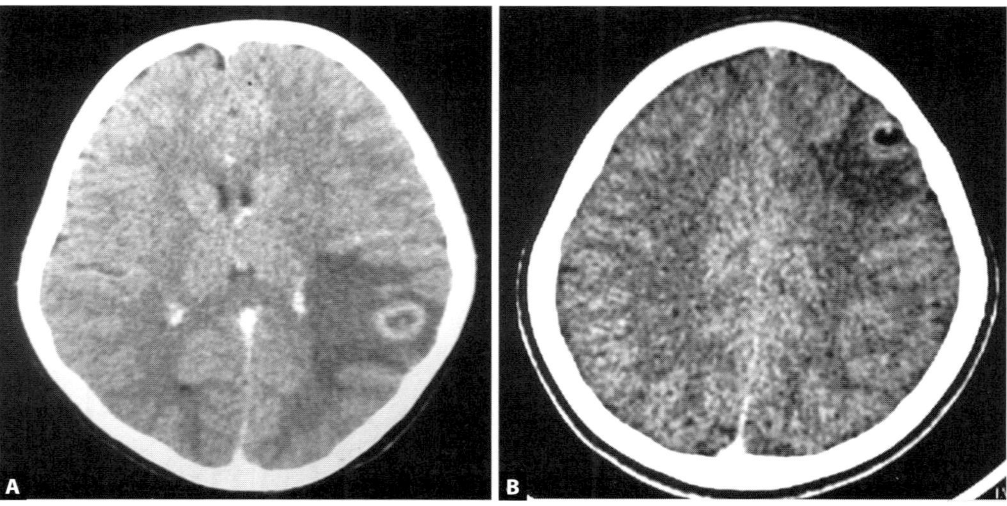

Figs 5.2.1A and B: CT scan: Ring-enhancing lesion with scolex in NCC

Table 5.2.1: Natural course of neurocysticercosis

Stages	*Pathology*	*CT features*
I. Vesicular phase	Viable/live larvae inside a translucent liquid filled cyst with thin membrane. No inflammation	Circumscribed, hypodense, unenhanced, cystic lesion No surrounding edema
II. Colloid stage	Host immune mechanism acts on cyst resulting in inflammation. Fluid becomes gelatinous, cyst wall thickens	Ring enhancing lesion with surrounding edema, scolex may or may not be seen
III. Granularnodular stage	Advanced inflammation due to dying larva. Cyst shrinks; fluid content is replaced by granulomatous tissue	Disc/coin-enhancing lesion with surrounding edema; no scolex
IV. Calcified stage	Calcification of gliotic scar that replaces the dead parasite	Calcified lesion No surrounding edema

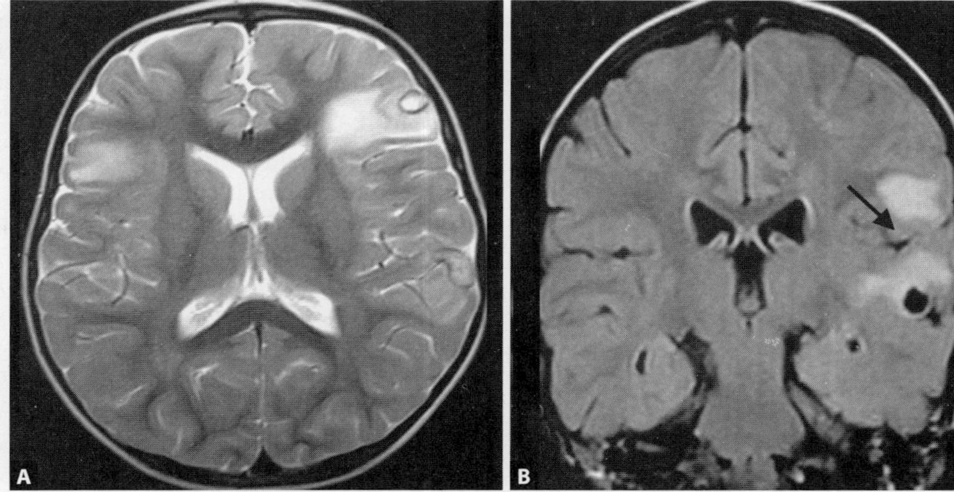

Figs 5.2.2A and B: (A) MRI T2W Image; (B) MRI FLAIR Image

more intraparenchymal brain calcification. It is hypothesized that in mild exposure the parasite dies in its early stages by action of the host immune system whereas a small proportion of patients with heavier egg challenges develop multiple viable cysts.

MAGNETIC RESONANCE IMAGING FEATURES

Magnetic resonance imaging (MRI) is superior to CT scan in revealing smallest lesions and the sensitivity is 95%. Neurocysticercosis is seen as hyperintense lesion with thin hypointense ring and surrounding edema in T2W image **(Fig. 5.2.2A)**. In FLAIR image, hyperintense lesion becomes suppressed, i.e. assumes black color **(Fig. 5.2.2B)**. Contrast study shows ring enhancement with or without scolex. Succinate/choline peak may be seen in magnetic resonance spectroscopy (MRS).

In tuberculoma, T2W image shows hyperintense lesion with hypointense core and surrounding edema. In FLAIR study, there is no suppression of lesion and appearance is similar to T2W images. The lesion shows ring enhancement with contrast study and the magnetic resonance spectroscopy (MRS) shows the characteristic lipid/lactate peaks.

Biopsy of lesion is not recommended but persistant and enhancing lesions must be subjected for biopsy.

CT SCAN VERSUS MRI

Visualization of scolex as eccentric dot on CT is characteristic of NCC. But this feature may not be seen always and smaller lesions are often missed by CT scan. Criteria for differentiating NCC from tuberculoma have been described but are not absolute and it may be difficult to differentiate smaller lesions with this criteria.

MRI is more sensitive in picking up NCC lesion of smaller size which are not visible in CT scan. Compared to CT scan, MRI has better sensitivity to differentiate tuberculoma from NCC. Even with MRI, it may become difficult. Preliminary experience with proton magnetic resonance spectroscopy shows promise in differentiating tuberculoma from NCC.

IMMUNOLOGICAL TESTS

The enzyme-linked immunosorbent assay ELISA test for cysticercus antibodies in serum and CSF is disappointing as the sensitivity (50%) and specificity (65%) are poor. False positive results due to past infection with *T. solium* and false negative result due to immune tolerance, inactive disease and localized antibody production in CSF could occur.

Enzyme-linked immuno-electro-transfer blot (EITB) assays are highly sensitive (98%) and specific (100%) in diagnosing neurocysticercosis. It uses purified glycoprotein antigen from *T. solium* and this test is less sensitive with single lesion and calcified lesions.

CSF ANALYSIS

When NCC or tuberculoma is restricted to brain parenchyma, CSF is normal.

If NCC involves meninges, there may be mononuclear pleocytosis, elevated protein with normal glucose level. Elevated eosinophil count in CSF has been reported. If tuberculoma co-exists with tuberculous meningitis then CSF is abnormal with lymphocytic pleocytosis, elevated protein and decreased glucose level.

CRITERIA FOR DIAGNOSIS OF BENIGN SECTL

The clinicoradiological picture forms the basis of diagnostic criteria for benign SECTL as proposed by Chandy et al. in 1991. All criteria must be satisfied for a diagnosis of benign SECTL.

Clinical Criteria

- Seizures (partial or generalized) should be the initial symptom
- There should be no features of persistently raised intracranial pressure.
- There should not be any progression of neurological deficit.
- Absence of an active systemic disease.

Radiological Criteria

- CT scan should only show a solitary, contrast-enhancing lesion.
- The lesion should measure less than 20 mm in maximal diameter.
- Edema may or may not be present, but is not severe enough to produce a shift of the midline structures.

These clinicoradiological criteria were found highly sensitive and specific in predicting benign outcome.

MANAGEMENT OF SECTL

The controversy in management persists, especially, when the treating physicians prefer to err in favor of tuberculosis rather than neurocysticercosis.

ALGORITHM FOR MANAGEMENT

Patients who do not have raised ICT, progressive neurological deficit, ancillary evidence of tuberculosis or malignancy should be treated with anticonvntsants alone as 50–75% of patients show spontaneous regression of lesion with AED treatment. A repeat CT scan is required after 3 months in symptom-free patients. Earlier CT scan is recommended, if seizures are uncontrollable or new signs and symptoms appear.

Further Management Depends on CT Result

- If the lesion is of same size or smaller than baseline, edema is less and patient is seizure free, anticonvulsants are continued.
- If the lesion shows enlargement but still less then 20 mm with no shift or ventricular compression, give a course of anti-parasitic drugs along with the anticonvulsants.
- If the lesion is greater than 20 mm with midline shift or gyral compression investigate and treat for tuberculosis.

CYSTICIDAL DRUGS

Its role in SECTL is controversial. Many studies have shown better resolution and fewer seizure recurrences with albendazole therapy. The advantages of albendazole over praziquantel

Flow chart 5.2.1: Treatment algorithm

Single-enhancing CT lesions with seizures → Start AED → Repeat CT scan after 3 months

- Lesion disappeared → Tapper off AED (Follow-up) → Seizures recurs → Restart AED 2–3 years
- Lesion persists
  - Same/smaller in size → Asymptomatic → AED alone
  - ↑ in size (≤20 mm) same size → Symptomatic → AED with albendazole therapy → Repeat CT scan after 3 months
    - Disappears
    - Persists asymptomatic → Continue AED → Follow-up clinical and neuroimaging until lesion disappears
    - Persists symptomatic > 20 mm in size → ATT is to be tried → Follow-up clinical and neuroimaging
- Lesion calcified → Continue AED (2–3 years)

Abbreviations: AED, antiepileptic drugs; ATT, antituberculous therapy.

are that it has better penetration into the CSF and its concentration is not affected by steroids.

ALBENDAZOLE THERAPY

Albendazole at a dose of 15 mg/kg/day in two divided doses for 28 days is preferred. The optimal duration of cysticidal therapy for less common forms such as giant cysts or subarachnoid lesions is not known but should be longer than for parenchymal NCC.

STEROID THERAPY

Corticosteroid usage has not be standardized and is given empirically for a variable duration of 5–28 days. Oral prednisolone is preferred at a dose of 1 mg/kg/day for 14 days and is started 2–3 days before starting cysticidal therapy and continued for 7–10 days along with cysticidal drug.

RECOMMENDATIONS FOR CYSTICIDAL DRUG

Viable cysts	Cysticidal drug and steroid
Enhancing lesion (Single/multiple)	AED, cysticidal drugs and steroid
Cysticercotic encephalitis	High dose steroid, osmotic diuretics, no cysticidal Drug is advised
Calcified lesion	Cysticidal drug is not advised

Treatment protocol for SECTL is given in **(Flow chart 5.2.1)**.

DURATION OF AED

AED may be continued until resolution of SECTL as monitored by CT/MRI and tapered off over next 12 weeks. If seizures are due to calcified parasite, then AED is to be continued for 2 years of seizures free period.

BIBLIOGRAPHY

1. Ahuja GK, Behari M, Goulatia RK, Jaikhani BL. Disappearing CT lesion in epilepsy. Is tuberculosis or cysticercosis the cause? J Neurol Neurosurg Psy. 1989;52:915-6.
2. Baranwal AK, Singhi PD, Khandelwal N, Singhi SC. Albendazole therapy in children with focal seizures and single small enhancing computerized tomographic lesions: A randomized, placebo-controlled, double blind trial. Pediatr Infect Dis J. 1998;17:696-700.
3. Chandy MJ, Rajshekhar V, Ghosh S. Single small-enhancing CT lesions in India patients with epilepsy: clinical, radiological and pathological considerations. J Neurol Neurosurgery Psychiatry. 1991;54:702-5.
4. Chopra JS, Sawhney IMS, Suresh N, Prabhakar S, Dhand UK, Suri S. Vanishing CT lesions in epilepsy. J Neurol Sci. 1992;107: 40-9.
5. Garcia HH, Nash TE, Takayanagui OM, White AC Jr, et al. Current Consensus Guidelines for Treatment of Neurocysticercosis. Clinical Microbiology Review. 2002;15:747-56.
6. Garg RK, Nag D. Single ring or disc enhancing computed tomographic lesion in Indian children and adolescents after first seizures (letter). Arch Pediatr Adolesc Med. 1997;157: 632-4.
7. Kalra V, Dua T, Kumar V. Efficacy of Albendazole and short-course dexamethasone treatment in children with 1 or 2 ring- enhancing lesions of Neurocysticercosis: A randomized controlled trial. J Pediatr. 2003;143:111-4.
8. Kumar N, Narayanaswamy AS, Singh KK. Ring enhancing CT lesion: A diagnostic dilemma. J Assoc Physicians India. 1995; 43:391-3.
9. Lotz J, Heuulett R, Alkert B, Bowen R. Neuro-cysticercosis Correlative Pathomorphology and MR imaging. Neuroradiology. 1988;30:35-41.
10. Mall RK, Agarwal A, Garg RK, Kar AM, Shukla R. Short course of prednisolone in Indian patients with solitary cysticercus granuloma and new-onset seizures. Epilesia. 2003;44:1397-401.
11. Murthy JMK, Subba Reddy YV. Prognosis of epilepsy associated with single CT enhancing lesion: a long-term follow-up study. J Neurol Sci. 1998;159:151-5.
12. Pal D, Carpio A, Sander J. Neurocysticercosis and epilepsy in developing countries. J Neurol Neurosurg Psychiatry. 2000;68: 137-43.
13. Rajshekhar V, Chacko G, Haran RP, Chandy MJ, Cnandi SM. Clinicoradiological and pathological correlations in patients with solitary cysticercus granuloma and epilepsy focus on presence of the parasite and oedema formation. J Neurol Neurosurg Phychiatry. 1995;59:284-6.

14. Rajshekhar V, Joshi DD, coanh NQ, Van de N, et al. Taenia solium cysticercosis in Asia: epidemiology, impact and issues. Acta Trop. 2003;87(1):53-60.
15. Sawheny IMS, Thussu A, Chopra JS. Single small enhancing CT lesions in epilepsy. In: Understanding a controversy. Acta Neurologica Scandinavia. 1991;44(4):204-10.
16. Schantz PM, Sarti E, Lancarte A. Community based Epidemiologocal Investigations of Cysticercosis due to Taenia solium: Comparison of serological screening tests and clinical findings in two populations in Mexico. Clin Infect Dis. 1994;18: 879.
17. Sethi PK, Kumar BR, Madan VS, Mohan V. Appearing and disappearing CT scan abnormalities and seizures. J Neurol Neurosurg. Phychiatry. 1985;48:866-9.
18. Sethi PP, Wadia RS, Kiyatwat DP, Ichaporia NR, Kothari SS, Sangle SA, Wadhwa P. Ring or disc enhancing lesions in epilepsy in India. J Trop Med Hyg. 1994;97:347-53.
19. Singhi PD, Jain V, Khandelwal N. Corticosteroid versus Albendazole for treatment of single small enhancing computed tomographic lesions in children with neurocysticercosis. J Child Neurol. 2004;19:323.
20. Srinivas HV. Disappearing CT lesions: clinical features. J Trop Geograph Neurol. 1992;2:88-91.
21. Tsang VC, Brand A, Boyer A. An Enzyme Linked Immuno Electro Transfer Blot assay by Glycoprotein antigens for diagnosing human Cysticercosis. J Infect Dis. 1989;159:50-9.
22. Varma A, Gaur KJ, The clinical spectrum of neurocysticercosis in the Uttaranchal region. J Assoc Physicians India. 2002;50: 1398-400.
23. Wadia RS, Makhale CN, Kelkar AV, Grant KB. Focal epilepsy in India with special reference to lesions showing ring or disc like enhancement on contrast computed tomography. J Neurol Neurosurg Psychiatry. 1987;50:1298-301.

5.3 Microbes in Meningitis: Laboratory Diagnosis

T Sivaraman

Reviewers: *MKC Nair, S Thangavelu, S Narmada*

INTRODUCTION

Meningitis in any age group is suspected based on history and clinical examination of the child showing signs of meningeal infection such as fever with seizure, neck stiffness, photophobia, altered sensorium and signs of increased intracranial pressure such as posturing, unequal pupil and abnormal respiratory pattern or apnea.

WHY LABORATORY DIAGNOSIS OF MENINGITIS IS IMPORTANT?

- The etiological organisms causing meningitis varies with the age from infancy to adolescence.
- To know the precise etiology as bacterial, viral, fungal or aseptic meningitis so that appropriate rational treatment can be started at the earliest. This improves the chance of intact neurological outcome in affected children with minimum morbidity and mortality.
- To determine the antibiotic to be given and the duration of treatment based on the organism grown in culture and drug sensitivity pattern.
- Precise diagnosis is also useful so as to initiate chemoprophylaxis and public health preventive measures in an epidemic condition like meningococcal meningitis (**Table 5.3.1**).

WHAT ARE THE FEASIBLE LABORATORY INVESTIGATIONS?

- CSF analysis.
- Blood culture—bacterial and fungal.
- Smear from petechiae in skin.
- Other tests like CRP, procalcitonin.

Table 5.3.1: Pathogens in meningitis

Age group	*Predominant pathogen*
Age 0–4 weeks	*S. agalactiae* *E. coli* K_1 *L. monocytogenes*
Age 4–12 weeks	*S. agalactiae* *E. coli* *H. influenzae* *S. pneumoniae* *N. meningitidis*
Age 3 months–18 years	*N. meningitidis* *S. pneumoniae* *H. influenzae*

- Complete blood count, differential count, blood sugar.
- Chest X-ray to find out foci of infection.

CSF ANALYSIS

Lab analysis of cerebrospinal fluid is the most important and investigation in diagnosis of meningitis.

All childrens with clinical suspicion of meningitis should have lumbar puncture done unless there are definite contraindications.

CONTRAINDICATIONS FOR LUMBAR PUNCTURE

- Signs of focally increased intracranial pressure like altered mental status, focal abnormalities on neurological examination or neuroimaging showing mass lesion, midline shift.
- Clinically significant cardiorespiratory compromise in neonates and older extremely sick patients.
- History or signs of bleeding disorder or platelet count less than 20,000
- Signs of local infection such pyoderma, crysipelas at lumbar puncture site.

COLLECTION AND TRANSPORT OF CSF FLUID

Strict aseptic precaution should be followed while collecting CSF samples and they should be immediately transported to lab so that chance of isolation of organism is maximized.

- Attenders should be especially trained and special attenders should be posted. Specimen should reach the lab within 10 minutes after collection.
- No transport media should be used if CSF can reach the lab within 20 minutes. Transport at ambient temperature. Sample should be never refrigerated.
  - CSF should be collected in 3 containers. First and second container to be sent to microbiology and third to be biochemistry lab.
  - If only 1 (or) 2 containers are available, both to be sent to microbiology lab. Minimum of 0.5–1 mL of CSF to be collected in each container. In practice, total volume of fluid is more important than the "tube" cultured.

ROLE OF TRANSPORT MEDIUM

- If delay is anticipated for inoculation of culture brain heart infusion broth (BHI) media can be used as a holding medium
- Brain heart infusion (BHI) media should be kept at room temperature. The inoculated BHI should be kept at the incubator within the candle jar.
- Subculture have to be made in appropriate media in the main lab.

CSF Analysis

- *Cytological analysis:*
  - Leukocytes cell count
  - Differential count
  - Gram stain, AFB, Indian ink, if clinically indicated
- *Biochemical analysis:*
  - CSF sugar
  - CSF proteins
- *Microbiological analysis:*
  - Isolation of organism
  - Demonstration of antigens
- *PCR:* Especially RT-PCR for viral infections.

Table 5.3.2: CSF findings in various types of meningitis

Condition	*Pressure (mmH_2O)*	*Leukocytes mm^3*	*Protein mg/dL*	*Glucose mg/dL*	*Others*
Normal	50–80	<5, lymphocytes	20–45	>50	
Bacterial meningitis	100–300 Elevated	100–10,000 Polymorphs predominate	100–500	Decreased <40	Gram staining useful
Viral meningitis	Normal 80–150	<1000 cells, lymphocyte predominate	50–200	Normal, reduced in mumps	PCR in diagnosing specific virus
Partially treated bacterial meningitis	Normal or elevated	5–10,000 Polymorphs or sometimes lymphocytes	100–500	Normal or decreased	Latex agglutination or PCR useful
TB meningitis	Usually elevated	100–500, lymphocytic predominance	100–3000, elevated in spinal block	<50 in most cases	GeneXpert assay of CSF and AFB staining
Fungal meningitis	Usually elevated	5–500 , lymphocyte predominance. None in cryptococcal meningitis	25–500	<50 in most cases	Indian ink preparation and fungal culture

Source: Nelson's Textbook of Paediatrics, 1st South Asian edition.

GRAM'S STAINING (FIG. 5.3.1)

- Gram stain may be negative in up to 60% of cases of bacterial meningitis even without prior antibiotics.
- Neither a normal Gram stain, nor a lymphocytosis excludes bacterial meningitis especially, if partially treated.
- Neutrophils may predominate in viral meningitis even after the first 24 hours. lymphocyte predominance occur later.
- CSF findings in bacterial meningitis may mimic those found in viral meningitis (particularly early on) **(Tables 5.3.2 to 5.3.4)**. It may be possible with modest accuracy to judge whether bacterial or viral is more likely based on CSF parameters. However if the CSF is abnormal the safest course is to treat as if it is bacterial meningitis.

Table 5.3.3: Morbid analysis of CSF

Clear	Normal or in aseptic meningitis
Turbid	Bacterial meningitis
Blood stained	Traumatic tap or subarachnoid bleed
Suspended particles	Contamination, antigen testing can be done but unsuitable for culture
Yellowish	In jaundice or high protein content

Table 5.3.4: Gram's staining

Observation	*Inference*
Predominant polymorphs	Bacterial meningitis
Predominant lymphocytes	TB or viral infection
Gram positive cocci pairs and chains	*Pneumococcus* and *Streptococcus*
Gram negative cocci	*N. meningitidis*
Gram negative bacilli	*H. influenzae* and other Gram negative bacteria

DEMONSTRATION OF THE ANTIGENS

Principle of Latex Agglutination

- Specific polysaccharide surface antigens present on organisms, a quantity of which diffuses into the body fluids. In meningitis, this antigens are present in CSF.
- This antigens can be detected by principle of specific antigen and antibody reactions. In the latex agglutination test, specific antibodies are coated with latex particles which shows clear clumping, if allowed to react with the specific antigens.

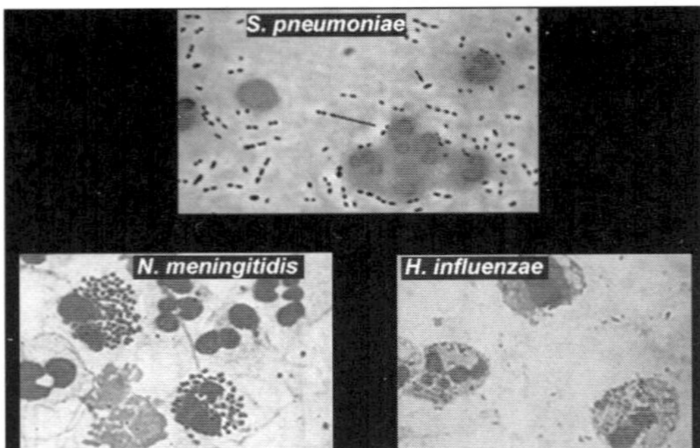

Fig. 5.3.1: Gram's staining (Direct smear)
(For color version, see Plate 6)

Antigens Detected

- *Group B Streptococcus, H. influenzae* type B, *S. pneumoniae, N. meningitidis* ACY W135, *N. meningitidis* B, *E. coli* K_1.

Antigen testing is useful if:

- Initial CSF Gram stain and culture are negative after 48 hours of incubation.
- Strong clinical evidence of meningitis but pretreated with antibiotics.
- Traumatic lumbar puncture.

CSF latex agglutination: Is a simple and rapid diagnostic test with 78–100% sensitivity for *H. influenzae*, 67–100% for *S. pneumoniae*, 69–100% for *S. agalactiae* and 50–93% for *N. meningitidis*.

POLYMERASE CHAIN REACTION

Principle

Amplification of virus specific DNA or RNA using PCR so that even small amount of infecting DNA can be found out.

It is especially useful in diagnosing viral infections of brain and also in bacterial meningitis.

- PCR is routinely available for *Neisseria meningitidis*, herpes simplex and enterovirus.
- With the advent of RT- PCR results are now available immediately.
- Enterovirus PCR should be requested on CSF from patients with clinical and/or CSF features of viral meningitis.
- HSV-PCR should be requested for patients with clinical features of encephalitis.
- Meningococcal PCR is particularly useful in patients with a clinical picture consistent with meningococcal meningitis, but who have received prior antibiotics.
- GeneXpert MTB very useful for diagnosing mycobacterial DNA and carries high specificity.

Bacterial PCR: When processed early, has a sensitivity of nearly 100%, specificity of 98%, positive predictive value of 98% and negative predictive value of 100%.

OTHER TESTS IN MENINGITIS

Blood culture: It is positive in 80–90% cases before antibiotic therapy, but rapidly becomes negative with antibiotic therapy. It should be done in all cases of suspected meningitis.

ACUTE PHASE REACTANTS

These are nonspecific markers of bacterial infection which can be used as corroborative evidence in addition to other lab tests.

C-reactive protein: In bacterial meningitis >50 mg/dL is common and normalizes within 1–2 days of antibiotic therapy; levels <10 mg/dL make the diagnosis highly unlikely.

CSF lactate: >4.2 mmol/L has high sensitivity (96%) and positive predictive value (100%) but has lower specificity and feasibility.

PROCALCITONIN

Although levels >5 µg/L are reportedly 99% sensitive and 83% specific for the diagnosis of bacterial infection its use is still limited, but falling levels from baseline value can be used to assess response to treatment.

IMPORTANT POINTS

- CSF analysis is the most important lab investigation for diagnosis of meningitis.
- Proper aseptic precaution during lumbar puncture and avoiding delay in diagnosis improves the culture positivity rate.
- Biochemical parameters and cell counts are unchanged till 48–72 hours in partially treated meningitis.
- Latex agglutination is useful in culture negative, partially treated meningitis. But negative test does not rule out meningitis.
- PCR especially RT-PCR is useful in diagnosing viral meningitis and meningoencephalitis especially caused by herpes simplex.
- CRP and procalcitonin are used to assess the response to treatment rather than relying on them for diagnosis.
- Inspite of negative lab reports, if strong clinical signs of meningitis are present better to treat the child for meningitis.

BIBLIOGRAPHY

1. Blazer S, Berant M, Alon U. Bacterial meningitis: effect of antibiotic treatment on cerebrospinal fluid. Am J Clin Pathol. 1983;80:386-7.
2. Kleigman, Stanton, St Geme, Scho (Eds). Nelson Textbook of Pediatrics First South Asian edn.
3. Lakeman FD, Whitley RJ. Diagnosis of herpes simplex encephalitis: application of polymerase chain reaction to cerebrospinal fluid from brain-biopsied patients and correlation with disease. National Institute of Allergy and Infectious Diseases Collaborative Antiviral Study Group. J Infect Dis. 1995;171: 857-63.
4. Maxson S, Lewno MJ, Schutze GE. Clinical usefulness of cerebrospinal fluid bacterial antigen studies. J Pediatr. 1994;125:235-8.
5. Rowley AH, Whitley RJ, Lakeman FD, et al. Rapid detection of herpes-simplex-virus DNA in cerebrospinal fluid of patients with herpes simplex encephalitis. Lancet. 1990;335: 440-1.
6. Swaiman KF, Ashwal S, Ferriero DM, Schor NF, (Eds). Swaiman's Pediatric Neurology, 5th edn. Philadelphia, 2012, WB Saunders.

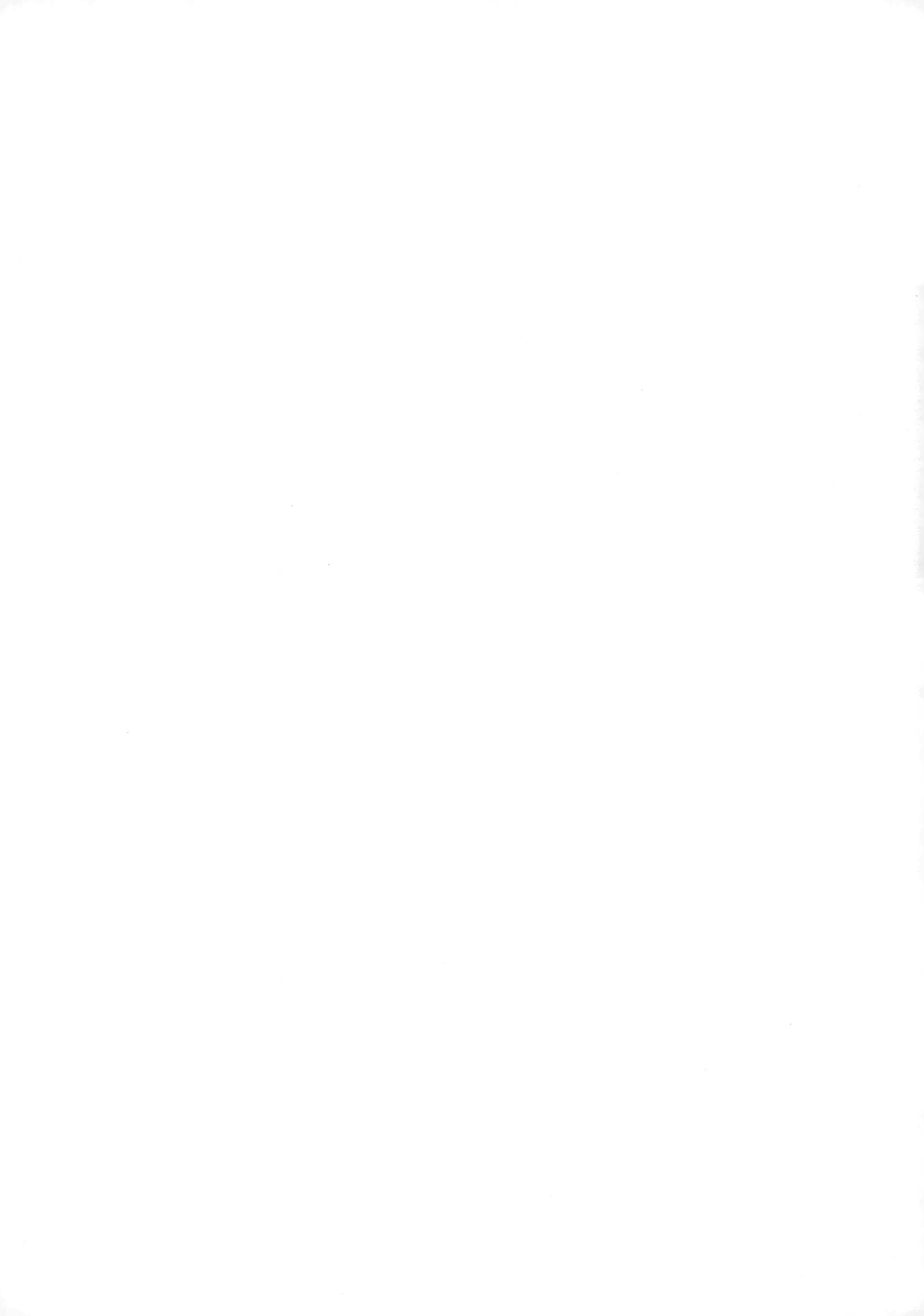

Cardiology

Reviewers: *PSN Menon, Alok Gupta, R Remesh Kumar, MKC Nair, S Thangavelu, S Narmada, K Nedunchelian, Jaydeep Choudhury, RV Dhakshayani*

6.1 X-ray in Pediatric Cardiology

Gnanasambandam Subramaniyan, Vadavil Suhas Das
Reviewers: *PSN Menon, Alok Gupta, R Remesh Kumar*

INTRODUCTION

X-ray is an essential tool of investigation in cardiology and has to be interpreted systematically in relation to the clinical profile of the patient. In this chapter, we will discuss about the technical adequacy, normal cardiac anatomy as seen in chest X-rays, image characteristics of the enlargements of various chambers of the heart, aortic arch and pulmonary vascularity. The radiological abnormalities seen in some common cardiac disorders are also briefly described.

TECHNICAL ADEQUACY

Rotation

The distance between medial ends of clavicles should be at equal distance from the adjacent posterior spinous process with the clavicles at the same level. Anterior ribs should be equidistant from the lateral margins of spine and posterior spinous process of vertebrae in a well-centered film. In postoperative patients with sternotomy, sternal wires appear to overlap the vertebral spine.

Rotation to the left will cause enlargement of left cardiac structures and rotation to the right will cause enlargement of right cardiac structures.

Exposure

With adequate exposure, the intervertebral disc spaces of the upper four (4) thoracic vertebrae are visualized through the cardiac silhouette. In an overexposed film, all intervertebral discs are visualized, which may mimic decreased pulmonary vascularity. In the underexposed film intervertebral discs are not visualized which may mimic increased pulmonary vascularity or pulmonary edema.

Inspiratory Film versus Expiratory Film

Cardiac silhouette is best visualized in an inspiratory film. In the inspiratory film, the 5th anterior intercostal space or the 9th posterior intercostal space is visualized above the diaphragm. An expiratory film overestimates cardiothoracic ratio and falsely mimics increased pulmonary vascular marking or pulmonary edema.

Anteroposterior versus Postero-Anterior Views

Table 6.1.1 details the various differences between the anteroposterior (AP) and postero-anterior (PA) views in a chest X-ray.

NORMAL CARDIAC ANATOMY IN CHEST X-RAY

Thymus

Thymus is an anterior mediastinal structure in the chest X-ray which mimics cardiomegaly in infancy but involutes with age.

Table 6.1.1: Differences between AP versus PA views in a chest X-ray

Characteristics	*PA view*	*AP view*
Film position	X-ray film anterior to the patient, close to heart	X-ray film behind the patient; away from heart; ↑ magnification
Distance from source	72 inches	40 inches
Position of patient	Erect	Supine (makes heart look bigger)
Position of scapula	Away from the lung fields	Overlies the lung fields

Abbreviations: AP, anteroposterior; PA, posteroanterior

- *Sail sign:* The right lobe of the thymus insinuates into the minor fissure.
- *Wave sign:* Thymic indentation of overlying ribs.

Heart Size

Cardiothoracic ratio in PA view (not applicable for AP view) is measured to assess cardiomegaly. It is the ratio between maximal cardiac dimensions (middle of spine to maximum cardiac border on right and left side) to the widest internal diameter of chest (at the level of dome of diaphragm). In neonates CT ratio of >0.6 indicates cardiomegaly and beyond infancy >0.5 indicates cardiomegaly. Since proper inspiratory film is taken less often in infancy, cardiothoracic ratio in infancy should be correlated clinically and if necessary with other views (lateral view).

An increase in transverse diameter of heart by 2 cm or more compared to a recent previous study is considered as significant increase in cardiac size even if the cardiothoracic ratio remains <0.5.

Cardiac Silhouette

PA view ***(Figs 6.1.1 and 6.1.2)***: Right border from above downwards is formed by superior vena cava and right atrium. The left border is formed by the aortic knob, main pulmonary artery, left atrial appendage and left ventricle.

Lateral view ***(Fig. 6.1.3)***: The borders are formed anteriorly by ascending aorta, main pulmonary artery, and right ventricle and posteriorly by left atrium, left ventricle and inferior vena cava.

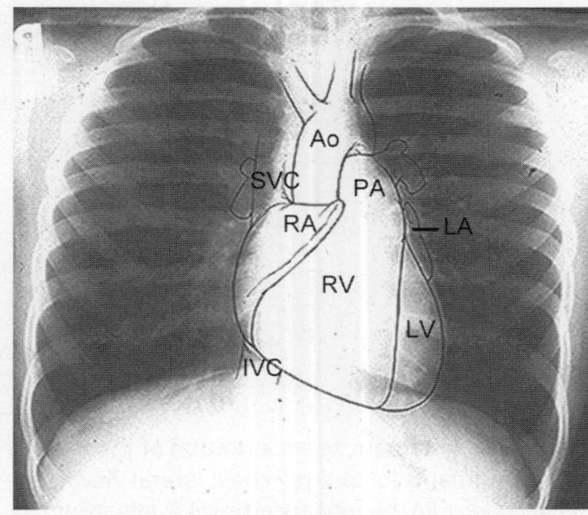

Fig. 6.1.1: Cardiac silhouette as visualized on PA view of chest X-ray

Abbreviations: Ao, aorta; SVC, superior vena cava; PA, pulmonary artery; RA, right atrium; RV, right ventricle; LA, left atrium; LV, left ventricle; IVC, inferior vena cava

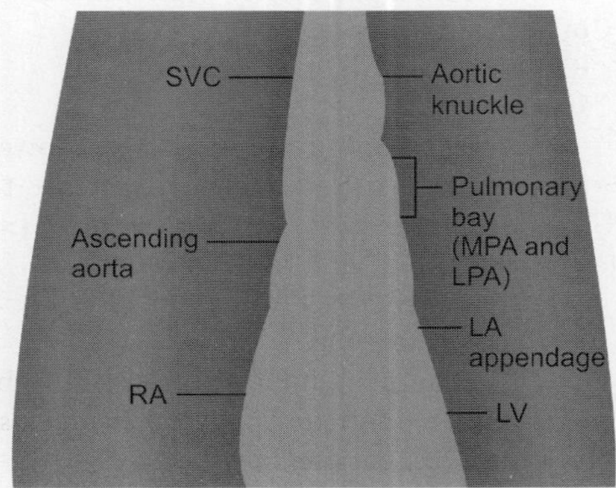

Fig. 6.1.2: Schematic representation of the various landmarks in a PA view of chest X-ray

Abbreviations: SVC, superior vena cava; RA, right atrium; LA, left atrium; LV, left ventricle; MPA, main pulmonary artery; LPA, left pulmonary artery

CARDIAC CHAMBER ENLARGEMENTS

Left Atrium Enlargement

- *PA view:*
  - *"Shadow within right atrial shadow"* or *"double-density sign"* occurs when the right side of the left atrium pushes behind the right cardiac shadow, indenting the adjacent lung and forming its own distinct silhouette
  - Widening of angle of carina to >75° (normal <60°)
  - Left atrial appendage is prominent.
- *Lateral view:* Abnormal bulge of the upper posterior cardiac border.

Left Ventricle Enlargement

- *PA view:* Apex dips into the left hemi-diaphragm forming an obtuse cardio-phrenic angle.

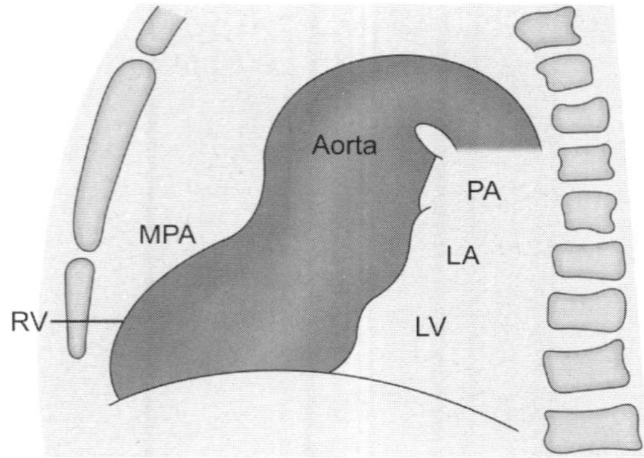

Fig. 6.1.3: Schematic representation of the various landmarks in an X-ray chest lateral view
Abbreviations: PA, pulmonary artery; LA, left atrium; LV, left ventricle; RV, right ventricle; MPA, main pulmonary artery.

- *Lateral view:* Lower posterior cardiac border will be shifted posteriorly with obliteration of retrocardiac space.
  Right Atrium (RA) Enlargement
- *PA view:*
  - Increased prominence of right lower cardiac silhouette. Mid-spine to maximum right heart border >4 cm (>5 cm in older children and adults)
  - RA border occupies more than 3 intercostal spaces
  - RA occupying more than 50% of right heart border (normally RA forms less than 50% of right heart border)
  - Dilated superior vena cava (SVC) due to increased right atrial pressure.

Right Ventricle Enlargement

- *PA view:* Cardiophrenic angle is acute with rounded apex which is above left hemi-diaphragm (in contrast to left ventricle apex which dips into diaphragm
- *Lateral view:* Obliteration of retrosternal space.

HEART POSITION

- *Levocardia:* Heart lies to the left side of chest.
- *Dextrocardia:* Heart lies to the right side of chest.
- *Situs solitus:* Morphological RA is right sided, morphological LA is left sided, hyparterial left upper lobe bronchus (bronchus below adjacent pulmonary artery), epiarterial right upper lobe bronchus (bronchus above adjacent pulmonary artery), right sided liver, left sided stomach and left sided spleen.
- *Situs inversus:* This is the mirror image of situs solitus.
- *Situs ambiguous with right isomerism* (bilateral right sidedness): Both atria are morphologically RA, both upper bronchi are eparterial and the spleen is absent (asplenia syndrome).
- *Situs ambiguous with left isomerism* (bilateral left sidedness): Both atria are morphologically LA; both upper bronchi are hyparterial with multiple small accessory spleens rather than a single, full-sized, normal spleen (polysplenia syndrome). *Both right isomerism and left isomerism are associated with midline liver.*

Aortic Arch

Sidedness of the aortic arch is determined by the indentation on the trachea. Left aortic arch produces indentation on the left side of the tracheal shadow, the right sided aortic arch produces indentation on the right side of the tracheal shadow and is usually at a higher level than the left arch.

Pulmonary Vascularity

Pulmonary vascularity may appear as:

- *Normal vascularity:* Pulmonary arteries (PAs) are vertical with sharp outline. Pulmonary veins are horizontal in lower lobes; they are vertical and lie lateral to arterial shadows in the upper lobes. PA branches are well seen in inner third and middle third of the lung fields and just seen in outer third of the lung fields, end on view of peripheral arteries are approximately the same size as the adjacent bronchi. *Right pulmonary artery (RPA) diameter equals the tracheal shadow in PA view and left pulmonary artery (LPA) equals the tracheal width in left lateral view.*

- *Increased pulmonary arterial flow (e.g. left to right lesions):* The main pulmonary artery (MPA), LPA and RPA are dilated; vascularity is well visualized in outer third of lung fields. Pulmonary arterial hypertension (PAH) results in peripheral pruning (Eisenmenger syndrome).
- *Decreased pulmonary arterial flow* (e.g. tetralogy of Fallot): MPA segment is concave; LPA and RPA are small with hyperlucent lung fields.
- *Pulmonary venous hypertension (PVHT)* (e.g. dilated cardiomyopathy, DCM): Margins of blood vessels appear thin and poorly defined. Increase in the venous pressure causes perivascular edema which constricts lower lobe veins and redistributes the flow into upper lobes (cephalization of veins/prominence in upper lobe). **Table 6.1.2** describes the grading of PVHT. **Table 6.1.3** describes the X-ray features of pulmonary arterial and pulmonary venous hypertension.

COMMON RADIOLOGICAL PATTERNS SEEN IN HEART DISEASES

Left to Right Shunts

Chest X-ray is unremarkable in small left to right shunts. **Table 6.1.4** lists the various radiological features seen in an X-ray chest in the three most common left to right shunts—atrial septal defect (ASD), ventricular septal defect (VSD) and patent ductus arteriosus (PDA).

Table 6.1.2: Pulmonary venous hypertension (PVHT) grading (Lary P Elliott's Classification)

Grade	*X-ray findings*
Grade 1	Cephalization
Grade 2	Interstitial edema (Kerley a, b and c lines, indistinct vessels, ground glass lung fields)
Grade 3	Alveolar edema
Grade 4	Hemosiderosis (longstanding PVHT)

Table 6.1.3: X-ray features of pulmonary arterial hypertension and pulmonary venous hypertension

Pulmonary arterial hypertension	*Pulmonary venous hypertension*
Well-defined margins of vascularity	Hazy margins
Both pulmonary vasculature and cardiac size increased significantly	Less cardiomegaly
Prominence of main pulmonary artery	Dilatation of pulmonary artery is delayed
End on view size of PA > bronchus	Kerley a, b and c lines
—	Prominence of upper lobe vessels and small basal vessels

Table 6.1.4: Radiological findings in left to right shunts

X-ray findings	*Atrial septal defect (ASD)*	*Ventricular septal defect (VSD)*	*Patent ductus arteriosus (PDA)*
Cardiothoracic ratio	+++	+	+
Right atrial enlargement	+	–	–
Left atrial enlargement	–	+	+
Right ventricle enlargement	++	+	–
Aorta	Small	Small	Dilated
Increased pulmonary blood flow (PBF)	++	++	++ (+/- left lung may appear more plethoric)

Table 6.1.5: Radiological findings in Eisenmenger syndrome

Radiological findings	*ASD (Pretricuspid)*	*VSD/PDA (Post-tricuspid)*
Peripheral pulmonary vascularity	Normal or decreased	Normal or decreased
Central pulmonary artery	Very large	Large
Heart size	Cardiomegaly	Normal

Abbreviations: ASD, atrial septal defect; VSD, ventricular septal defect; PDA, patent ductus arteriosus.

Complete endocardial cushion defect: Cardiomegaly involving all four chambers with increased pulmonary vascular markings and prominence of main pulmonary artery will be present. Pulmonary oligemia is seen if associated with pulmonic stenosis.

Partial anomalous pulmonary venous return (PAPVR or Scimitar syndrome): Cardiomegaly involving right atrium, right ventricle, prominence of main pulmonary artery and increase in pulmonary vascular markings. A crescent-shaped vertical shadow (*Scimitar-Turkish sword*) can be seen in front of the right lower lung due to dilated superior vena cava.

Eisenmenger syndrome: This is characterized by peripheral pruning of vessels. **Table 6.1.5** lists the differentiating features of pretricuspid (ASD) shunt from post-tricuspid shunts (e.g. VSD/PDA and aorta-pulmonary window).

Obstructive Lesions

Pulmonary stenosis: Main pulmonary artery (MPA) and left pulmonary artery (LPA) appear prominent (poststenotic dilatation). Right pulmonary artery (RPA) may appear normal due to its anatomy. Cardiomegaly is seen if cardiac failure develops.

Aortic stenosis: Cardiomegaly with left ventricle configuration in moderate and severe aortic stenosis.

Coarctation of aorta: Cardiomegaly with pulmonary edema or pulmonary venous congestion is noted in moderate and severe coarctation. Rib notching (scalloping and focal necrosis) in children more than 4–5 years of age is noted in inferior borders of the ribs on the posterior side of 3rd–8th ribs.

- *3 sign (PA view):* Due to prominent aortic knob and left subclavian artery proximal to the coarctation, indentation from coarctation and poststenotic aortic dilatation below the coarctation.
- *E sign* is seen with barium swallow due to the indentation of esophagus by the dilated aorta proximal and distal to coarctation.

Cyanotic Heart Diseases

Tetralogy of Fallot

- Heart size is normal or smaller than normal with decreased pulmonary vascular marking.
- Concave main pulmonary arterial segment (hypoplasia of main pulmonary artery) with upturned apex.
- Elevation of apex of heart due to right ventricular hypertrophy and concave contour along the left cardiac border causes the characteristic boot-shaped heart (Coeur *en Sabot).*
- Right atrium enlargement and associated right aortic arch in 20% of children with tetralogy of Fallot (TOF).
- Unilateral decrease in pulmonary blood flow when associated with absent LPA/RPA or peripheral pulmonary artery stenosis.
- Unilateral increase in blood flow following Blalock-Thomas-Taussig (BTT) shunt.
- Reticular or lacy network pattern in lung fields if associated with major aorto-pulmonary collateral arterial system (MAPCAS).

TOF with absent pulmonary valve: Right pulmonary artery and left pulmonary artery are markedly dilated with ischemic peripheral lung fields.

Transposition of great arteries (TGAs): Cardiomegaly with increased pulmonary vascular marking and narrow pedicle (egg on side appearance).

Tricuspid Atresia

- Cardiomegaly with LV configuration.
- Decreased pulmonary vascularity when associated with pulmonary stenosis.
- Increased pulmonary pattern when pulmonary stenosis/right ventricular outflow tract obstruction is absent.
- When associated with juxtaposed RA appendage, the right cardiac border is straight.

Total Anomalous Pulmonary Venous Connection

- Moderate to marked cardiomegaly involving right atrium and right ventricle present with increase in the pulmonary vascular markings.
- *Snowman sign* or figure of eight configuration in supracardiac total anomalous pulmonary venous connection (TAPVC) noted in older infants.

Truncus arteriosus (TA): Triad of cardiomegaly, increased pulmonary vascular marking and a right sided aortic arch (in 50% of cases) in a cyanotic child favors truncus arteriosus. MPA segment is concave.

Ebstein anomaly: Marked cardiomegaly with small main pulmonary artery segment and ischemic lung fields.

Rheumatic Heart Disease

Mitral stenosis: Left atrium and right ventricle enlargement, prominent main pulmonary arterial segment with features of pulmonary venous hypertension (*straightening of left cardiac border due to prominent pulmonary artery and left atrial appendage*) (**Table 6.1.3**).

Mitral regurgitation: Left atrium and left ventricle enlargement in moderate and severe mitral regurgitation with features of pulmonary venous hypertension.

Aortic regurgitation: Cardiomegaly with left ventricle configuration; dilated ascending aorta and prominent aortic knob.

Pericardial Effusion

Large pericardial effusion presents with gross cardiomegaly (water bottle configuration) and a narrow pedicle with poor differentiation of cardiac chambers. Cardiophrenic angle is acute with oligemic lung fields.

CONCLUSION

- It must be emphasized that X-ray interpretation is never done in isolation and should always be correlated with clinical profile of the patient.
- Technical adequacy of X-ray film should be assessed before interpretation.
- X-ray interpretation should never be done in isolation and should always be correlated with the clinical profile of the patient.
- Features of peripheral pulmonary vascularity can be picked up only by X-rays compared to other diagnostic modality like echocardiogram.

BIBLIOGRAPHY

1. AE Rubio, Lewin MB. Ventricular septal defect. In: Allen HD, Driscoll DJ, Shaddy RE, Feltes TF (Eds). Moss and Adams Heart Disease in Infants, Children and Adolescents, 8th edn. Philadelphia; Lippincott Williams & Wilkins; 2013. pp. 713-21.
2. Bernstein D. Acyanotic congenital heart disease: obstructive lesions: pulmonary valve stenosis with intact ventricular septum. In: Kleigman RM, Stanton BMD, St Geme J, Schor NF (Eds). Nelson Textbook of Paediatrics, 20th edn. Philadelphia; Elsevier, 2015;2:2199-202.
3. Chow JS, Cleveland RH. Normal pediatric chest. In: Cleveland RH (Ed). Imaging in Pediatric Pulmonology, 1st edn. New York; Springer. 2011. pp. 21-9.
4. Geggel RL, Flyer DC. Mitral valve and left atrial lesions. In: Keane JF, Flyer DC, Lock JE (Eds).

Nadas Pediatric Cardiology, 2nd edn. Philadelphia; Saunders Elsevier. 2007. pp. 697-710.
5. Gordon Culham JA, Mawson JB. Chest radiography in pediatric cardiovascular disease. In: Coley BD (Ed). Caffey's Pediatric diagnostic imaging, 12th edn. Philadelphia; Elsevier Saunders; 2013;684-8.
6. Sachdeva R. Atrial septal defect. In: Allen HD, Driscoll DJ, Shaddy RE, Feltes TF (Eds). Moss and Adams Heart Disease in Infants, Children and adolescents, 8th edn. Philadelphia; Lippincott Williams & Wilkins; 2013. pp. 678-89.
7. Spicer RL, Ware SM. Diseases of the pericardium. In: Kleigman RM, Stanton BMD, St Geme J, Schor NF (Eds). Nelson Textbook of Paediatrics, 20th edn. Philadelphia; Elsevier. 2015;2. pp. 2279-81.
8. Tandon R. Usefulness of thoracic roentgenogram. In: Tandon R (Ed). Bedside Approach in the Diagnosis of Congenital Heart Disease, 2nd edn. New Delhi; BI Churchill Livingston Pvt. Ltd; 2011. pp. 69-86.

6.2 Laboratory Backup in Kawasaki Disease and Rheumatic Fever

Gnanasambandam Subramaniyan, J Ritchie Sharon Solomon, Vadavil Suhas Das, Gopala Krishnan
Reviewers: *MKC Nair, S Thangavelu, S Narmada*

KAWASAKI DISEASE DIAGNOSTIC CRITERIA

Case definition of classic Kawasaki disease (KD) requires the presence of fever for at least 5 days and four of the five principal clinical features listed below:[1]

- Changes in the extremities, including erythema and/or indurative edema and later (2nd week of illness) membranous desquamation starting in the subungual regions
- Polymorphous exanthema (but not including bullous or vesicular lesions)
- Bilateral nonexudative conjunctival injection
- Changes in lips and oral cavity (but not including discrete oral lesions)
- Cervical lymphadenopathy, usually unilateral and large (≥1.5 cm).

Patients with fever but fewer than four principal clinical features can be diagnosed as having Kawasaki disease when coronary artery disease is detected by 2-D echocardiography.

SUPPLEMENTAL LABORATORY FINDINGS (NOT REQUIRED FOR DIAGNOSIS)

- Anemia (normochromic, normocytic and self-limited)
- White blood cell (WBC) count ≥ 15,000/mm^3 (neutrophilia and immature forms)
- Thrombocytosis > 450,000/mm^3 (usually in 2nd and 3rd week of illness)
- Elevated acute phase reactants: CRP, ESR, α-1 antitrypsin
- Elevated liver enzymes (Serum transaminases, gamma glutamyltranspeptidase)
- Hypoalbuminemia<3 g/dL
- Hyponatremia
- Abnormal plasma lipids
- Sterile pyuria (urine ≥ 10 WBC/hpf)
- Pleocytosis in cerebrospinal fluid.

INCOMPLETE KAWASAKI DISEASE

Any child presenting with fever >5 days and not fulfilling the diagnostic criteria for classic

KD may have some of the abovementioned laboratory findings. In such scenario, the diagnosis of incomplete Kawasaki disease should be considered and echocardiography should be obtained since 15% of cases present with coronary artery lesion.[2]

Diagnostic algorithm for incomplete KD is shown in **Flow chart 6.2.1**.

Atypical Kawasaki disease: Patients who have problems such as renal involvement, cholecystitis, and hydrops of gallbladder, etc. that are generally not seen in KD.

CLINICAL FEATURES

There is usually a prodrome of upper respiratory or gastrointestinal symptoms before the onset of acute phase of KD. The acute phase begins with abrupt onset of high grade remittent fever along with skin rash, conjunctival injection, reddening and fissuring of lips, erythema of the buccal mucosa, strawberry tongue, nonsuppurative cervical lymphadenitis and erythema and edema of hands and feet.

The acute phase is followed by a subacute phase, which occurs from the 2nd to the 4th week of illness. Desquamation starts during this phase and starts in the subungual region and spreads to the palms and soles. There may be hepatomegaly, hydrops of gallbladder, transient jaundice and elevated liver enzymes.

Patients who are untreated or those who are treated with aspirin only have febrile course lasting for 1–3 weeks.

LAB ABNORMALITIES

- Leukocytosis with increased numbers of neutrophils and bands can occur during the acute period. Leukopenia is rare.
- There is elevation of acute phase reactants during the acute stage.
- Transient anemia can occur particularly when active inflammation is prolonged.
- Thrombocytosis usually happens during the 2nd and 3rd weeks of the illness. Both elevated platelet count and acute phase reactants will gradually subside by 6th–8th week of the illness.
- Thrombocytopenia is seen rarely in the acute stage and may be a sign of disseminated intravascular coagulation.
- Severe hemolytic anemia is rare but may be related to intravenous immunoglobulin (IVIG) infusion.[3]
- Lipid profile is markedly altered in acute KD with decreased plasma cholesterol, highdensity lipoprotein and apolipoprotein A1.[4]
- Mild-to-moderate elevations in serum transaminases occur in ≤40% of patients and mild elevation of serum bilirubin levels in 10%.[5]
- Plasma gamma glutamyltranspeptidase is elevated in 67% of patients.[6]
- Hypoalbuminemia is common and is associated with more severe and prolonged acute disease.
- Sterile pyuria is probably due to urethritis. CSF shows evidence of aseptic meningitis with predominance of mononuclear cells as well as normal glucose and protein levels.[7]

Kawasaki disease is unlikely if platelet counts and acute phase reactants (ESR and CRP) are normal after day 7 of illness. Low WBC count, lymphocyte predominance and low platelet count in absence of disseminated intravascular coagulation suggest a viral etiology.

Incomplete KD is more common in young infants who are at a substantial risk of developing coronary abnormalities than compared to older children. Hence, accurate diagnosis and timely treatment is of paramount importance. Though laboratory findings are not diagnostic, they are useful in diagnosis of suspected case of incomplete KD.

CARDIAC INVOLVEMENT IN KD

Cardiovascular manifestations are the leading cause for long-term morbidity and mortality. It can involve pericardium, myocardium, endocardium, valves and coronary arteries.

During acute phase, signs of myocarditis may develop such as sinus tachycardia, gallop rhythm and muffled heart sounds. These findings are generally self-limited and improve with IVIG treatment. Innocent flow murmur or pansystolic murmur of mitral regurgitation may be heard. Pericardial effusions are uncommon and rarely measure >1 mm.[8] Pericardial tamponade is very rare.[9] Coronary artery involvement may range from mild features of coronary arteritis to aneurysm and coronary occlusion.

ELECTROCARDIOGRAM IN KD

Electrocardiogram (ECG) may show prolonged PR interval or nonspecific ST and T-wave changes. Large aneurysms may lead to acute myocardial infarction manifested as ST segment elevation and inversion of T-waves.

ECHOCARDIOGRAPHY IN KD

Evaluation of coronary arteries should be performed at diagnosis to establish a baseline and in some cases to aid in diagnosis. Echocardiography is a valuable tool during the acute and subacute stages of KD to evaluate coronaries. During the acute stage of KD features suggestive of coronary arteritis may be seen before development of aneurysms. Perivascular brightness, ectasia and lack of tapering of the coronary arteries are suggestive of coronary arteritis. Decrease in left ventricular function, mild mitral regurgitation[8] and pericardial effusion may be seen. Mild diffuse coronary artery dilatation and enhanced perivascular brightness may be seen in 30–50% of patients in acute stage of KD. Without IVIG treatment, these lesions may become aneurysmal 1–3 weeks from onset of illness (average 10 days).

As per the Japanese national Kawasaki disease surveillance data incidence of coronary artery aneurysms is between 10% and 17.9%.[10] Coronary artery aneurysms tend to develop most frequently in the proximal segments of left anterior descending artery and right coronary artery and less common in left main coronary artery.

Based on internal diameter of aneurysm, they are classified as:[11,12]

- *Small aneurysm:* < 5 mm
- *Medium aneurysm:* 5–8 mm
- *Giant aneurysm:* > 8 mm

The Japanese Ministry of Health criteria[13] *term coronary arteries as abnormal if:*

- Internal lumen diameter >3 mm in children <5 years of age (or)
- Internal lumen diameter >4 mm in children ≥5 years of age (or)
- Internal diameter of a segment measures ≥1.5 times that of its adjacent segment (or)
- Coronary lumen is clearly irregular.

Based on Z scores,[14] *the following cut-off points have been proposed:*

- *Small aneurysm:* Z-score ≥ 2.5 to < 5.0
- *Large aneurysm:* Z-score ≥ 5.0 to < 10.0
- *Giant aneurysm:* Z-score ≥ 10.

DIAGNOSIS OF INCOMPLETE KAWASAKI DISEASE

The algorithm that can be used as a guide to evaluate a patient with suspected incomplete KD is given in **Flow chart 6.2.1**.

HARADA SCORE

Risk score at the time of diagnosis of a child with KD to determine the risk of future coronary aneurysms.[15,16] Intravenous gamma globulin is given to children who fulfill 4 of the following criteria, assessed within 9 days of onset of illness:

- White blood cell count >12,000/mm^3
- Platelet count <350,000/mm^3
- CRP >3 mg/dL
- Hematocrit <35%
- Albumin <3.5 g/dL
- Age ≤12 months
- Male sex.

If risk factors <4 but continuing acute symptoms, the risk score is reassessed daily. It is used in few centers in Japan to determine whether IVIG treatment will be used.

In North America and also in our institution, we give IVIG for all children diagnosed with KD.

Flow chart 6.2.1: Algorithm for evaluation of suspected incomplete Kawasaki disease[1]

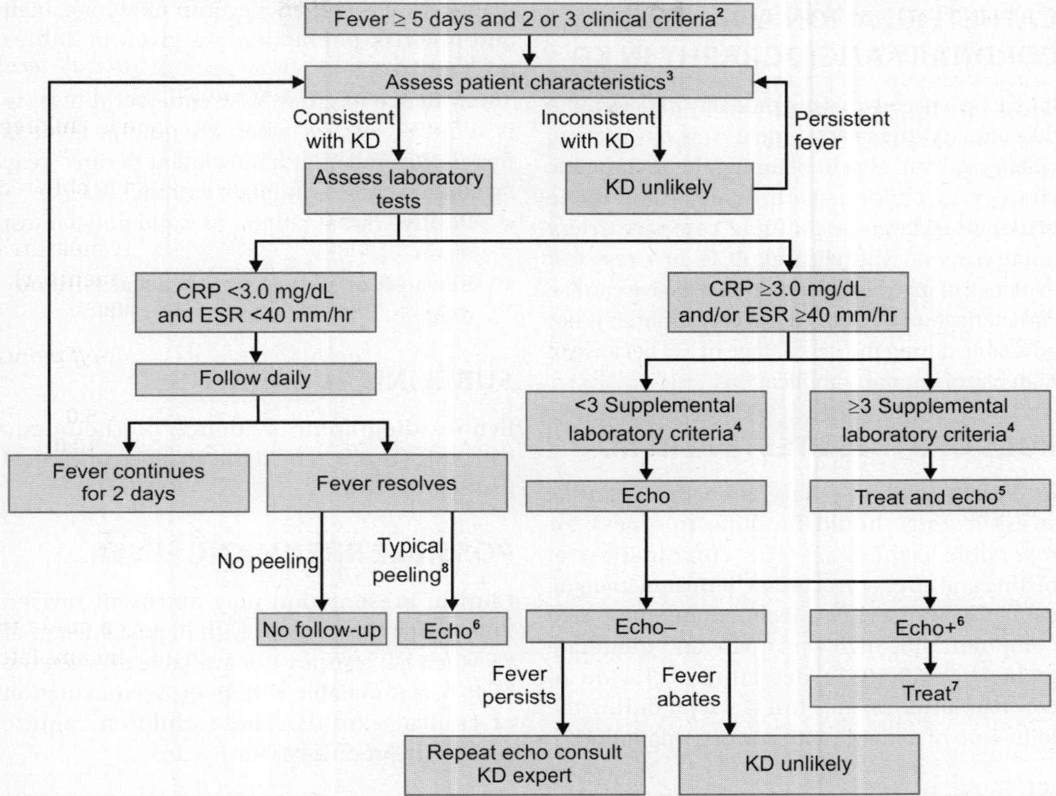

[1] In the absence of a gold standard for Kawasaki disease diagnosis, this algorithm cannot be evidence based but rather represents the informed opinion of the experts committee. Consultation with an expert should be sought anytime assistance is needed.

[2] Infants ≤ 6 months old with fever for ≥7 days without any explanation should undergo laboratory testing, and if evidence of systemic inflammation is found, echocardiography should be performed, even if the infants have no clinical criteria.

[3] Patient characteristics suggestive of Kawasaki disease (Principal Symptoms). Characteristics suggestive of a disease other than Kawasaki disease include exudative conjunctivitis, exudative pharyngitis, discrete intraoral lesions, bullous or vesicular rash, or generalized adenopathy. An alternative diagnosis should be considered.

[4] Supplemental laboratory criteria include albumin ≤ 3.0 g/dL, anemia, elevation of alanine aminotransferase, platelet count ≥ 450,000/mm^3 after 7 days, WBC count ≥ 15,000/mm^3, and WBC in urine ≥ 10/high-power field.

[5] Treatment can be undertaken before performing echocardiography.

[6] The echocardiogram is considered positive for the purpose of this algorithm if any of the following 3 conditions are met: (1) z-score of LAD or RCA ≥ 2.5; (2) the coronary arteries meet the Japanese Ministry of Health criteria for aneurysms; and (3) ≥3 other suggestive features exist, including perivascular brightness, lack of tapering, decreased LV function, mitral regurgitation, pericardial effusion, or z-scores in LAD or RCA of 2–2.5.

[7] If the echocardiogram is positive, treatment should be given to children within 10 days of fever onset and those with fever beyond day 10 with clinical and laboratory signs (CRP, ESR) of ongoing inflammation.

[8] Typical peeling begins under the nail bed of the fingers and then the toes.

Abbreviations: KD, Kawasaki disease; white blood cell; CRP, C-reactive protein; ESR, erythrocyte sedimentation rate. Reproduced from Newburger JW, et al. Pediatrics 2004;114:1708-33, with permission of American Academy of Pediatrics.

ROLE OF CARDIAC CATHETERIZATION AND CORONARY ANGIOGRAPHY IN KD

It may be a useful imaging modality to determine the coronary artery status (aneurysms, obstruction, collaterals) and also in planning the therapeutic strategy in children with echocardiographic evidence of large or multiple coronary artery aneurysms or with clinical, ECG, or stress test evidence of myocardial ischemia. Elective cardiac catheterization for delineation of coronaries is not advisable during the acute stage of KD because of high risk of arterial complications.[17]

ROLE OF STRESS TESTING IN KD

In patients with coronary aneurysms cardiac stress testing should be done to assess for reversible ischemia.[17] The combination of resting and stress myocardial perfusion imaging using thallium 201 or a technetium-99m based compound has high sensitivity and moderate to low specificity in detecting occlusion of coronary arteries. This test is useful during the follow-up of patients with coronary pathology.

INVESTIGATIONS: RHEUMATIC FEVER REVISED JONES CRITERIA[18,19]

Diagnosis:

Initial ARF	2 Major manifestations or 1 major plus 2 minor
Recurrent ARF	2 Major or 1 major and 2 minor *With*

evidence of preceding group A streptococcal infection.

The major and minor criteria for the diagnosis of rheumatic fever in moderate, high and low-risk population are given in **Tables 6.2.1 and 6.2.2**.

Evidence of group A streptococcal disease is required except when rheumatic fever is first discovered after a long latent period[20] (e.g. Sydenham chorea, indolent carditis).

- Positive throat culture or rapid antigen test result
- Elevated or rising streptococcal antibody titer.

SUBCLINICAL CARDITIS

Echocardiographic evidence of rheumatic valvulitis **(Box 6.2.1)** in the absence of clinical features of carditis.

POSSIBLE RHEUMATIC FEVER

Clinical presentation may not fulfill revised Jones criteria in a child with high suspicion of RF when lab tests are not available or when the history is unreliable with poor documentation of clinical carditis. These children require secondary prophylaxis for 1 year.

THROAT CULTURE

Throat culture remains the gold standard for confirmation of group A streptococcal infection.

RAPID ANTIGEN DETECTION TESTS

Highly specific but not sensitive, hence a positive rapid antigen test confirms a streptococcal infection.[21-23,26]

Table 6.2.1: Major and minor criteria for the diagnosis of rheumatic fever in moderate and high-risk populations*

Major criteria	*Minor criteria*
• Carditis—Clinical and/or subclinical	• Monoarthralgia#
• Arthritis# (Polyarthritis or monoarthritis or polyarthralgia)	• Fever (≥38°C)
• Chorea	• ESR ≥30 mm in the first hour and/or
• Erythema marginatum	• CRP ≥3.0 mg/dL
• Subcutaneous nodules	• Prolonged PR interval

Abbreviations: ESR, erythrocyte sedimentation rate; CRP, C-reactive protein.
* See footnote of Table 6.2.2.
# See footnote of Table 6.2.2.

Table 6.2.2: Low-risk populations*	
Major criteria	*Minor criteria*
• Carditis—Clinical and/or subclinical • Arthritis# (Polyarthritis only) • Chorea • Erythema marginatum • Subcutaneous nodules	• Polyarthralgia# • Fever (≥38.5°C) • ESR ≥60 mm in the first hour and/or • CRP ≥3.0 mg/dL • Prolonged PR interval

Abbreviations: CRP, C-reactive protein; ESR, erythrocyte sedimentation rate.
(Prolonged PR interval is not considered as minor criteria if carditis is a major criterion)
Normal upper range – PR Interval: 3–12 yrs-0. 16 sec; 12–14 y- 0.18 sec; >17 y-0. 20 sec
* Low-risk populations are those with ARF incidence ≤2 per 100 000 school-aged children or all-age rheumatic heart disease prevalence of ≤1 per 1000 population per year.
# Polyarthralgia, which should be considered as a major manifestation in moderate—to high—risk populations after exclusion of other causes. Joint manifestations can only be considered in either the major or minor categories but not both in the same patient.

Box 6.2.1: Morphological findings on echocardiogram in rheumatic valvulitis[19]

Acute mitral valve changes
- Annular dilation (Chordal elongation)
- Chordal rupture resulting in flail leaflet with severe mitral regurgitation
- Anterior (or less commonly posterior) leaflet tip prolapse
- Beading/nodularity of leaflet tips

Chronic mitral valve changes: not seen in acute carditis
- Leaflet thickening
- Chordal thickening and fusion
- Restricted leaflet motion and calcification

Aortic valve changes in either acute or chronic carditis
- Irregular or focal leaflet thickening
- Coaptation (leaflet approximation) defect
- Restricted leaflet motion
- Leaflet prolapse

If a rapid antigen detection test result is negative, obtain a throat culture in patients with suspected rheumatic fever.

ANTIBODY TITER TESTS

Antibody titer tests used include:
- Antistreptolysin O (ASO) test
- Antistreptococcal DNase B (ADB) test
- Antistreptococcal hyaluronidase (AH) test.

ASO is a test used to detect streptococcal antibodies directed against streptococcal lysin O. An elevated titer of > 1:250 indicates a previous streptococcal infection. It is usually more elevated after a pharyngeal than skin infection, while the ADB is typically elevated regardless of the site of the infection.

The antibody tests must be interpreted with caution in areas with high rates of streptococcal infection and ARF, as relatively high titers are commonly encountered in the population. These tests are of greater utility in areas with lower prevalence (e.g. in most Western countries).[27-29]

ACUTE-PHASE REACTANTS

Acute-phase reactants, the erythrocyte sedimentation rate (ESR), and C-reactive protein (CRP) levels are usually elevated at the onset of ARF and serve as a minor manifestation in the Jones criteria. These tests are nonspecific, but they may be useful in monitoring disease activity.[24,25]

ELECTROCARDIOGRAM

The most common finding on electrocardiography is a prolongation of the PR interval a nonspecific finding which may not indicate carditis. Rarely second- or third-degree heart block may be present. In patients with chronic rheumatic heart disease,

Box 6.2.2: Doppler findings in rheumatic valvulitis[19]

- Pathological mitral regurgitation (all 4 criteria met)
- Seen in at least 2 views
- Jet length ≥2 cm in at least 1 view
- Peak velocity >3 m/s
- Pansystolic jet in at least 1 envelope
- Pathological aortic regurgitation (all 4 criteria met)
- Seen in at least 2 views
- Jet length ≥1 cm in at least 1 view
- Peak velocity >3 m/s
- Pan diastolic jet in at least 1 envelope

electrocardiography may show left atria enlargement secondary to mitral stenosis/regurgitation.[24]

CHEST RADIOGRAPHY

Chest radiography can reveal cardiomegaly and congestive heart failure in patients moderate and severe carditis.

ECHOCARDIOGRAPHY

Echocardiography may demonstrate valvular regurgitant lesions in patients with ARF who do not have clinical manifestations of carditis. This does not qualify as carditis in the most recent Jones diagnostic criteria, as the clinical implications of subclinical carditis remain unclear, but some experts believe the diagnostic criteria for ARF should be modified to allow for specific abnormalities found only on echocardiograms to be included.[30]

Valvular stenotic lesions, especially of the mitral valve, can be observed in rheumatic heart disease.

In the absence of mitral valve disease involvement, isolated echocardiographic disease of the aortic valve is uncommon in patients with rheumatic heart disease.[31]

Early in the course of acute rheumatic fever, mitral or aortic valve morphology may be normal on echocardiogram while Doppler shows regurgitation **(Box 6.2.2)**. These findings can also be seen in chronic rheumatic heart disease.

BLOOD CULTURES

In selective cases, blood cultures are obtained to rule out infective endocarditis, disseminated gonococcal infection, etc. Various other studies may be needed to rule out other illnesses in the differential diagnoses. Common tests would include rheumatoid factor, antinuclear antibody (ANA), and Lyme serology.

REFERENCES

1. Newburger JW, Takahashi M, Gerber MA, et al. Diagnosis, treatment, and long-term management of Kawasaki disease: a statement for health professionals from the Committee on Rheumatic Fever, Endocarditis, and Kawasaki Disease, Council on Cardiovascular Disease in the Young, American Heart Association. Circulation. 2004;110:2747-71.
2. Rowley AH, Gonzalez-Crussi F, Gidding SS, et al. Incomplete Kawasaki disease with coronary artery involvement. J Pediatr. 1987;110:409-13.
3. Comenzo RL, Malachowski ME, Meissner HC, Fulton DR, Berkman EM. Immune hemolysis, disseminated intravascular coagulation, and serum sickness after large doses of immune globulin given intravenously for Kawasaki disease. J Pediatr. 1992;120:926-8.
4. Newburger JW, Burns JC, Beiser AS, Loscalzo J. Altered lipid profile after Kawasaki syndrome. Circulation. 1991;84:625-31.
5. Burns JC, Mason WH, Glode MP, Shulman ST, Melish ME, Meissner C, et al. Clinical and epidemiologic characteristics of patients referred for evaluation of possible Kawasaki disease. United States Multicenter Kawasaki Disease Study Group. J Pediatr. 1991;118:680-6.
6. Ting EC, Capparelli EV, Billman GF, Lavine JE, Matsubara T, Burns JC. Elevated gamma-glutamyltransferase concentrations in patients with acute Kawasaki disease. Pediatr Infect Dis J. 1998;17:431-2.
7. Dengler LD, Capparelli EV, Bastian JF, Bradley DJ, Glode MP, Santa S, et al. Cerebrospinal fluid profile in patients with acute Kawasaki disease. Pediatr Infect Dis J. 1998;17:478-81.
8. Printz BF, Sleeper LA, Newburger JW, et al. Noncoronary cardiac abnormalities are associated with coronary artery dilation and with laboratory inflammatory markers in acute Kawasaki disease. J Am Coll Cardiol. 2011;57:86-92.

9. Ozdogu H, Boga C. Fatal cardiac tamponade in a patient with Kawasaki disease. Heart Lung. 2005;34:257-9.
10. Belay ED, Maddox RA, Holman RC, et al. Kawasaki syndrome and risk factors for coronary artery abnormalities: United States, 1994–2003. Pediatr Infect Dis J. 2006;25:245-9.
11. Dajani AS, Taubert KA, Gerber MA, Shulman ST, Ferrieri P, Freed M, et al. Diagnosis and therapy of Kawasaki disease in children. Circulation. 1993;87:1776-80.
12. Dajani AS, Taubert KA, Takahashi M, Bierman FZ, Freed MD, Ferrieri P, et al. Guidelines for long-term management of patients with Kawasaki disease. Report from the Committee on Rheumatic Fever, Endocarditis, and Kawasaki Disease, Council on Cardiovascular Disease in the Young, American Heart Association. Circulation. 1994;89:916-22.
13. Research Committee on Kawasaki Disease. Report of Subcommittee on Standardization of Diagnostic Criteria and Reporting of Coronary Artery Lesions in Kawasaki Disease. Tokyo, Japan: Ministry of Health and Welfare; 1984.
14. Manlhiot C, Millar K, Golding F, et al. Improved classification of coronary artery abnormalities based only on coronary artery z-scores after Kawasaki disease. Pediatr Cardiol. 2010; 31:242-9.
15. Harada K, Yamaguchi H, Kato H, Nishibayashi Y, Ichiro S, Okazaki T, et al. Indication for intravenous gammaglobulin treatment for Kawasaki disease. In: Takahashi M, Taubert K (Eds). Proceedings of the Fourth International Symposium on Kawasaki disease. Dallas, Tex: American Heart Association; 1993. pp. 459-62.
16. Harada K. Intravenous gamma-globulin treatment in Kawasaki disease. Acta Paediatr Jpn. 1991;33:805-10.
17. De Ferranti SD, Newburger JW. Kawasaki disease. Moss and Adams' heart disease in infants, children and adolescents. 2008;2:1287-97.
18. Shrivastava S. Rheumatic heart disease: is it declining in India? Indian Heart J. 2007;59: 9-10.
19. Gewitz MH, et al. Revision of the Jones Criteria for the diagnosis of acute rheumatic fever in the era of Doppler Echocardiography: a scientific statement from the American Heart Association. Circulation; 1806-18.
20. Rheumatic fever and rheumatic heart disease. Report of a WHO Study Group. World Health Organization, Geneva, 1988 (Technical Report Series No. 764).
21. Prevention of rheumatic fever. Report of a WHO Expert Committee. World Health Organization, Geneva, 1966 (Technical Report Series No. 342).
22. Strasser T, et al. The community control of rheumatic fever and rheumatic heart disease: report of a WHO international cooperative project. Bulletin of the World Health Organization; 1981;59(2):285-94.
23. Joint WHO/ISFC meeting on rheumatic fever/ rheumatic heart disease control with emphasis on primary prevention, Geneva, 7–9 September 1994. Geneva, World Health Organization, 1994 (WHO/CVD 94.1).
24. The WHO global programme for the prevention of RF/RHD. Report of a onsultation to review progress and develop future activities. Geneva, World Health Organization, 2000 (WHO/ CVD/00.1).
25. Narula J, et al. R Tandon, R. K. Rheumatic fever and Rheumatic heart disease:the last 50 years. The Indian Journal of Medical Research; 2013. pp. 643-58.
26. American Academy of Pediatrics, Committee on Infectious Diseases. Red Book: Report of the Committee on Infectious Diseases, 27th edn. Elk Grove Village, Ill: American Academy of Pediatrics; 2006.
27. Kaplan EL, Rothermel CD, Johnson DR. Antistreptolysin O and anti-deoxyribonuclease B titers: normal values for children ages 2 to 12 in the United States. Pediatrics. 1998;101:86-8.
28. Shet A, Kaplan EL. Clinical use and interpretation of group A streptococcal antibody tests:a practical approach for the paediatrician or primary care physician. Pediatr Infect Dis J. 2002;21:420-6.
29. Kaplan EL, Huew BB. The sensitivity and specificity of an agglutination test for antibodies to streptococcal extracellular antigens: a quantitative analysis and comparison of the streptozyme test with anti-streptolysin O and antideoxyribonuclease B tests. J Pediatr. 1980; 96:367-73.
30. Jones criteria updates 1992. Circulation 87. Circulation, 1993.
31. Marijon E, Ou P, Celermajer DS, Ferreira B, Mocumbi AO, Sidi D, et al. Echo cardiographic screening for rheumatic heart disease. Bull World Health Organ, 2008 Feb. Jones TD. Diagnosis of rheumatic fever. JAMA. 1944;126:481.

6.3 Timing of Intervention in Congenital Heart Diseases

Gnanasambandam Subramaniyan, J Ritchie Sharon Solomon
Reviewers: *K Nedunchelian, Jaydeep Choudhury, RV Dhakshayani*

INTRODUCTION

Nearly 180,000 children are born with heart defects each year in India. 60,000–90,000 suffer from critical cardiac lesions requiring early intervention and 10% of the infant mortality is related to congenital heart disease (CHD). Inappropriate timing can lead to increased complexity of surgical procedure and poor outcome and more often a treatable condition may become inoperable due to undue delay.

ATRIAL SEPTAL DEFECT

The most common type of atrial septal defect (ASD) is ostium secundum ASD, which is in the central part of atrial septum in the region of fossa ovalis. Other types are ostium primum ASD, sinus venosus ASD and coronary sinus ASD.

Spontaneous closure of ostium secundum ASD detected during neonatal period occurred in all the defects that were < 3 mm, in 80% of defects that were 5–8 mm and in none of the defects that were greater than 8 mm. Closure of the defect is indicated when there is a large shunt with Qp: Qs ≥ 1.5 (pulmonary blood flow: systemic blood flow). Diastolic murmur in tricuspid area, ECG evidence of right ventricle (RV) volume overload, chest X-ray evidence of cardiomegaly or increased pulmonary vascular markings and echocardiographic evidence of right ventricular enlargement and/or paradoxical septal motion are indicative of a large shunt across the atrial septal defect; ASDs with Qp: Qs< 1.5 need not be closed and have to be followed up.

Though children with large defects may be asymptomatic, elective closure is advised in order to prevent long-term complications. Elective closure between 2 and 5 years of age is recommended in asymptomatic patients with large shunt. Patients with large shunts presenting later in life need evaluation of pulmonary vascular reactivity and the net left to right shunt before contemplating closure. Routine follow-up of these patients through adulthood is advised. Symptomatic ASD in infancy (congestive heart failure, severe pulmonary artery hypertension) is seen in about 8–10% of cases. Associated lesions (e.g. anomalous pulmonary venous drainage, left ventricular inflow obstruction) need to be ruled out in such cases. Early closure is recommended in such symptomatic infants. In sinus venosus type of ASD surgical closure may be delayed to 4–5 years of age. Device closure of ostium secundum type of ASD is generally feasible in children more than 10 kg with good margins around the defect.

VENTRICULAR SEPTAL DEFECT

These defects are classified based on their size as follows:

- *Large/unrestrictive ventricular septal defect (VSD)* (>50% of the aortic valve annulus and interventricular gradient <20 mm Hg by echocardiographic Doppler) results in nearly systemic systolic pulmonary artery pressures. The right ventricular systolic pressure is usually systemic and the degree of left to right shunt depends on the pulmonary vascular resistance.

- *Moderate sized VSD* (>33% of aortic annulus but <50% of the annulus and interventricular gradient >20 mm Hg. Right ventricular pressure is ½ to 2/3 systemic and there is mild elevation of pulmonary arterial pressure with near normal pulmonary vascular resistance. Volume overload causes dilatation of left atrium and ventricle.
- *Small/restrictive VSD* (<1/3 of aortic annulus and high interventricular gradient). Right ventricular systolic pressure, pulmonary arterial pressure and pulmonary vascular resistance are normal.

These defects are classified based on their location as—subarterial (outlet, subpulmonic, supracristal or infundibular), perimembranous, inlet and muscular.

Spontaneous closure of large VSD is uncommon. Size of VSD may decrease in few cases. Most (75–80%) small perimembranous and small muscular type of VSDs will close spontaneously within two years of life. Untreated infants with large VSD can succumb to congestive cardiac failure within 6 months of life.

Infants with large VSD in congestive cardiac failure with failure to thrive, despite optimal medical therapy should be operated as soon as possible. Large VSD with hyperkinetic pulmonary arterial hypertension (PAH) should be operated in 3–6 months of age.

Moderate sized VSD can be intervened by 1–2 years of age or earlier if there is one episode of life threatening lower respiratory tract infection or failure to thrive. In small sized VSDs with left to right shunt (Qp: Qs)>1.5:1, intervention may be needed by 2–4 years.

In small outlet VSDs with aortic valve prolapse and no aortic regurgitation, closure is advised by 2–3 years of age irrespective of the size of defect and quantum of left to right shunt. Small outlet VSD without aortic valve prolapse can be followed up once in every 1 or 2 years for development of aortic valve prolapse.In small outlet VSDs with any degree of aortic regurgitation, surgery is indicated whenever aortic regurgitation is detected.

Small perimembranous VSDs with aortic prolapse with no/mild aortic regurgitation require 1–2 yearly follow-up to assess for any increase in aortic regurgitation. In small perimembranous VSDs with aortic cusp prolapse and moderate aortic regurgitation, surgery is indicated whenever aortic regurgitation is detected.

In small VSDs with one episode of infective endocarditis, early VSD closure is advised.

Structural remodeling at pulmonary vascular bed leading to elevated pulmonary vascular resistance appears inevitable in patients with high flow defects operated the age of 2 years. Whenever baseline pulmonary vascular resistance (PVR) is high and when overall operability seems to be doubtful based on clinical and radiological findings, it is better not to attempt complete closure. Patients with unoperated VSD and elevated baseline PVR who are Eisenmengerized may have a better long-term prognosis compared to those who undergo complete closure and later have significant residual PAH.

Direct VSD closure is done in most cases. Pulmonary artery banding is done initially in few cases with very large VSD or multiple (Swiss cheese) VSD. In selected cases, device closure can be done successfully.

PATENT DUCTUS ARTERIOSUS

Whenever medical therapy is unsuccessful or not possible, surgical or catheter device closure can be performed. In large and moderate sized patent ductus arteriosus (PDA) with congestive cardiac failure and pulmonary arterial hypertension, early closure by 3–6 months is advised. Moderate PDA with no congestive cardiac failure can be closed by 6 months to 1 year. Small PDA can be closed by 12–18 months of age. Silent PDA (no murmur clinically and only diagnosable by echocardiography) need not be intervened.

For preterm babies with hemodynamically significant PDA, indomethacin, ibuprofen or oral paracetamol can be given if not contraindicated.

Transcatheter therapy using coils or PDA closure devices is feasible even in small babies in selected cases.

Surgical closure can be done in cases not suitable for device closure.

ATRIOVENTRICULAR SEPTAL DEFECTS

These defects are classified as follows:

- *Partial atrioventricular septal defects (AVSD):* Ostium primum ASD with right and left AV valve annuli and left AV valve cleft
- *Transitional AVSD:* Partial AVSD with small inlet VSD
- *Complete AVSD:* Ostium primum ASD with large inlet VSD and common.

AV Valve with Single Annulus

Intermediate AVSD: Type of complete AVSD with distinct right and left AV valve orifices despite only one common annulus.

AVSDs can be balanced or unbalanced based on how the AV junction is shared by the ventricles. In balanced ventricles, the AV inlet is shared by both ventricles and suitable for biventricular repair. Unbalanced AVSD need to be managed along single ventricle pathway.

Complete and intermediate AVSDs have the physiology and clinical features of both ASD and VSD. Partial and transitional AVSDs have the clinical picture of a large ASD.

In infants with complete AVSD with congestive cardiac failure not responding to medical therapy, surgery is advised as soon as possible. Complete AVSD with controlled heart failure, complete surgical repair (closure of interatrial and interventricular communication, construction of two separate competent AV valves) is advised by 3–6 months of age. Surgical options are palliative PA banding or complete repair with single patch or double patch technique.

Partial AVSD can be operated by 2–3 years of age (closure of interatrial communication and repair of cleft anterior mitral leaflet). Significant AV regurgitation may need early surgery.

Infants with Down syndrome with complete AVSD develop pulmonary vascular obstructive disease earlier than nonsyndromic infants and hence need to be operated early.

COARCTATION OF AORTA

Infants with significant coarctation present with heart failure and usually require immediate and aggressive management. Medical management of such infants include initial stabilization with ionotropic support, diuretics and prostaglandin E1 (PGE1) infusion to improve ductal patency to enable lower body tissue perfusion. Later single stage repair in newborns with coarctation and intracardiac anomalies is a relatively safe option in many centers.

Coarctation repair is recommended at 1–3 years of age in asymptomatic children without severe upper extremity hypertension.

Generally patients with left ventricular dysfunction, congestive heart failure or severe upper limb hypertension at any age require immediate intervention. Balloon dilatation can be done in cases with discrete coarctation. Restenosis after an initial successful angioplasty is common in infants less than 6 months of age. Emergency balloon dilatation/stenting is a temporary bail out option in infants who are very ill for surgical repair. Balloon dilatation with stent deployment can be considered in children >10 years of age, if required. Intervention is not indicated if Doppler gradient across coarctation segment is <20 mm Hg with normal left ventricular function.

AORTIC STENOSIS

Severity of aortic stenosis (AS) is classified based on echocardiographic Doppler as follows:

- *Mild AS:* Aortic V_{max} (maximum velocity)—2–2.9 m/sec or mean gradient : <20 mm Hg
- *Moderate AS:* Aortic V_{max}—3–3.9 m/sec or mean gradient: 20–39 mm Hg
- *Severe AS:* Aortic V_{max}—≥ 4m/sec or mean gradient ≥ 40 mm Hg

Neonates with critical aortic stenosis needs initial stabilization with PGE1 infusion and ionotropic support. Once they are stabilized balloon valvuloplasty can be done. In neonates balloon dilatation is indicated when the baby is symptomatic or there is evidence of left ventricular dysfunction or mild left ventricular hypoplasia or if Doppler gradient is >75 mm Hg. Infants and older children with left ventricular dysfunction require immediate intervention by balloon dilatation, irrespective of gradients. In those with normal ventricular function, balloon dilatation is advised if any one of the following is present: (a) peak gradient >80 mm Hg and mean gradient >50 mm Hg; (b) ST-T changes with peak gradient >50 mm Hg; (c) symptoms due to AS with peak gradient of > 50 mm Hg.

Subvalvar aortic stenosis needs surgical intervention if peak gradient is > 64 mm Hg or more than mild aortic regurgitation is present.

In supravalvar aortic stenosis surgical management is the treatment of choice. Indications for surgery are not well-defined and most centers use pressure gradient criteria similar to those in valvar aortic stenosis.

VALVAR PULMONARY STENOSIS

- Mild stenosis is characterized by right ventricular pressure less than half the left ventricular pressure or peak valve gradient of <35–40 mm Hg.
- Moderate stenosis has right ventricular pressure greater than half but <75% of LV pressure or the peak valve gradient is 40–60 mm Hg.
- Severe stenosis is defined by RV pressure is ≥75% of the LV pressure or a gradient >60–70 mm Hg

Asymptomatic patients with severe obstruction should be treated semielectively with valvuloplasty. Children with moderate obstruction should undergo valvuloplasty, if the right ventricular pressure is 50% systemic or higher. No intervention is needed for mild obstruction. Presence of right ventricular dysfunction requires immediate intervention, irrespective of gradient.

TETRALOGY OF FALLOT

Management of cyanotic spells and correction of iron deficiency anemia is important. Beta blockers should be given in dose range of 1–4 mg/kg/day in 2–3 divided doses.

Most centers perform elective repair of tetralogy of Fallot (TOF) in asymptomatic infants between 3 and 12 months of age. Current trend is that the age of complete repair is moving towards the lower end of the range in many large centers.

Complete repair includes VSD closure, aggressive resection of infundibular muscle and augmentation of RV outflow tract. RVOT outflow patch may be sufficient in some infants, whereas transannular patch is needed if the pulmonary artery annulus and main pulmonary artery are more than two to three standard deviations below normal. Most centers preferentially perform TOF repair via transatrial and transpulmonary approach, thereby avoiding transannular patch whenever possible so that pulmonary valve remains competent.

Relative indications for shunt (systemic artery to pulmonary artery) in the early neonatal period are severely hypoplastic pulmonary arteries, anomalous coronary artery across the RVOT (anomalous left anterior descending artery from right coronary artery), early cyanotic spells or associated noncardiac anomalies. Modified Blalock Taussig (BT) shunt is done using a prosthetic graft interposed between the subclavian/innominate artery and pulmonary artery. Classical BT shunt involved end to side anastomosis of the subclavian artery to pulmonary artery. Pott shunt is done between descending aorta and left pulmonary artery. Waterson shunt is done between ascending aorta and pulmonary artery. Systemic to pulmonary artery shunt is done in babies less than 3 months of age with significant cyanosis or an episode of spell. In babies, greater than 3 months of age, shunt or complete repair can be done based on the anatomy and surgical expertise.

VENTRICULAR SEPTAL DEFECT WITH PULMONARY ATRESIA

Babies with confluent and adequate sized branch pulmonary arteries with duct dependent pulmonary circulation presenting early, will need systemic to pulmonary artery shunt. In babies presenting after 3 months, Glenn shunt (cavopulmonary shunt) or systemic to pulmonary artery shunt can be performed as interim procedure and right ventricle to pulmonary artery conduit can be done at a later age. Unifocalization or interruption of unnecessary aortopulmonary collaterals is done based on its communication with pulmonary arterial tree.

TOF PHYSIOLOGY CONDITIONS WHERE TWO VENTRICLE REPAIR IS POSSIBLE

For example, DORV/VSD/PS, TGA/VSD/PS.

Infants who present with significant cyanosis very early would require a systemic artery to pulmonary artery shunt and if they present after 3 months, either a Glenn shunt or systemic artery to pulmonary artery can be done. Complete repair can be done at 1–2 years of age if RV to PA conduit is not required. If RV to PA conduit is required then it is better to delay complete repair as much as the child's symptom status allows.

TOF PHYSIOLOGY CONDITIONS WHERE TWO VENTRICLE REPAIR IS NOT POSSIBLE

For example, DORV/VSD/PS, TGA/VSD/PS, DORV/with non-routable VSD/PS, Tricuspid atresia/PS, Single ventricle/PS.

When two ventricular corrections are not possible, staged palliative surgeries along the single ventricle pathway is done. Before 3 months, systemic artery to pulmonary artery shunt is done to provide adequate pulmonary blood flow. Beyond the first 4–6 months of life, the bidirectional cavopulmonary connection (bidirectional Glenn shunt) provides long-term palliation.

Children who are stable with mild cyanosis can either undergo a direct Fontan at 3–4 years of age or a initial Glenn surgery after 3 months of age followed by Fontan at 3–4 years of age. Infants with significant cyanosis (SaO_2<70%) presenting before 3 months would need a systemic to pulmonary artery shunt initially followed by a staged Fontan surgery (Glenn shunt after 6 months of age followed by Fontan at 3–4 years of age.

UNIVENTRICULAR HEART/ ADMIXTURE LESIONS WITH INCREASED PULMONARY BLOOD FLOW WHERE TWO VENTRICULAR REPAIR IS NOT POSSIBLE (TRICUSPID ATRESIA, SINGLE VENTRICLE, DORV WITH NON-ROUTABLE VSD) WITH NO PULMONARY STENOSIS

All univentricular heart with increased pulmonary blood flow conditions need staged palliative surgeries along single ventricle pathway. Surgeries are staged in such a way that the child is finally a suitable surgical candidate for Fontan surgery. Timing of the palliative surgical procedures is important to protect the integrity of both the pulmonary vascular bed and the myocardium. Initially, pulmonary artery banding is recommended for patients with univentricular AV connection without pulmonary stenosis. Uncontrollable congestive heart failure, excessive pulmonary blood flow and severe pulmonary hypertension should prompt pulmonary artery banding in early infancy (4–8 weeks of age) to prevent the development of pulmonary vascular obstructive disease.

TRANSPOSITION OF GREAT ARTERIES

Balloon atrial septostomy (BAS) will enable adequate shunting of oxygenated blood and help in initial stabilization of a severely hypoxic neonate with transposition of great arteries (TGA)/intact ventricular septum (IVS) and restrictive ASD. It may be helpful in TGA/VSD and/or PDA, when surgery is delayed for a few weeks. As early arterial switch is possible in many tertiary level cardiac centers, many centers have chosen to perform a BAS only in babies with profound hypoxemia, or when corrective surgery must be delayed due to some reason. In routine cases, when baby is maintaining acceptable oxygenation with a PDA, a native septal communication and PGE1 infusion, baby is directly taken for arterial switch operation.

Definitive anatomic repair is accomplished by arterial switch operation. A critical physiologic challenge to anatomic repair is the functional adequacy of the left ventricle (LV), which preoperatively faces the pulmonary circulation and postoperatively must instantly cope with the increased systemic workload. As many babies are detected antenatally or shortly after birth, an "unprepared" or "regressed" left ventricle is increasingly uncommon. Adequate left ventricular muscle mass for successful systemic function is usually present in early infancy in patients with TGA/IVS. LV is also prepared in cases of TGA with associated anomalies like large VSD or dynamic left ventricular outflow obstruction. Definitive early (neonatal) one-stage arterial repair is presently preferable to early palliation with pulmonary artery banding and later arterial switch surgery.

In TGA with intact ventricular septum, optimum age for arterial switch operation is 3–4 weeks. In babies presenting after 3–4 weeks of age, assessment of LV by ECHO is of paramount importance. If LV is regressed, a rapid two stage arterial switch (PA banding followed by arterial switch) or atrial switch is possible based on institutional practice. In TGA with VSD, arterial switch operation is advised before 3 months of age.

Physiological repair/atrial switch operation (Senning/Mustard operation) is done in babies who present late with regressed LV or in those who have associated problems that preclude arterial switch operation.

TOTAL ANOMALOUS PULMONARY VENOUS CONNECTION

The various types are supracardiac, cardiac, infracardiac/infradiaphragmatic and mixed type. Management depends on whether pulmonary venous drainage is obstructive or not.

In obstructive type of total anomalous pulmonary venous connection (TAPVC), emergency TAPVC repair is advised. In nonobstructive type of TAPVC, TAPVC repair can be done beyond the neonatal period, if baby is stable. In children presenting at an older age, elective TAPVC repair can be done if pulmonary vascular resistance is in operable range.

TRUNCUS ARTERIOSUS

Infants with truncus arteriosus are at risk of developing pulmonary vascular obstructive disease at an early age, and this has driven the major impetus for early surgical correction.

Successful correction during early infancy, includes total repair with right ventricle to pulmonary artery conduit. If infant is stable with controlled heart failure, it is done by 6–12 weeks. Pulmonary artery banding may be done in cases when total repair is not possible. Small right ventricular to pulmonary artery conduit eventually must be replaced with a larger one, but reoperation for conduit replacement alone carries a low risk. Parents should be counseled about the need for repeat surgeries for conduit obstruction.

BIBLIOGRAPHY

1. Bulbul ZR, Bruckheimer E, Love JC, Fahey JT, Hellenbrand WE. Implantation of balloon expandable stents for coarctation of the aorta: implantation data and short term results. Cathet Cardiovasc Diagn. 1996;39:36-42.
2. Consensus on Timing of Intervention for Common Congenital Heart Diseases. Working group on management of congenital heart diseases in India. Indian Pediatr. 2008:45:117-26.
3. Cotton RB, Stahlman MT, Berder HW, Graham TP, Catterton WZ, Kovar I, et al. Randomized trial of early closure of symptomatic patent ductus arteriosus in small preterm infants. J Pediatr. 1978;93:647-51.
4. Driscoll D, Allen HD, Atkins DL, Brenner J, Dunnigan A, Franklin W, et al. Guidelines for evaluation and management of common congenital cardiac problems in infants, children, and adolescents. A statement for healthcare professionals from the Committee on Congenital Cardiac Defects of the Council on Cardiovascular Disease in the Young, American Heart Association. Circulation. 1994;90: 2180-8.

5. Ebert PA, Turley K, Stanger P. Surgical treatment of truncus arteriosus in the first 6 months of life. Ann Surg. 1984;200:451-6.
6. El-Khuffash AF, Molloy EJ. Influence of a patent ductus arteriosus on cardiac troponin T levels in preterm infants. J Pediatr. 2008;153:350-3.
7. El-Khuffash AF, Slevin M, Mc Namara PJ, Troponin T. N-terminal pro-natriuretic peptide and a patent ductus arteriosus scoring system predict death before discharge or neurodevelopmental outcome at 2 years in preterm infants. Arch Dis Child Fetal Neonatal Ed. 2011;96:F133-7.
8. Fiore AC, Fischer LK, Schwartz T. Comparison of angioplasty and surgery for neonatal aortic coarctation. Ann Thorac Surg. 2005;80:1659-64.
9. Freedom RM, Benson LN, Smallhorn JF. Subaortic stenosis, the univentricular heart, and banding of the pulmonary artery: an analysis of the courses of 43 patients with univentricular heart palliated by pulmonary artery banding. Circulation. 1986;73:758-64.
10. Giannopoulos NM, et al. Early results after transatrial/transpulmonary repair tetralogy of Fallot. Eur J Cardiothorac Surg. 2002;22:582-6.
11. Hammerman C, Bin-Nun A, Markovitch E. Ductal closure with paracetamol: a surprising new approach to patent ductus arteriosus treatment. Pediatrics. 2011;128:e1618-21.
12. Hayashi G, Kurosaki K, Echigo S. Prevalence of arrhythmias and their riskfactors mid- and long-term after the arterial switch operation. Pediatr Cardiol. 2006;27:689-94.
13. Heymann MA, Berman W Jr, Rudolph AM. Dilatation of the ductus arteriosus by prostaglandin E1 in aortic abnormalities. Circulation. 1979;59:169-73.
14. Jonas RA. Early primary repair of tetralogy of Fallot. Semin Thorac Cardiovasc Surg Pediatr Card Surg Annu; 2009. pp. 39-47.
15. Kilman JW, Williams TE Jr, Breza TS. Reversal of infant mortality by early surgical correction of coarctation of the aorta. Arch Surg. 1972;105:865-8.
16. Lemmers PMA, Molenschot MC, Evens J. Is cerebral oxygen supply compromised in preterm infants undergoing surgical closure for patent ductus arteriosus? Arch Dis Child Fetal Neonatal Ed. 2010;95:F429-34.
17. Nicholson IA, Nunn GR, Sholler GF. Simplified single patch technique for the repair of atrioventricular septal defect. J Thorac Cardiovasc Surg. 1999;118:642-6.
18. Prieto LR, Latson LA. Pulmonary stenosis. Moss and Adams' heart disease in infants, children and adolescents. In: Hugh D Allen,Howard P Gutgesell, Edward B Clark, David J Driscoll, (Eds). Lippincott Williams & Wilkins Philadelphia, 2008; pp. 913-25.
19. Rabinovitch M, Haworth SG, Castaneda AR, Nadas AS, Reid LM. Lung biopsy in congenital heart disease: a morphometric approach to pulmonary vascular disease. Circulation. 1978;58:1107-22
20. Radzik D, Davignon A, van Doesburg N, Fournier A, Marchand T, Ducharme G, et al. Predictive factors for spontaneous closure of atrial septal defects diagnosed in the first 3 months of life. J Am Coll Cardiol. 1993;22:851-3.
21. Roche SL, Greenway SC, Redington AN. Tetrology of Fallot with pulmonary stenosis and tetralogy of Fallot with absent pulmonary valve. In: Moss and Adams' heart disease in infants, children and adolescents. In: Hugh D Allen, Howard P Gutgesell, Edward B Clark, David J Driscoll, (Eds). Lippincott Williams & Wilkins Philadelphia, 2008. pp. 978-80.
22. Rubay JE, Sluysmans T, Alexandrescu V. Surgical repair of coarctation of the aorta in infants under one year of age: long-term results in 146 patients comparing subclavian flap angioplasty and modified end-to-end anastomosis. J Cardiovasc Surg (Torino). 1992;33:216-22.
23. Rubio AE, Lewin MB. Ventricular septal defects. Moss and Adams' heart disease in infants, children and adolescents, Hugh D Allen, Howard P Gutgesell, Edward B Clark, David J Driscoll, (Eds). Lippincott Williams & Wilkins Philadelphia, 2008. pp. 713-4.
24. Sandhu SK, Beekman RH, Mosca RS. Single-stage repair of aortic arch obstruction and associated infracardiac defects in the neonate. Am J Cardiol. 1995;75:370-3.
25. Starr JP. Tetrology of Fallot: Yesterday and today. World J Surg. 2010;34:658-68.
26. Warnes CA, Williams RG, Bashore TM, Child JS, Connolly HM, Dearani JA, et al. ACC/AHA 2008 guidelines for the management of adults with congenital heart disease: a report of the American College of Cardiology/American Heart Association Task Force on Practice Guidelines (Writing Committee to Develop Guidelines on the Management of Adults with Congenital Heart Disease). Developed in Collaboration with the American Society of Echocardiography, Heart Rhythm Society, International Society for Adult Congenital Heart Disease, Society for Cardiovascular Angiography and Interventions, and Society of Thoracic Surgeons. J Am Coll Cardiol. 2008;52:e1–e121.

6.4 Kawasaki Disease: Therapy Revisited

VV Varadarajan

Reviewers: *K Nedunchelian, Jaydeep Choudhury, RV Dhakshayani*

Kawasaki disease (KD) is the second most common cause of vasculitis in children. It has become the leading cause of cardiac disease in the developed countries. The therapy of KD has undergone changes over the last three decades which will be discussed here.

The clinical course of Kawasaki disease can be divided into four phases namely the acute, subacute, convalescent and chronic phase.

The acute phase lasts for two weeks, characterized by the classical clinical features and cardiac manifestations like valvulitis, pericarditis and myocarditis. The sub-acute phase lasting for the next two weeks is remarkable as the child is at the risk of developing aneurysms and sudden death, if untreated. The convalescent phase clinically invisible following the control of symptoms lasts till the acute phase reactants return to normal. The chronic phase is only for patients who have developed the coronary involvement requiring follow-up.

There is no specific diagnostic test available for Kawasaki disease. According to American Heart Association, the diagnostic criteria include fever of more than five days with any four of the following five:

1. Polymorphous nonvesicular rash
2. Nonexudative bulbar conjunctivitis
3. Changes in the lips and oral cavity—erthema of lips and pharyngeal mucosa, cracking of lips, strawberry tongue
4. Changes in the extremity-erythema of palms and soles, edema of hands and feet, periungual peeling of fingers and toes
5. Acute nonpurulent cervical adenitis (> 1.5 cm, usually unilateral).

There are certain terminologies which require clarification before we proceed on to the management proper. The term "Atypical Kawasaki disease" is used whenever unusual complications like lung infiltrates, renal failure are seen. The term "incomplete Kawasaki disease" is used when only two or three of the clinical criteria are satisfied. But their laboratory parameters support systemic inflammation or echocardiographic findings suggested by the Japanese Ministry of Health.

Laboratory criteria supporting Kawasaki disease include albumin < 3 g/dL, C-reactive protein >6, ESR > 40 mm/hour, Elevated SGPT, leukocytosis >15000 cells/mm^3, normo chromic, normo cytic anemia for age, sterile pyuria (>10 white cells/hpf).

The echocardiographic criteria suggested by the Japanese Ministry of Health are given further.

Z score of LAD (*left anterior descending* coronary artery) or RCA (right coronary artery)—more than 2.5 standard deviation of the coronary size appropriate for the body surface area or coronary artery aneurysm.

Internal lumen diameter:

- >3 mm in children < 5 years
- > 4 mm in children > 5 years

A segment of coronary artery measuring >1.5 times that of an adjacent segment and any 3 of the following:

- Perivascular brightness of CA
- Lack of tapering of CA
- Decreased LV function
- Mitral regurgitation
- Pericardial effusion.

ACUTE PHASE MANAGEMENT

Aim of the acute phase management is to reduce the inflammation of the coronary artery and myocardium. The drugs that are frequently used in this phase are aspirin and intravenous immunoglobulin.

Aspirin was used for several years in an anti-inflammatory dose of 80–100 mg/kg given in four divided doses. The duration of therapy varied from center to center—48–72 hours after the child becoming afebrile to 14 days (the end of the acute phase). The side effects ranged from sensory neural hearing loss to Reye syndrome. Hence, the dose of aspirin was reduced to 30–50 mg/kg per day during the acute phase.[1] This was followed by low dose therapy. 3–5 mg/kg per day till the patient showed no evidence of coronary changes or 8 weeks till the platelet count returned to normal. Recent studies show that aspirin is effective only in the control of fever and acute phase reactants, but has no relevance to coronary artery lesions.

The efficacy of intravenous immunoglobulin in reducing the prevalence of the coronary artery anomaly is well established. The mechanism of action proposed include:

- Modulation of cytokine production
- Neutralization of bacterial super antigen
- Suppression of antibody synthesis
- Fc receptor blockade
- Reduction of immune response leading to TNF alpha expression.

The dosage recommendation of IV IgG varies (a variety of regimens are being used in Japan and USA). Two meta-analysis have revealed a dose response effect with high doses given as a single infusion over 12 hours (2 g/kg). Resistance to IV IgG is reported when given before five days. Ideal time proposed is between 5–7 days of the illness to prevent coronary changes.

The side effects of IV IgG infusion include rash, fever, nausea, hypotension, high solute load, hemolysis, headache and potential risk of transmission of blood-borne pathogens.

MANAGEMENT OF RESISTANT KAWASAKI DISEASE

By definition, persistence of fever or recrudescence of fever after 48 hours of administration of IV IgG qualifies the Kawasaki disease to be called resistant. The incidence of resistant Kawasaki reported varies from center to center (9.4–38%).

Factors which can predict primary non responders include, age below one year, male sex, longer duration of pretreatment illness. The lab characteristics like abnormal echo, elevated ESR and CRP, hyponatremia, hypoalbuminia, elevated SGPT and low Hb and high platelet count.

Studies done by various workers have shown a sensitivity between 77 and 86%, but specificity in the range of 67–76% with a high negative predictive value.

In resistant[2] Kawasaki disease, retreatment with a second dose of IV IgG is initially tried; this is followed by a pulse therapy with methyl prednisolone (30 mg/kg per day) for three days in refractory cases.[3] This can be followed up with two weeks of oral prednisolone. This modality of treatment is associated with decreased risk of coronary artery lesions.[3]

Other drugs that are tried in refractory Kawasaki disease include Infliximab (5 mg/kg) which is a monoclonal antibody to TNF alpha (which is implicated in the causation of inflammatory changes in coronary artery). Has a good effect in reducing the fever and C-reactive protein, but not in preventing the coronary artery changes. The major side effect is anaphylaxis and immune suppression. The minor side effects are headache and nausea.

STEROID IN KAWASAKI DISEASE

The role of steroids was questionable in 1984 when Kato et al. suggested that steroids may worsen coronary artery lesions. But the pendulum has swung in favor of steroids when Okada et al. in 2003 and Hara et al. published in 2009[4] that methyl prednisolone and IV IgG were effective and safe in the initial management of Kawasaki disease.

The side effects of steroids include hypertension, bradycardia, hypothermia, secondary infection, thrombosis, GI bleed, hyponatremia, hyperkalemia and hyperglycemia.

The other modalities of treatment in refractory Kawasaki include plasmapheresis (tried only in a small number of patients–risky not routinely recommended), ulinastatin (a human trypsin inhibitor) and abciximab (a platelet glycoprotein receptor inhibitor used in children with large aneurysms). Cytotoxic agents like methotrexate and cyclosporine have also been tried with oral steroids in rare instances.

CHRONIC PHASE MANAGEMENT OF KAWASAKI DISEASE

This is purely in the domain of a pediatric cardiologist and the aim of the management is in preventing myocardial ischemia and infarction in those children with established coronary changes. The drugs employed include low dose aspirin, dipyridamole, clopidrogel, warfarin and low molecular weight heparin.

RISK STRATIFICATION IN KAWASAKI DISEASE[5]

Level 1

- No coronary artery changes detected at any stage
- No intervention required beyond 8 weeks after onset of the illness.

Level 2

- Transient coronary dilatation which regresses within 8 weeks:
  - No intervention beyond 8 weeks after the onset of the illness
  - Risk assessment and counseling at 3–5 years.

Level 3

- Isolated small aneurysm in one coronary artery
  - Long-term antiplatelet therapy until regression
  - Annual ECG and echocardiogram
  - Biennial stress test with myocardial perfusion imaging if child is more than 10 years
  - Angiography if ischemia implicated.

Level 4

- One large coronary artery aneurysm
  - Same as above with cardiac cath and coronary angiography at 6–12 months after recovery from acute illness.

Level 5

- Patient with coronary artery obstruction confirmed by angiography
  - Long-term antiplatelet therapy with or without warfarin
  - Beta adrenergic blockers
  - ECG and Echo once in 6 months
  - Annual stress test
  - Therapeutic option of grafting or catheter intervention.

CONCLUSION

About 15–25% of untreated children with Kawasaki disease can develop coronary artery aneurysms. Treatment with IV Ig reduces this risk to 5%. For patients with refractory Kawasaki disease; methylprednisolone can be given even after the second dose of IV IgG. Several studies employing methylprednisolone with IV IgG in the initial management are in vogue. Placebo-controlled double blind studies are required to prove the best modality of therapy. Long-term management of children with Kawasaki disease should be tailored according to the degree of coronary involvement.

REFERENCES

1. Hsichk S, Weng KP, Lin CC, Huang TC, Lee CL, Huang SM, et al. Treatment of Kawasaki disease: aspirin's role in febrile stage revisited. Pediatrics. 2004;114(6):689-93.
2. Shinohara M, Sone K, Tomomasa T, Morikava A. Corticosteroids in the treatment of the acute phase of Kawasaki disease. J Pediatr. 1999;135:465-9.
3. Inoue Y, Okada Y, Shinohara M, Kobayashi T, Tomomasa T, Takeuchi K, et al. A multicenter prospective randomized trial of corticosteroids in primary therapy for Kawasaki disease: clinical course and coronary artery outcome. J Pediatr. 2006;149:336-41.

4. Okada Y, Shinohara M, Kobayashi T, Inoue Y, Tomomasa T, Kobayashi, et al. Kawasaki Disease Study Group. Effect of corticosteroids in addition to intravenous gamma globulin therapy on serum cytokine levels in the acute phase of Kawasaki disease in children. J Pediatr. 2003;143:363-7.
5. Newburger JW, Takahashi M, Gerber MA, Gewitz MH, Tani LY, Burns JC, et al. Diagnosis, treatment, and long-term management of Kawasaki disease: a statement for health professionals from the Committee on Rheumatic Fever, Endocarditis, and Kawasaki Disease, Council on Cardiovascular Disease in the Young, American Heart Association. Pediatrics. 2004;114(6):1708-33.

Pulmonology

Reviewers: *PSN Menon, Alok Gupta, R Remesh Kumar, MKC Nair, S Thangavelu, S Narmada Ashok*

7.1 The X-ray Chest in the Diagnosis of Respiratory Distress

G Vijayalakshmi, Balakrishnan Natarajan
Reviewers: *PSN Menon, Alok Gupta, R Remesh Kumar*

INTRODUCTION

One of the most common symptoms that a pediatrician encounters in clinical practice is respiratory distress. This single problem has a variety of causes. A simple X-ray of the chest and abdomen is sufficient to come to a diagnosis in most situations. No other imaging modality is usually necessary. At times, it seems prudent to obtain an X-ray straightaway rather than wasting too much time on clinical examination. For example, the X-ray may reveal a diaphragmatic hernia in a gasping neonate who can be immediately referred to the pediatric surgeon or the X-ray in a child with dyspnea and fever may show pneumonia or a complication like pyopneumothorax prompting the need for a chest tube. This will guide the pediatrician to the medical or surgical nature of the problem and start appropriate treatment.

The chest X-ray **(Fig. 7.1.1)** in a child almost always includes the abdomen. Not only does the small size of the child make it possible for the abdomen also to be included in the same film but also many abdominal conditions causing respiratory symptoms and vice versa can be detected. One has to study every part included in a chest X-ray, not only the heart and lungs. The trachea is in the midline or a little to the right. Most of the heart is seen on the left. Both lungs should be equal in volume and equal in translucency or aeration. Within the lungs, normal bronchovascular markings should be seen. The bones, domes of diaphragm, the costophrenic and cardiophrenic angles, gas-filled bowel in the abdomen and other soft tissues are to be noted.

COMMON RESPIRATORY ABNORMALITIES SEEN IN X-RAY CHEST

Respiratory distress syndrome (RDS) is a peculiar condition of the preterm newborn, where both lungs are not aerated and the lungs are white. The alveoli are collapsed due to lack of surfactant but air freely flows in and out of the airways. Hence the air bronchogram is very well seen even in the peripheral small airways **(Fig. 7.1.2)**.

Figure 7.1.3 shows an X-ray of a newborn with respiratory distress. The X-ray shows hazy parenchymal shadowing in both lungs. The clinical dilemma here is between *aspiration pneumonia* and *transient tachypnea of the newborn (TTN)*. The latter is due to slow clearance of normal pulmonic fluid while aspiration pneumonia is a more serious problem in a gasping hypoxic neonate. It is not possible to differentiate between the two. The baby has to be maintained on supportive measures for 24 hours. A repeat X-ray the next day will show full resolution of shadows in TTN while it will persist in pneumonia as no pathology can disappear so quickly. Unlike RDS, parenchymal shadowing in TTN is not bilaterally symmetric.

Loss of air within the alveoli results in loss of blackness in the lung. **Figure 7.1.4** shows a white triangular opacity conforming to the shape of the right upper lobe. **Figure 7.1.5** also shows a similar triangular shadow. The difference is in the features of volume loss seen in **Figure 7.1.5**. The trachea is much to the right and the minor fissure shows a convex pull upwards which points to a *collapse*. **Figure 7.1.4**

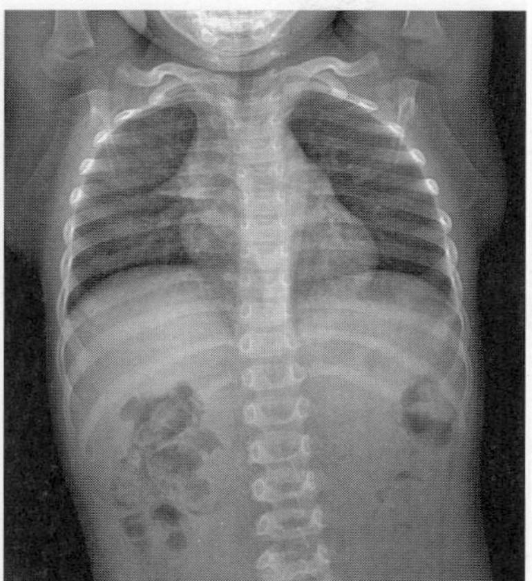

Fig. 7.1.1: Normal chest. Note the sail-shaped thymus

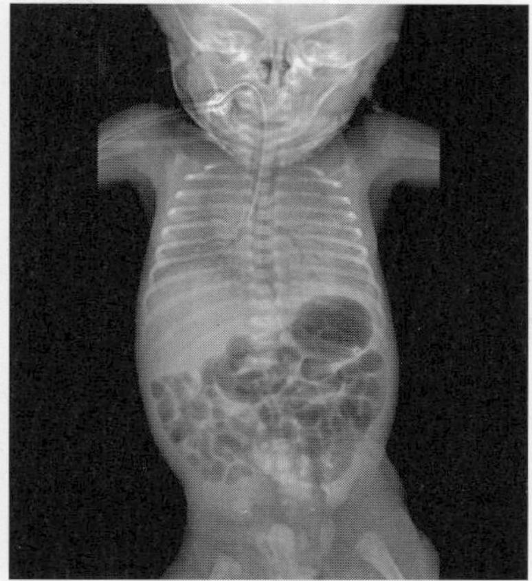

Fig. 7.1.2: Respiratory distress syndrome

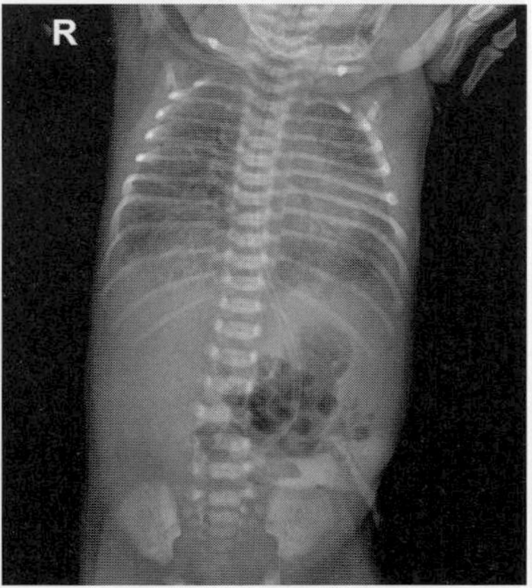

Fig. 7.1.3: Delayed expulsion of pulmonic fluid

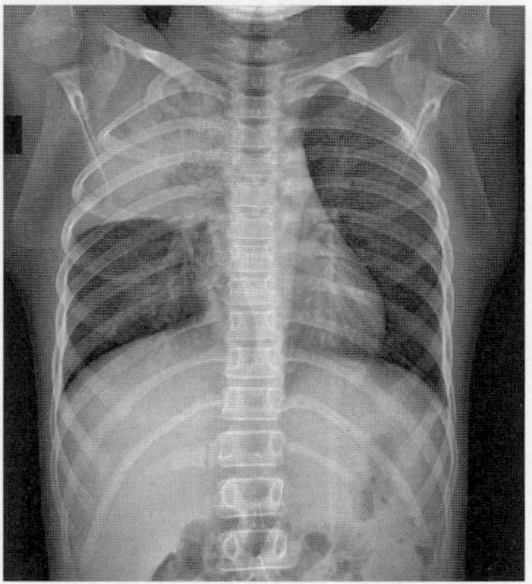

Fig. 7.1.4: Consolidation—right upper lobe

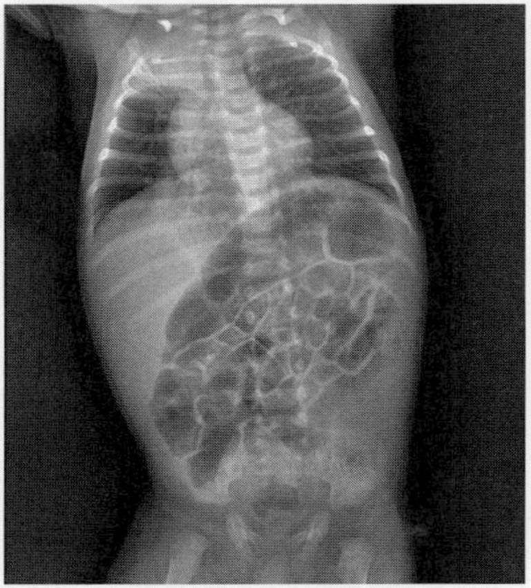

Fig. 7.1.5: Collapse—right upper lobe

indicates *consolidation* as there is no volume loss because the alveoli are not collapsed but filled with exudate. The air bronchogram can be present in both.

Figure 7.1.6 is a classical left lower lobe or *retro-cardiac collapse* where there is a triangular opacity seen behind the heart. There is no volume loss in this X-ray because of *compensatory emphysema* of the upper lobe. If the entire lung loses air, the whole hemithorax becomes opaque. The white hemithorax in **Figure 7.1.7** is consolidation of the left lung as there are no signs of volume loss while **Figure 7.1.8** is that of collapse of the left lung as there are signs of volume loss. The trachea which represents

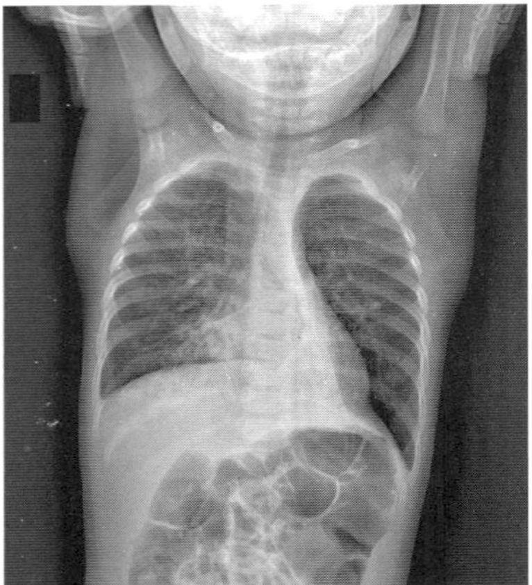

Fig. 7.1.6: Retrocardiac collapse

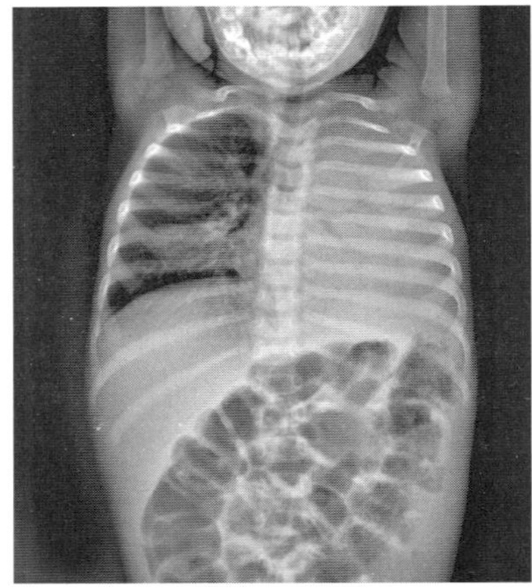

Fig. 7.1.7: Consolidation—left lung

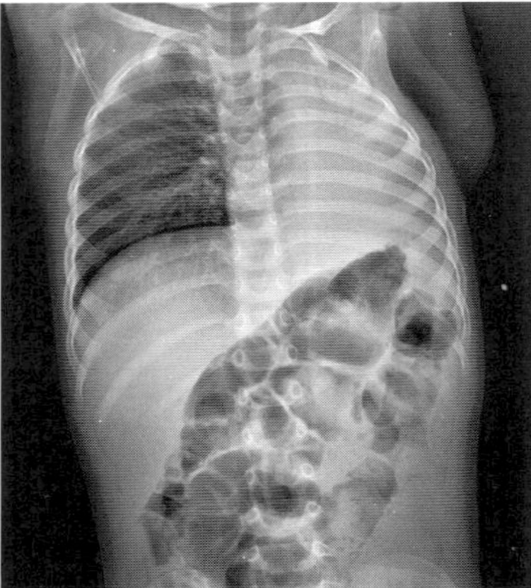

Fig. 7.1.8: Collapse—left lung

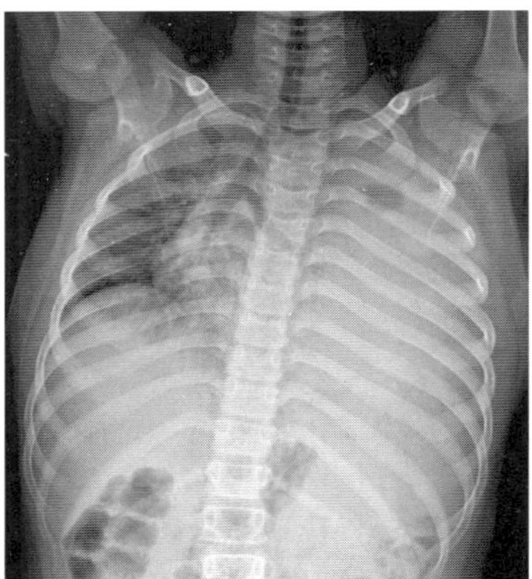

Fig. 7.1.9: Pleural fluid—left

the upper mediastinum is pulled to the left. The heart which is of the lower mediastinum is seen entirely on the left. Other signs of volume loss that should be remembered are elevation of the diaphragm and crowding of ribs.

Figure 7.1.9 is also an opaque left hemithorax but shows increase in volume as is seen by a push of the mediastinum to the opposite side. This is the unmistaken *pleural fluid.* It has to be remembered that a mass is also opaque. An ultrasound of the chest will help in clearing the doubt. If there is air mixed along with pleural fluid as in the common *pyopneumothorax,* then the color of the hemithorax is grey which is a mixture of black air and white fluid **(Fig. 7.1.10)**.

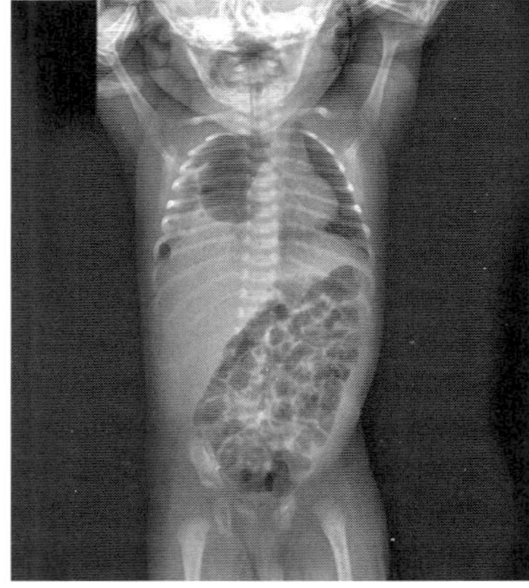

Fig. 7.1.10: Pyopneumothorax—right. Note grey color in the right hemithorax

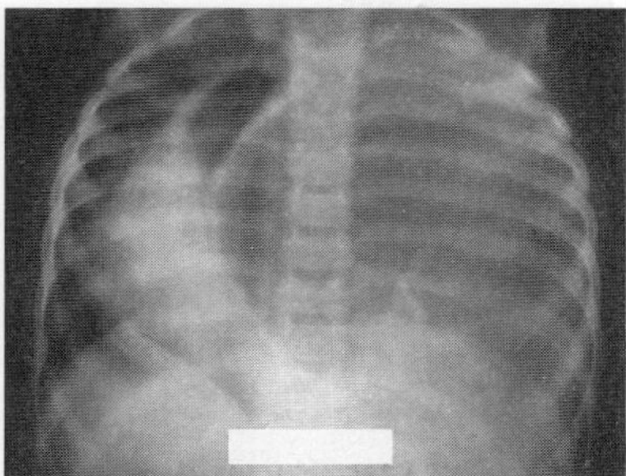

Fig. 7.1.11A: Delayed diaphragmatic hernia

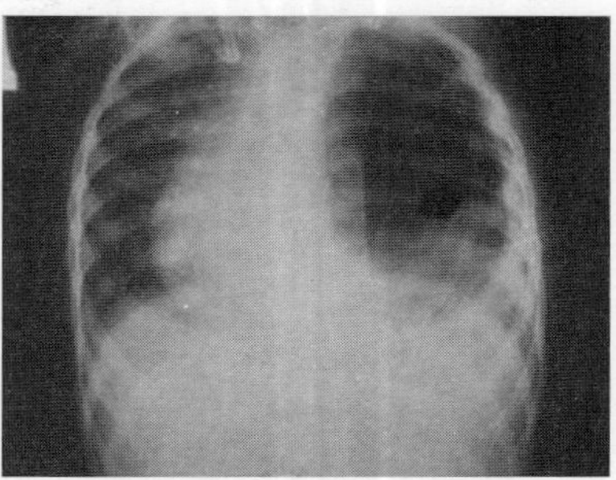

Fig. 7.1.11B: Delayed diaphragmatic hernia with nasogastric tube

Sometimes there is grey hemithorax with gross mediastinal shift to the opposite side **(Fig. 7.1.11A)**. Clearly there is some increase in content in the left hemithorax which is a mixture of air and fluid. If the child has high fever, it will point to infective etiology and help to make a diagnosis of pyopneumothorax. However, the child may have had partial treatment with antibiotics and antipyretics. If the collapsed lung is seen, then we can safely think of pyopneumothorax and go ahead with a chest tube. But if it is not seen and if the child is in acute distress, one should entertain a diagnosis of *delayed diaphragmatic hernia.* A history of trauma if available is helpful, but most of the time the trauma is too trivial to be considered worth mentioning. A quick repeat of the X-ray after positioning a nasogastric tube will solve the problem **(Fig. 7.1.11B)**. The tube will be seen coiled in the hemithorax indicating that it is the stomach that has moved into the thorax. The defect in the diaphragm is a congenital one and stays sealed by the fundus of the stomach till some minor trauma drives the stomach and some bowel loops into the thorax. When in doubt, remember a repeat X-ray after a simple insertion of a nasogastric tube will save much embarrassment—respiratory and otherwise.

Occasionally, there is a lucent hemithorax with shift of the mediastinum to the opposite side. This means there is excess black air on that side. This air may have accumulated in the pleural cavity as in *pneumothorax* or within the lung itself as in *emphysema.* If there are no vascular markings, it is pneumothorax; while in emphysema, there are bronchovascular markings which are normal but widely spaced. The lucent hemithorax in **Figure 7.1.12** is emphysema. The upper lobe alone is emphysematous as is evident by the herniation across the midline in the upper chest while the compressed lower lobe with the crowded bronchovascular markings is seen in the lower chest near the spine. This is *congenital lobar emphysema.* **Figure 7.1.13A** is lobar emphysema of the middle lobe with compressed upper and lower lobes. Other lobes, which are compressed, have to be identified to diagnose lobar emphysema. If not well-seen in the X-ray, CT scan **(Fig. 7.1.13B)** has to be done. **Figure 7.1.14** is *compensatory emphysema* as the right lung is destroyed showing multiple cysts of varying size in a white background.

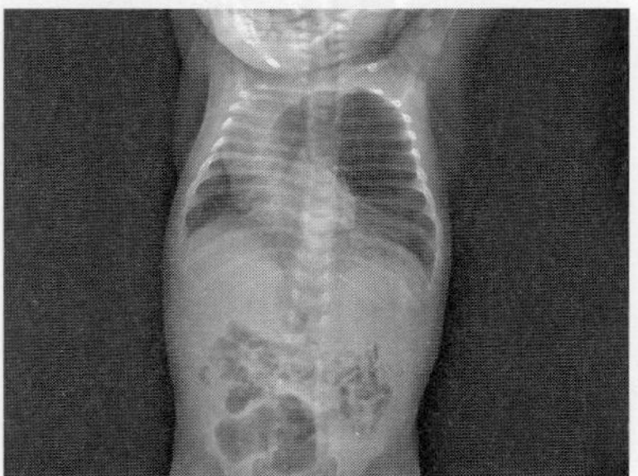

Fig. 7.1.12: Congenital lobar emphysema—left upper lobe

Another important cause for unilateral lucent hemithorax is *obstructive emphysema* **(Fig. 7.1.15)**. The obstructing foreign body is usually organic and, therefore, not seen

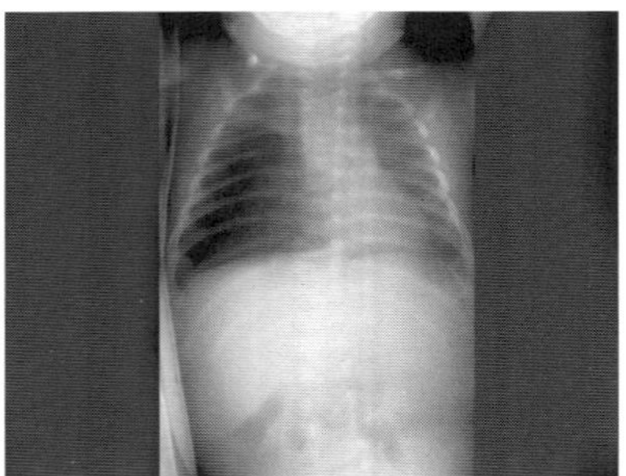

Fig. 7.1.13A: Congenital lobar emphysema—middle lobe

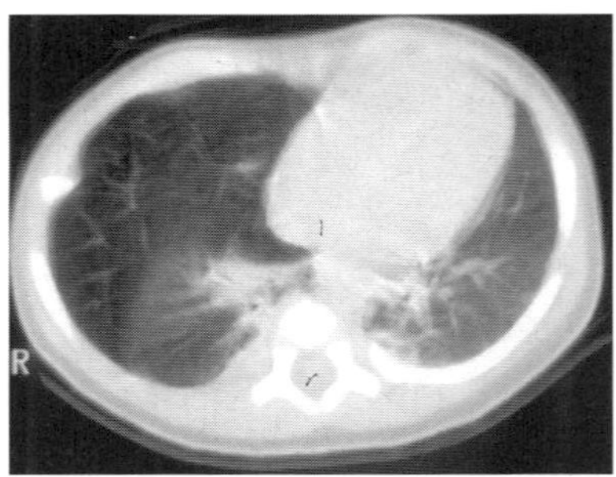

Fig. 7.1.13B: Congenital lobar emphysema—CT image. Note the compressed lower lobe posteriorly

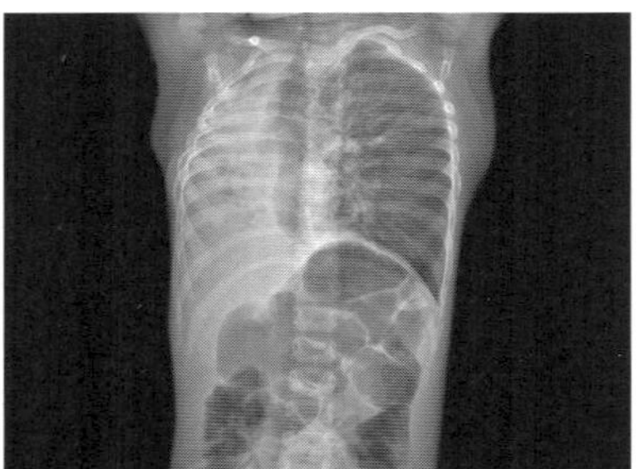

Fig. 7.1.14: Compensatory emphysema—left

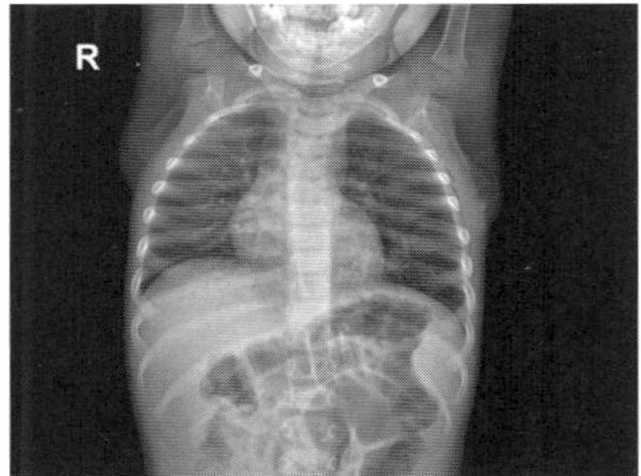

Fig. 7.1.15: Obstructive emphysema—left

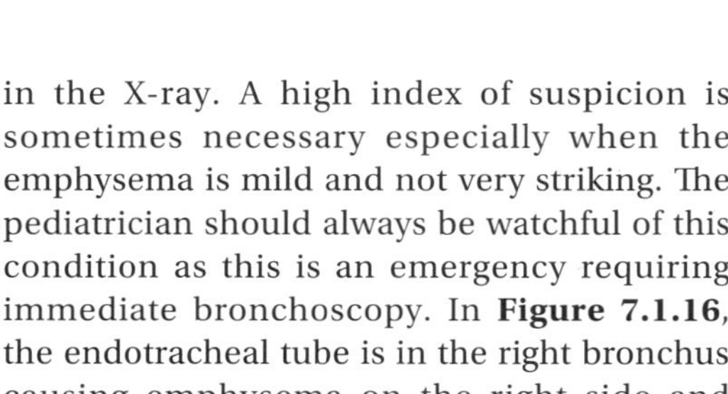

in the X-ray. A high index of suspicion is sometimes necessary especially when the emphysema is mild and not very striking. The pediatrician should always be watchful of this condition as this is an emergency requiring immediate bronchoscopy. In **Figure 7.1.16**, the endotracheal tube is in the right bronchus causing emphysema on the right side and partial collapse of the left lung.

In emphysema, normal bronchovascular markings are seen. These show normal dichotomous branching and taper towards the periphery. In **Figure 7.1.17**, the lucent hemithorax on the right has many markings that run across haphazardly. This is *congenital cystadenomatoid malformation*. It may involve the entire lung or a lobe. CT scan will help to identify the compressed normal lobe.

Apart from more air accumulating in the lung or in the pleural cavity, it can also percolate into the mediastinum causing respiratory distress. In **Figure 7.1.18** the *pneumomediastinum* has lifted the thymus away from the heart. Normally the thymus is not seen separately and the heart shadow in the child is referred to as the cardiothymic shadow. Similarly, the diaphragm is not normally seen separately from the heart. In pneumomediastinum, air tracks in between the diaphragm and the heart causing the 'continuous diaphragm sign' **(Fig. 7.1.19)**.

The chest and abdomen in **Figure 7.1.20** shows all the bowel loops in the chest with only the stomach remaining in the abdomen (*Congenital diaphragmatic hernia*). The mediastinum is displaced to the opposite side because of the additional content in that hemithorax. **Figure 7.1.21A** also shows bowel loops in the thorax with shift of the mediastinum to the opposite side. But it is seen that the stomach has also ascended into the hemithorax unlike (**Fig. 7.1.20**). Further there is a definite convex upper border above which normal lung is seen. This is *eventration of diaphragm*. However, thin and flimsy the diaphragm, it will never reach the apex of the hemithorax. In diaphragmatic hernia bowel loops pass through the defect

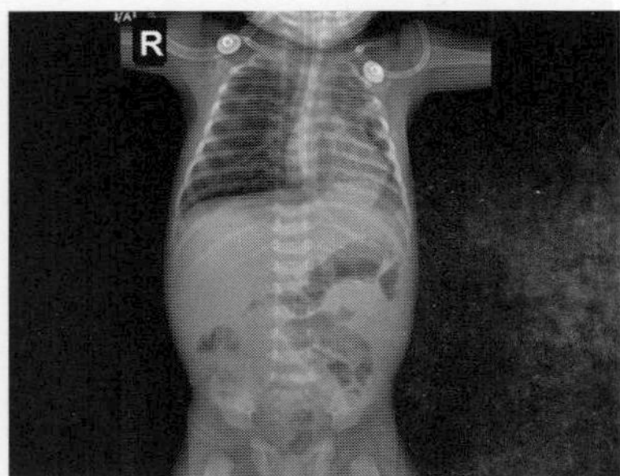

Fig. 7.1.16: Hyperaeration due to endotracheal tube in right bronchus. Note also the pneumothorax on the right

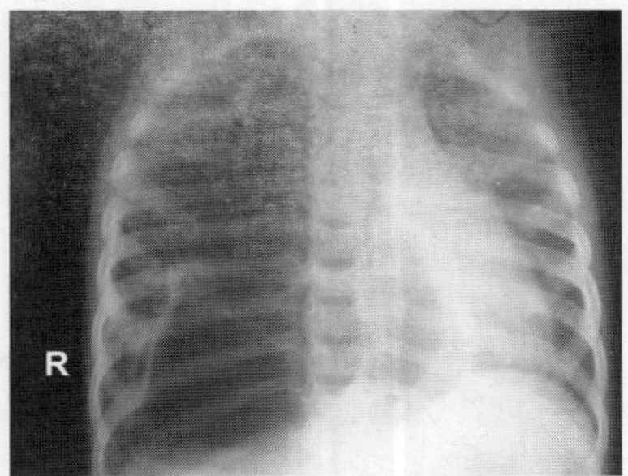

Fig. 7.1.17: Congenital cystadenomatoid malformation—right

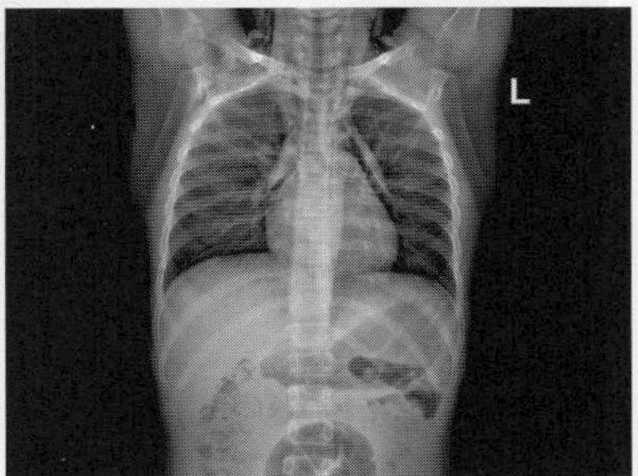

Fig. 7.1.18: Pneumomediastinum—spinnaker sail sign

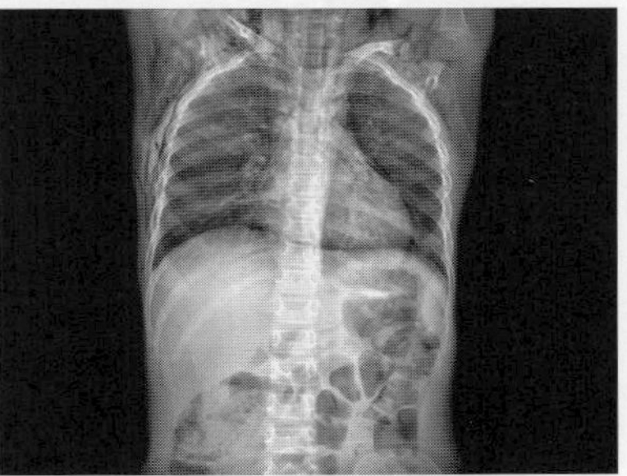

Fig. 7.1.19: Pneumomediastinum—continuous diaphragm sign

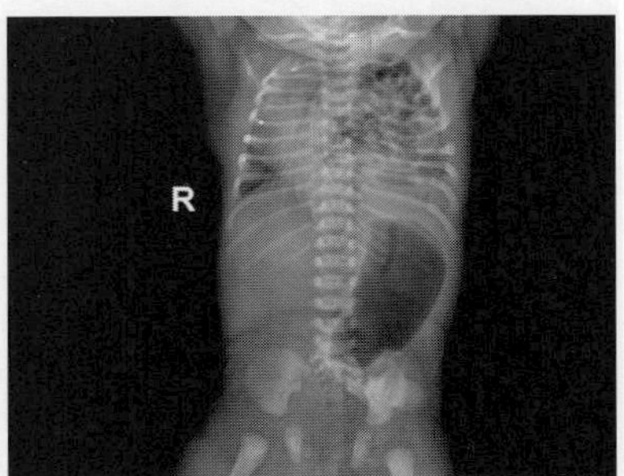

Fig. 7.1.20: Congenital diaphragmatic hernia—left

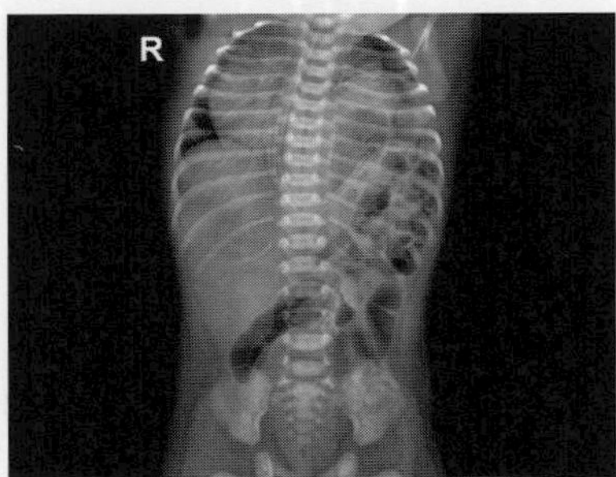

Fig. 7.1.21A: Eventration of diaphragm—left

in the diaphragm and are stopped only by the upper limit of the hemithorax. **Figure 7.1.21B** is eventration on the right. The liver is in the right hemithorax.

Other important sites that are to be checked in the hemithorax are the costophrenic and cardiophrenic angles which are the seats of certain abnormalities. There is a round opacity in the right cardiophrenic angle in **Figure 7.1.22A**. The differential diagnosis

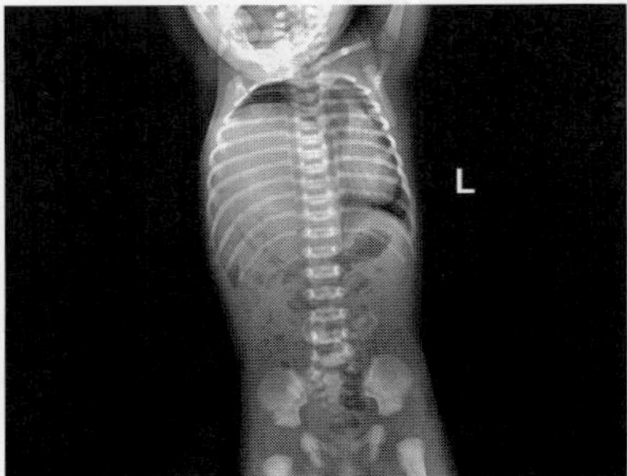

Fig. 7.1.21B: Eventration of diaphragm—right

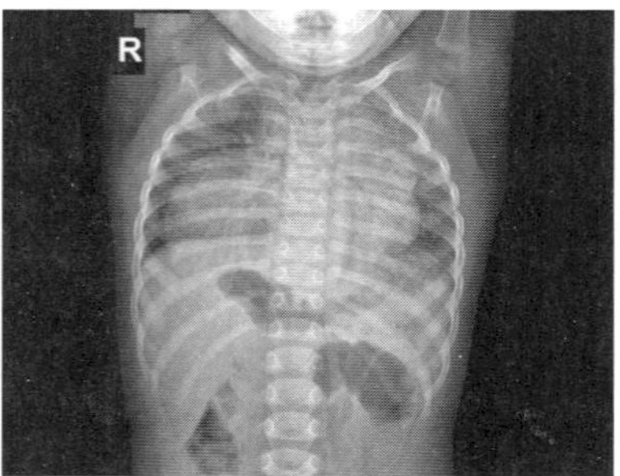

Fig. 7.1.22A: Cardiophrenic angle opacity—hiatus hernia

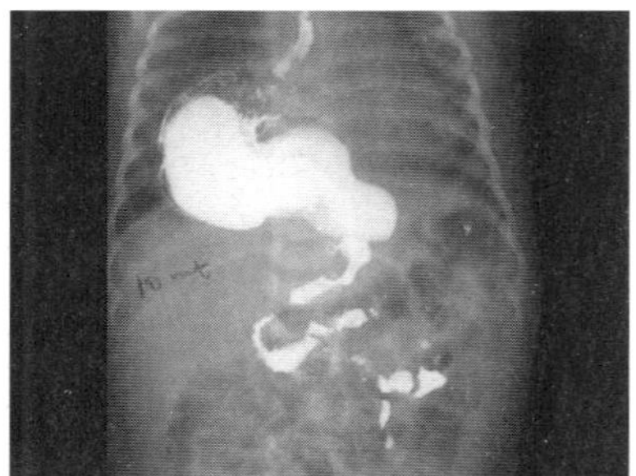

Fig. 7.1.22B: Hiatus hernia—barium study

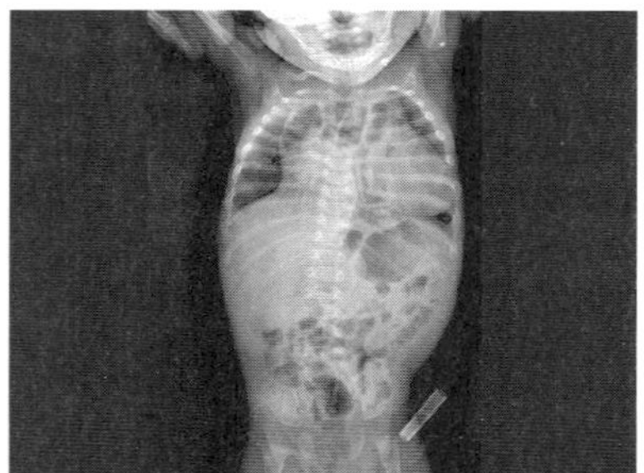

Fig. 7.1.23A: Morgagni hernia

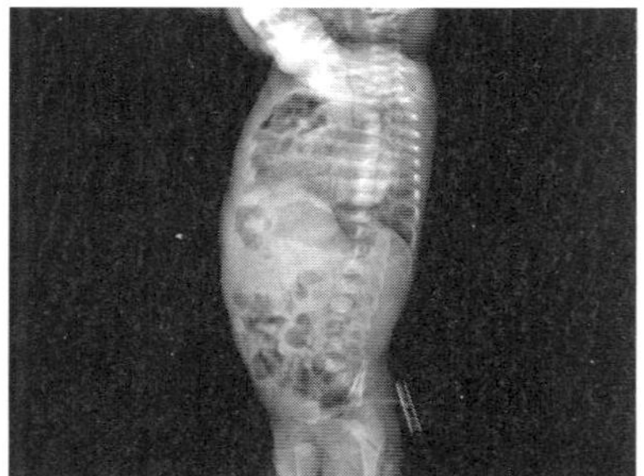

Fig. 7.1.23B: Morgagni hernia—lateral film

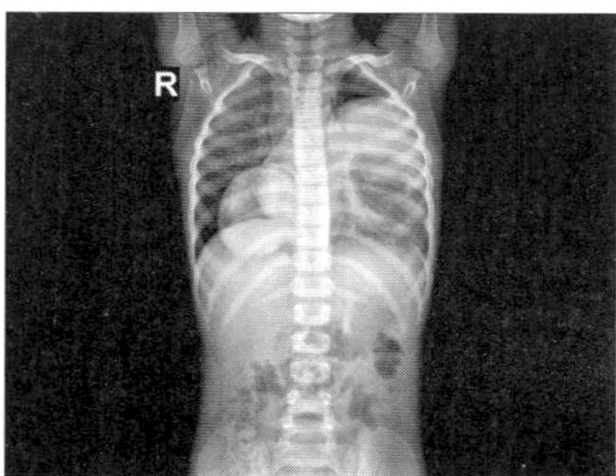

Fig. 7.1.24A: Hydatid cysts

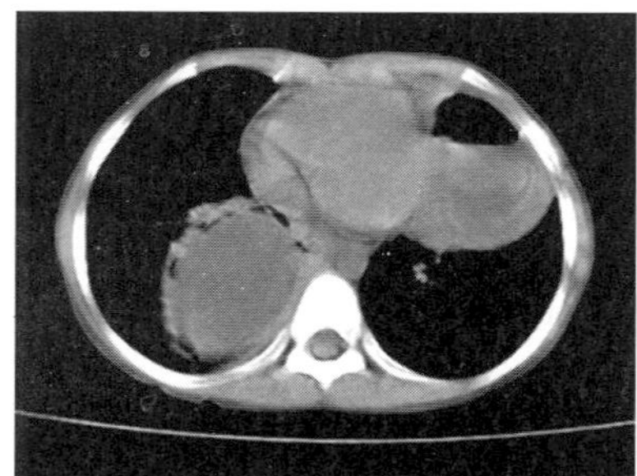

Fig. 7.1.24B: Hydatid cysts—meniscus sign

includes lesions from within the lung like *abscesses* and some other lesions like pleuropericardial cysts, hiatus hernia and Morgagni hernia from neighboring structures. Of these, *hiatus hernia* is very common. A simple barium meal as in **Figure 7.1.22B** will set aside all doubts when the fundus of the stomach is shown within the round opacity. **Figure 7.1.23A** shows a blunted cardiophrenic angle and many round cystic shadows in the mediastinum. A lateral chest view **(Fig. 7.1.23B)** shows all the loops in the anterior chest. This is *Morgagni hernia* where the transverse colon and some bowel loops escape into the thorax through an antero-medial defect in the diaphragm.

The round shadow in the cardiophrenic angle in **Figure 7.1.24A** is well-defined and opaque. There is another large similar lesion on the left with air within. These are multiple *hydatid cysts*. They may get secondarily infected and

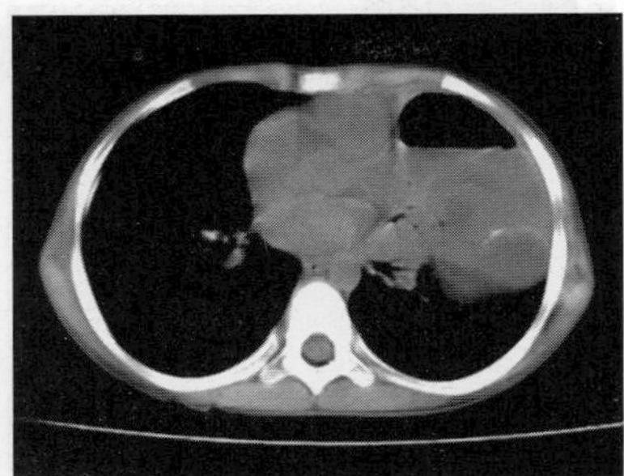

Fig. 7.1.24C: Hydatid cysts—floating lily sign

present acutely. CT scan delineates the lesions clearly. The cyst on the right shows a thin sliver of air that has insinuated between the cyst wall and the lung **(Fig. 7.1.24B, meniscus sign)**. As more and more air gets in, the cyst wall collapses and moves away from the roof giving rise to the floating lily sign **(Fig. 7.1.24C)**. There are multiple daughter cysts seen within along with even a short thin, curved line of calcification.

CONCLUSION

The chest X-ray is a valuable tool in the diagnosis of respiratory distress and an intelligent evaluation of the X-ray will give a quick diagnosis that will decide on the right course of action immediately, especially in a clinical scenario of respiratory distress where time is precious. CT scan is sometimes required for confirmation of the diagnosis.

BIBLIOGRAPHY

1. Ananda Kesavan TM. IAP Textbook of Pediatric Radiology (Indian Academy of Pediatrics National Publication House, Gwalior). New Delhi; Jaypee Brothers Medical Publishers, 2013.
2. Carty H, Brunelle F, Stringer DA, Kao CS (Eds). Imaging Children. Elsevier Churchill Livingstone, New York; 2005.
3. Swischuk LE (Ed). Imaging of the Newborn Infant and Child Lippincott Williams & Wilkins; 2004.

7.2 Tests for Microbiological Diagnosis in Childhood TB

NC Gowrishankar

***Reviewers:** MKC Nair, S Thangavelu, S Narmada Ashok*

Every year more than 9 million people suffer from TB and India accounts for more than 25% of global tuberculosis (TB) burden. Tuberculosis prevalence per lakh population has reduced from 465 in year 1990 to 211 in 2013. In absolute numbers, prevalence has reduced from 40 lakhs to 26 lakhs annually. Tuberculosis mortality per lakh population has reduced from 38 in year 1990 to 19 in 2012. In absolute numbers, mortality due to TB has reduced from 3.3 lakhs to 2.4 lakhs annually. This has been possible after Revised National Tuberculosis Control Programme (RNTCP) has streamlined the methodology for diagnosis and treatment. In children the crux of the problem is getting body fluids for a microbiological diagnosis of tuberculosis unlike adults. In this overview the microbiologic diagnostic tools for TB in children is discussed.

In order to diagnose TB in children, one has to meticulously follow this order of a good history including history of contact with tuberculosis in the adult members of the family or neighborhood and proper clinical examination before proceeding onto investigation. The basis of doing investigation is either to directly detect the TB bacilli or indirectly by the host response to TB bacilli. The direct tests can be phenotypic tests which detect the whole bacteria or genotypic tests which detect the nucleic acid fragments of TB bacilli **(Table 7.2.1)**. If the treating pediatrician is able to understand this concept, then tests for microbiologic diagnosis

Table 7.2.1: Lab diagnosis of TB

Direct tests		*Indirect tests*
Phenotype tests	Genotype tests	Mantoux tests IGRA tests
AFB smear AFB culture	Genexpert TB Line probe assay test	

in TB becomes very easy. All the body fluids except blood can be used for a microbiological confirmation for tuberculosis.

For demonstration of acid-fast bacilli (AFB), one has to get a sputum sample which can be challenging as less sputum production and lack of sufficient tussive force in children are the main stumbling blocks. This can be overcome by inducing sputum using 3% hypertonic saline nebulization followed by chest physiotherapy to loosen up secretion and then samples are collected from throat or nasopharynx with collector attached to suction at one end and catheter/tube to the other. The suction catheter provokes cough and the secretions coughed up are collected via suction. It is well-tolerated, safe and effective in both older infants and very young children. The yield of one induced sputum is equal to the same yield as that of three gastric aspirates. Two samples need to be tested as per RNTCP guidelines.

If sputum sample is unavailable, then gastric aspirate (GA) is done. Nasogastric tube is inserted 3-4 hours after dinner and the GA sample is taken early in the morning before the child wakes up as waking up induces gut peristalsis. If aspirate is less than 5 mL then a saline wash with 15-30 mL is done and gastric contents aspirated. The contents are immediately transferred to laboratory. GA can be done as an ambulatory procedure with 4-6 hours fasting but some loss of yield will be there.

DIRECT TESTS—PHENOTYPE TESTS

AFB Smear

Once the body fluid is obtained, both AFB stain and culture, have to be done. For AFB smear to be positive 10,000 AFB/mL has to be present.

Table 7.2.2: Interpretation of AFB stain results

Examination	*Result*	*Grading*
>10 AFB/oil immersion field	Positive	3+
1–10 AFB/oil immersion field	Positive	2+
10–99 AFB/100 oil immersion field	Positive	1+
1–9 AFB/100 oil immersion field	Positive	Scanty
No AFB in 100 oil immersion field	Negative	Negative

The AFB stain result has to be reported as given in **Table 7.2.2**. Ziehl-Neelsen staining is the method used as it is available everywhere while fluorescent microscopy technique is available in few places. With fluorescent microscopy and auromine rhodamine staining, it is easier to identify the AFB which will be seen as a yellow fluorescence against a dark background. It reduces the operator time and increases the sensitivity of the microscopy. Also traditional ZN stain can be performed over the fluorescent stain if confirmation is required. LED lights are replacing the conventional light source in dark field microscopy which not only reduces the operator cost but also can be adapted to battery operation especially when continuous power supply cannot be ensured. Though smear examination can be easily done, it neither has the ability to discriminate reliably between the mycobacterial species nor does it have the ability to differentiate live and dead bacilli as well as non-tuberculous mycobacteria. Automation of microscopy enhances the consistency of results and efficiency of process and reduces human resources required. The automated staining system loads the stained slides onto fluorescent microscope, focuses automatically, captures images digitally and classifies smears as positive or negative based on computerized algorithms.

AFB Culture

Positive culture is the 'gold standard test' for the diagnosis of tuberculosis.

Table 7.2.3: Liquid culture and characteristics

Test	*Advantages*	*Limitations*
Radiometric BACTEC 460 TB culture	Early results compared to solid culture	Need for disposal of radiolabelled products
MGIT 960 detection systems	Machine monitors growth every hour	Costlier than other liquid cultures
Microscopic observation drug susceptibility testing	Less costly than MGIT	Technically demanding and operator dependence

- *Traditional solid media:* This can be either egg based—LJ media or agar based—7H10 and 7H11 Middlebrook medium. Slow turnaround time is the drawback wherein one expects faster result especially in the era of multidrug resistant TB.
- *Liquid culture media:* Based on the indicators used, there are different types of liquid cultures **(Table 7.2.3)**. Most of the liquid culture mediums are automated and are endorsed by the World Health Organization (WHO). Liquid medium (e.g. Middlebrook 7H9), with use of various growth-indicator methods is able to detect even small growth of mycobacteria. This may be by detecting oxygen concentration changes indicated by fluorescence (e.g. MGIT 960), colorimetric (e.g. BacT/ALERT), microscopical (e.g. tuberculosis microscopical observation drug susceptibility test kit), detecting radioactivity as growth index (e.g. BACTEC 460), and pressure changes (e.g. VersaTREK) can help in getting positive cultures earlier than traditional culture using LJ medium. Each of the liquid cultures has some advantages and disadvantages. The main advantage for the liquid culture medium is shorter turnaround time unlike the solid media.

Detection Systems

- *Radiometric BACTEC 460 TB culture:* This is a liquid culure technique which uses radiometric indicator. In this culture method radiolabeled C^{14} palmitic acid is used in 7H12 medium. This method detects the presence of mycobacteria in the culture based on their metabolism rather than the visible growth. When mycobacteria grows in the culture, it utilizes the radiolabeled C^{14} palmitic acid and produces^{14} CO_2 which is measured by the BACTEC system and reported as Growth Index. The results will be available in less than half the time needed for regular culture. Also when sufficient growth index is observed, drug susceptibility test also can be performed. But the need for disposal of radiolabelled products has allowed this test to be superseded by the other liquid culture test (MGIT).
- *MGIT 960 detection system:* This is an automated system with liquid culture using fluorescent growth indicator. The system monitors for the growth of *MTb* every hour. The growing mycobacteria deplete the dissolved oxygen and allows the indicator to fluoresce brightly under 365 nm UV light. The machine monitors and reads the tubes every hour. It takes around 15–16 days for the results in this system.
- *Line probe assay (LPA), lateral flow assay or nucleic acid hybridization:* If there is growth in liquid culture medium it should be differentiated from nontuberculous mycobacteria by doing line probe assay (LPA), lateral flow assay or nucleic acid hybridization as there is increased risk of cross-contamination in liquid cultures. Also drug sensitivity testing is the ideal step after every positive culture as our country has shown more MDR TB cases. For developing countries with poor resources, drug susceptibility tests can be done directly from the samples from subjects or indirectly from the growth in cultures.
- *Microscopic observation drug susceptibility testing (MODS), nitrate reductase assay and colorimetric redox indicator assay:* These are used for screening those suspected to have

drug resistance. In MODS, the sample is inoculated into wells of tissue culture plate containing liquid growth media. Some wells contain rifampicin and isoniazid at critical concentrations facilitating simultaneous detection of growth and drug resistance. Growth by visual inspection using inverted microscope is cheaper but labor intensive and operator dependent. But as is the norm drug resistance has to be confirmed from a reference lab as per requirement of MDR treatment protocol.

- *Loop-mediated isothermal amplification tests (LAMP):* This is a constant temperature method for amplification of nucleic acids eliminating the need for thermal cycler. High concentrations of amplified DNA can be generated and the test allows detection of fluorescence or turbidity by naked eye. The disadvantages include complexity of the procedure, number of steps involved and the potential for cross-contamination. It does not perform well in pauci-bacillary clinical specimens as in childhood TB.

GENOTYPE TESTS

Nucleic Acid Amplification Tests

In nucleic acid amplification tests detection of amplified specific target RNA/DNA sequence is done by nucleic acid probe. Though it can detect nucleic acid, it cannot differentiate dead and live organisms. It is expensive and a very high degree of quality control is required to avoid false-positive results. It is a rapid procedure with a high sensitivity, i.e. 1–10 bacilli/mL sputum can be detected within hours. It can be either in-house or commercial. In-house polymerase chain reaction (PCR) tests are highly dependent on the operator and strict quality control has to be maintained to avoid cross-contamination.

Among the commercial ones, the US FDA has approved three nucleic acid amplification tests; of which, Xpert MTB/RIF test (Genexpert TB) is available in India. It is a cartridge based nucleic acid amplification test (CBNAAT). The test is an automated one which simultaneously identifies *MTb* and rifampicin resistance. Also the test is unaffected by patient HIV status. It is simple to perform with minimal training, highly specific but the sensitivity for sputum smear-negative TB in children remains low. All body fluids except blood can be used as the sample. It uses hemi-nested real-time PCR assay to amplify an *MTb* specific sequence of the *rpoB* gene, which is probed with molecular beacons for mutations within the rifampin-resistance determining region. It takes about 105 minutes for the test to be completed after loading the cartridge into the machine. As it is fully automated except for the first step of loading, the patients' sample into the cartridge, the chances for cross-contamination are very minimal or absent. It is now being done free of charge in the national reference labs in the country and the results are sent to the treating pediatrician by short message service (SMS) and email, making it as a very easily done point of care test.

The sample handling and extraction of DNA which are the traditional stumbling blocks in nucleic acid amplification test (NAAT) are being overcome by advances in nucleic acid amplification technology. Newer NAAT include Truenat MTB, EasyNAT Diagnostic Kit, VereMTB assay. Truenat MTB (Molbio Diagnostics, India) is a miniaturized chip-based real-time PCR which can run on handheld battery-operated device and give results in less than an hour. The sputum is processed by battery-operated sample preparation device which extracts nucleic acids using nanoparticle based protocol. The sensitivity and specificity are similar to Xpert MTB/RIF. EasyNAT Diagnostic Kit for M. Tb complex (Ustar Biotechnologies, China) is an isothermal amplification kit with a 60 minutes amplification reaction step and a 30 minutes visual detection using lateral flow device.

INDIRECT TESTS

Mantoux Test (Tuberculin Skin Test)

It is the most commonly done test. Though it is a very old test, it is still the first test advised along with other investigation while evaluating a child with possibility of TB diagnosis.

As India is a high burden country for TB, it is always necessary to use the lowest strength of Mantoux as higher strengths will lead to higher chance of a positive reaction. The ideal strength (Tuberculin Unit–TU) of Mantoux fluid should be 1 TU or 2 TU. It should never be beyond 5 TU. Also it is necessary to look for the size of the induration and not the erythema. An induration of 10 mm or more is a positive reaction. In children who are immunocompromised or on immunosuppressive medications, an induration of 5 mm or more is taken as a positive test. The treating pediatrician should always make it a point to read and document the Mantoux reading by themselves, thus avoiding or overcoming chances of error. But a positive test does not differentiate between an infection and a disease. False negative results can occur in post-viral (measles, varicella, influenza) state, immunocompromised children, and those children on corticosteroid therapy. False positive results can occur in non-tuberculous mycobacteria (NTM) and if test is repeated at the same site unknowingly (booster effect).

Interferon Gamma Release Assay Test

A recent addition in the TB diagnostics is interferon gamma release assay (IGRA) test. This test measures the amount of interferon gamma produced by the activated T-lymphocytes after stimulation by specific antigens of *Mycobacterium tuberculosis* [Early secretory antigen target 6 (ESAT6), Culture filtrate protein 10 (CFP10)] by ELISA method (Quantiferon-TB Gold) or ELISPOT assay (T-SPOT TB). The quantiferon TB gold test incubates whole blood with the *MTb* specific antigen and the amount of interferon gamma released is measured after a period of time and measures IFN gamma production with an enzyme-linked immunosorbent assay (ELISA), while the T-SPOT TB test measures the number of IFN gamma producing peripheral mononuclear cells. The child's blood will be incubated. The child needs to visit the lab only once for giving blood for testing unlike Mantoux, where the child needs to visit the second time for Mantoux reading after 48 to 72 hours. The test is unaffected by previous BCG vaccination and by most nontuberculous mycobacteria.

Available data suggest that TST and IGRAs have similar accuracy for detection of TB infection or the diagnosis of disease in children. The testing lab should provide both qualitative and quantitative results. Qualitative results are reported as positive, negative or indeterminate/borderline. Quantitative results are reported as numerical values which include a response to TB antigen and 2 controls. But the biggest disadvantage is cost factor. Though IGRA can be of help in immunocompromised conditions including HIV, because of the high cost involved and the need for expensive equipment, RNTCP does not endorse the use of IGRA in Tb diagnostics.

False positive IGRA can happen repeatedly in individuals infected with *M. Kansasii, M. marinum* and *M. szulgai*. Performance of IGRA in immunodeficiencies or those receiving immunosuppressive treatment is overall poor. Several robust meta-analyses on performance of IGRA as a supportive tool for diagnosis of active TB has found that IGRA performs no better than Mantoux test. Also performance of IGRA is worse in young children compared with adults but the precise underlying mechanisms remain uncertain with incomplete immune maturation playing a significant role. The factors which are associated with indeterminate IGRA include malnutrition, chronic renal disease, autoimmune conditions, malaria and co-existing helminth infections. The reproducibility of IGRA is suboptimal when serial testing is performed, i.e. with unexplained conversions from positive to negative and vice versa. With Mantoux test, a large amount of longitudinal data is available and the predictive value for development of active TB is known but data in relation to IGRA, particularly in children, still remain relatively limited.

RECENT ADVANCES

- *c-TB test:* A new skin test based on recombinant early secreted antigen target (ESAT-6) and culture filtrate protein (CFP-10) is being developed which is likely to achieve greater specificity than Mantoux test. It is well-tolerated and adverse events are rare. It can be performed at primary care/community level with no specific need for laboratory infrastructure. Also the healthcare professionals can be made familiar with test method easily as it is identical to Mantoux test. The anticipated cost of this test is lower than IGRA-based testing.

- *Gas sensor array electronic nose (E-Nose):* This test has the potential to detect different *Mycobacterium* species in headspaces of cultures and sputum samples. The array uses 14 sensors to profile a "smell" by assessing change in each sensor's electrical properties, when exposed to specific odor mixture but the potential value in TB diagnosis in children is still being evaluated.
- *Mycobacterial antigen detection in urine:* Urine Lipoarabinomannan (LAM): This test detects *M. tuberculosis* glycolipid by ELISA in the urine of child suspected to have *MTb* but does not differentiate *MTb* from NTM. The sensitivity is best in immune compromised patients with HIV infection but pediatric studies are limited.
- *Volatile organic acids:* Detection of disease by smell is an ancient practice. Volatile organic compounds (VOCs) as TB diagnostic targets have been based on the ability of trained African giant pouched rats to detect *M. tuberculosis* in human sputum specimens through smell. VOC arises from *M. tuberculosis* metabolism and human tissue injury. This method of detection of VOC will require relatively expensive instruments and its performance in those with pauci-bacillary disease is quite poor. Moreover, it does not have the ability to detect extrapulmonary TB and hence it is not expected to perform well in children.

BIBLIOGRAPHY

1. Chiang SS, Swanson DS, Starke JR. New Diagnostics for Childhood Tuberculosis.Infect Dis Clin N Am. 2015. *http://dx.doi.org/10.1016/j.idc.2015.05.011.*
2. Chiappini E, Lo Vecchio A, Garazzino S, et al. Recommendations for the diagnosis of pediatric tuberculosis. Eur J Clin Microbiol Infect Dis. DOI 10.1007/s10096-015-2507-6.
3. Graham, et al. Evaluation of Tuberculosis Diagnostics in Children: 1. Proposed Clinical Case Definitions for Classification of Intra-thoracic Tuberculosis Disease. Consensus From an Expert Panel.The Journal of Infectious Diseases. DOI: 10.1093/infdis/jis008.
4. Turkova A, Welch SB, Paton JY, et al. Management of paediatric tuberculosis in leading UK centres unveiling consensus and discrepancies. Int J Tuberc Lung Dis. 2014;18(9):1047-56.
5. V Singh, Kaur S. Diagnosis of Tuberculosis—Newer Investigations. Indian Journal of Practical Pediatrics. 2012;14(3):273-83.

Gastroenterology

Reviewers: *PSN Menon, Alok Gupta, R Remesh Kumar, K Nedunchelian, Jaydeep Choudhury, RV Dhakshayani*

8.1 Liver Enzymes and Hepatitis Markers: How to Interpret?

Dheivamani Nirmala

Reviewers: *PSN Menon, Alok Gupta, R Remesh Kumar*

LIVER ENZYMES

Liver has to perform different biochemical, synthetic and excretory functions and no single biochemical test can detect the global functions of liver. A liver enzyme is a protein that helps to speed up a chemical reaction in the liver. Liver enzymes have been measured as part of liver function tests though strictly they do not measure the functions of the liver.

The liver enzymes have been used as a screening test for liver diseases, to assess the pattern of disease and severity and in the follow-up of patients during recovery from liver diseases. The limitations of their use are due to the poor sensitivity (e.g. they may be normal in certain liver diseases) and specificity (e.g. they may be altered in diseases affecting other organs also) though at times abnormal liver enzymes may be the only indication of liver dysfunction.

Clinically significant liver enzymes include:

- Those which detect hepatocellular necrosis/biochemical activity (e.g. aminotransferases), and
- Those which detect cholestasis (e.g. alkaline phosphatase and gamma glutamyltranspeptidase).

Aminotransferases

Aspartate aminotransferase (AST, formerly known as serum glutamic oxaloacetic transaminase, SGOT) and alanine aminotransferase (ALT, formerly known as serum glutamic-pyruvic transaminase, SGPT) are the most frequently utilized and specific indicators of hepatocellular necrosis. They usually catalyze the transfer of α-amino group to α-keto group.

Aspartate aminotransferase (AST) is a mitochondrial enzyme present in liver, cardiac muscle, skeletal muscle, kidneys, brain, pancreas, lungs, leukocytes and erythrocytes whereas alanine aminotransferase (ALT) is a cytosolic enzyme which is more specific for liver damage and present in higher concentration in liver than in heart or skeletal muscle and normal values of these enzymes range from 5 to 35 IU/L.

The rise in liver enzymes may be severe (> 20 times, 1000 IU/L) in viral hepatitis, drug or toxin-induced hepatic necrosis and circulatory shock; moderate (3–20 times) in acute and chronic hepatitis, neonatal hepatitis, and acute biliary tract obstructions or mild (1–3 times) in sepsis, extrahepatic biliary atresia (EHBA), myositis, Duchenne muscular dystrophy and even after vigorous exercise. **Table 8.1.1** lists the conditions where liver enzymes are elevated without an underlying liver disease whereas **Table 8.1.2** lists liver diseases in which liver enzymes are not elevated.

Table 8.1.1: Conditions with elevated liver enzymes without liver disease
1. Primary muscle disease
2. Macro-AST in which AST complexes with immunoglobulin, usually IgG
3. Celiac disease
4. Thyroid dysfunction (hyper- and hypothyroidism)
5. Adrenal insufficiency

Abbreviation: AST, aspartate aminotransferase

Table 8.1.2: Liver disease without elevated liver enzymes
1. Hemochromatosis
2. Methotrexate-induced hepatic injury
3. Chronic hepatitis C virus infection
4. Post-jejunoileal bypass

Level of enzyme elevation shows poor correlation with regard to the extent of necrosis and is of little value in predicting the outcome. Similarly decreasing enzyme level though may indicate recovery can also be due to massive destruction when it indicates poor prognosis.

The ratio of AST and ALT (AST/ALT) may be useful to differentiate certain conditions. The normal ratio is less than or equal to 1 and a ratio of more than 2 is seen commonly in alcoholic hepatitis probably due to pyridoxine deficiency. In acute Wilson's disease, the ratio is usually more than 4. One should remember that a higher ratio may also be seen in cirrhosis due to any cause because of reduced plasma clearance of AST.

Low levels of aminotransferases have been seen in patients on long-term hemodialysis and also in uremia and the cause is probably secondary to either dialysate or pyridoxine deficiency.

Alkaline Phosphatase

This enzyme is found histochemically in the microvilli of bile canaliculi and on the sinusoidal surface of hepatocytes. Normal value ranges from 45 to 115 IU/L and usually due to overproduction and leakage into blood. These enzymes are usually seen in the diseases of the liver, bone, kidney, intestine, placenta and tumors and most of the circulating alkaline phosphatase originates from either liver or bone.

Physiologically high values are seen in childhood and puberty due to bone growth. Though highest levels of alkaline phosphatase occur in cholestatic disorders; other causes for increase include infiltrative liver diseases, abscesses, granulomatous liver disease and amyloidosis. Low levels of alkaline phosphatase can occur in hypothyroidism, pernicious anemia, zinc deficiency and congenital hypophosphatasia.

Gamma-glutamyl Transpeptidase

Gamma-glutamyl transpeptidase (GGT) is a membrane bound glycoprotein and normal value ranges between 0 and 30 IU/L. Elevated serum level is due to overproduction and leakage into blood. In addition to liver, the enzyme is also expressed in the kidney, spleen, pancreas, heart, lung and brain except bones and therefore, useful in the exclusion of bone diseases. The newborns may have high levels of GGT 5–8 times the upper limit of normal. One should also remember that this enzyme is inducible by certain drugs such as anticonvulsants and depressed by female sex hormones.

Serum GGT is high in all cholestatic disorders and cannot differentiate between intrahepatic and extrahepatic causes. Low levels of GGT is found in certain cholestatic disorders like progressive familial intrahepatic cholestasis (PFIC) types I and II and inborn errors of bile acid metabolism where GGT has been useful to differentiate these conditions from other causes of cholestasis.

Other Enzymes

Other enzymes to detect cholestasis are 5'-nucleotidase and leucine-aminopeptidase; but are not put to use commonly.

Enzymes like glutamate dehydrogenase, isocitrate dehydrogenase, lactate dehydrogenase and sorbitol dehydrogenase have also been found to be raised in hepatocellular necrosis but have not been found to be clinically significant.

The factors mentioned in **Flow chart 8.1.1,** are to be considered whenever you approach a child with elevated liver enzymes irrespective of the presence or absence of symptoms.

VIRAL HEPATITIS MARKERS

Viral hepatitis is a common form of liver disease. It is caused by a diverse group of hepatotropic agents that lead to liver inflammation and cell death. Five hepatitis viruses have been well-characterized: hepatitis A (HAV), B (HBV), C (HCV), D (HDV), and E (HEV). Other viruses that cause hepatitis include cytomegalovirus (CMV), Epstein-Barr virus (EBV), and human immunodeficiency virus (HIV). Hepatitis may also be due to other diseases or medications.

Flow chart 8.1.1: Interpretation of altered liver enzymes

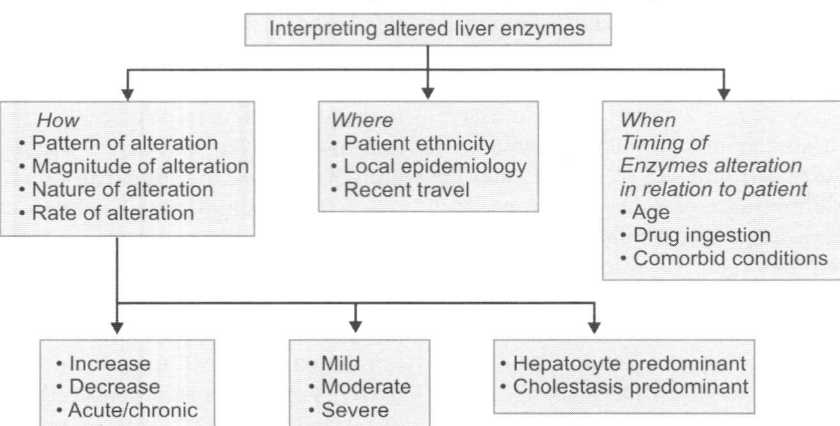

Clinical manifestations vary widely between different forms of viral hepatitis. HAV infection manifests as acute or asymptomatic disease; has no chronic carrier state and seldom causes serious sequelae although some patients may develop acute fulminant liver failure. HBV, HCV, and HDV infections can also cause asymptomatic or acute infection, but often establish chronic infection resulting in significant morbidity and mortality. Chronic infection with HBV or HCV may lead to liver cirrhosis and hepatocellular carcinoma (HCC). HDV is a "defective" virus in that it can replicate only in the presence of HBV infection. **Table 8.1.3** provides a short summary of the clinical spectrum of various types of viral hepatitis.

Diagnosis of Viral Hepatitis

- *Serologic tests* include immunoassays for antibodies and antigens. Reference levels are available to assess the presence and severity of infection, immune status, disease status and the need for treatment.
- *Nucleic acid-based tests* including real-time polymerase chain reaction (PCR) and transcription-mediated amplification (TMA), are used to detect viremia (confirm infection or document resolution of infection) and measure viral load (assess prognosis, need for treatment and treatment response).
- *Genotyping tests* including hybridization and sequencing-based assays are used to determine HBV subtype (for epidemiological purposes) and HCV genotype (to assess prognosis and inform treatment decisions) and also to identify the presence of HBV or HCV mutations associated with resistance to antiviral agents.

Being commonly used, only serologic tests are elaborated in detail here. Multiple tests may be required to appropriately characterize an individual's viral hepatitis infection. **Tables 8.1.4** and **8.1.5** summarize the use and interpretation of some of the major serologic and molecular tests available for diagnosis and disease management.

Diagnosis of Chronic Hepatitis

Early diagnosis of chronic hepatitis is relevant with reference to hepatitis B and C and one should remember that hepatitis C is chronic at diagnosis and acute hepatitis C is virtually not known.

Hepatitis B

Table 8.1.6 summarizes the interpretation of various hepatitis B markers used in the diagnosis of chronic hepatitis B infection.

Table 8.1.3: Clinical spectrum of viral hepatitis

Virus	*Transmission route*	*Incubation period*	*Mortality*	*Likelihood of carrier state*	*Likelihood of chronic disease*	*Associated with HCC*
HAV	Fecal-oral	2–6 wk	1%	None	None	No
HBV	Parenteral, perinatal, sexual	4–26 wk	1–2% (3,000/yr)	10% (adults) 90% (infants)	1–10%	Yes
HCV	Parenteral, perinatal, possibly sexual	2–23 wk	1–5% (12,000/yr)	50%-80%	80–90%	Yes
HDV	Parenteral, sexual, perinatal	6–26 wk	2–20%	Variable	80% in superinfection	Yes
HEV	Fecal-oral	2–9 wk	1%	Rare	Rare	No

Abbreviations: HAV, hepatitis A virus; HBV, hepatitis B virus; HCV, hepatitis C virus; HDV, hepatitis D virus, HEV, hepatitis E virus; HCC, hepatocellular carcinoma.

Table 8.1.4: Available markers and interpretation of Individual test results in the diagnosis of acute and chronic viral hepatitis*

Marker	*Interpretation*
HAV	
HAV IgM	A reactive result indicates current or recent infection
	A negative result indicates absence of infection
HAV total Ab	The presence of total HAV antibody in the absence of HAV IgM antibody indicates immunity against HAV infection
HBV	
HBsAg	A reactive result indicates that a person has HBV infection and is infectious
HBcAb, Total	Presence indicates past or present HBV infection
HBcIgM	Presence usually indicates HBV infection within the preceding 4–6 months (i.e. acute infection)
HBeAb	Presence indicates resolving infection or response to therapy
HBsAb	Presence indicates recovery and immunity against HBV infection
HBV DNA	Presence indicates active infection
HDV	
HDV Ab, Total	Reactive results, coincident with the presence of HBsAg indicate past or current HBV/HDV coinfection or superinfection
HDV IgM	Reactive results coincident with the presence of HBsAg indicate past or current HBV/HDV coinfection or superinfection
	Negative results in the presence of positive HDV total antibody indicates resolved infection
HCV	
HCV Ab	Reactive antibody results (with confirmatory HCV RNA results) indicate active infection
	False-positive HCV antibody results may occur in cases of alcoholic liver disease, autoimmune chronic active hepatitis, or improper sample storage and testing conditions
HCV RNA	Positive results indicate current infection
	A negative result indicates absence of current infection

Note: *Interpretation of viral markers for hepatitis E is similar to hepatitis A, hence not separately mentioned.

Table 8.1.5: Interpretation of serologic and nucleic acid testing for acute viral hepatitis

Hepatitis virus	*HAV IgM*	*HBsAg*	*HBV DNA*	*HBc IgM*	*HBc Total*	*HCV Ab*	*HCV RNA*	*HDV Ab*	*HDV RNA*
A	+	–	–	–	–	–	–	–	–
B	–	+	+	+	–	–	–	–	–
B with D coinfection	–	+	+	+	–	–	–	+	+
B with D superinfection	–	+	+	–	–	–	–	+	+
C	–	–	–	–	–	+	+	–	–

Table 8.1.6: Interpretation of hepatitis B markers in chronic hepatitis B

Marker	*HBV Infection status*						
	Susceptible	*Successful vaccination*	*Resolved (Immune)*	*Acute (Early)*	*Acute (Resolving)*	*Chronic (Low infectivity)*[a]	*Chronic (High infectivity)*
HBsAg	–	–	–	+	+	+	+
HBc Total Ab	–	–	+	+	+	+	+
HBV DNA	–	–	–[b]	+	-[b]	±	+
HBcIgMAb	–	–	–	+	±	–	–
HBeAg[c]	–	–	–	+	±	–	?
HBeAb[c]	–	–	+	–	±	±	–
HBsAb	–	+	+	–	–	–	–

[a] Includes inactive HBsAg carrier state.
[b] Very low levels may be detected with highly sensitive assays.
[c] In mutant HBV infection, HBeAg is absent and HBeAb may test positive even when HBV DNA is positive.

Hepatitis D

Nonreactive hepatitis D virus (HDV) antibody results are consistent with absence of HDV infection. Presence of HDV IgG and IgM is consistent with current or past HDV coinfection or superinfection. HDV IgG and IgM levels are typically high and long-lasting in chronic HDV infection. HDV IgM tends to disappear with resolution of infection while HDV IgG persists. Thus, negative HDV IgM in a patient with positive total antibody results indicate resolved HDV infection. Positive HDV RNA results in patients with HDV antibodies indicate active infection, whereas negative results indicate resolved infection.

Hepatitis C

Nonreactive hepatitis C virus (HCV) antibody results indicate absence of infection. However, individuals with suspected recent exposure (<6 months previously) should either receive HCV RNA testing or undergo follow-up antibody testing. HCV RNA testing might also be considered for immunocompromised individuals. Reactive HCV antibody results need to be confirmed with HCV RNA testing (or an alternate method). Positive HCV RNA results are consistent with current infection and negative results indicate absence of current infection. In patients with reactive antibody results who are negative for HCV RNA, repeat HCV RNA testing can be considered if the patient has suspected recent (<6 months) exposure or clinically suspected hepatitis.

MOLECULAR ASSAYS

Both quantitative and qualitative assays are available for HCV RNA and HBV DNA. For the assay plasma or serum must be separated from cells within 6 hours and plasma can be stored at 4°C for several days or –70°C for long-term. Results of different assays may (HBV) or may not (HCV) be interchangeable. Quantitation of RNA or DNA may be reported as copies/mL or IU/mL. Conversion factor for copies/mL to IU/mL is not the same for different assays measuring the same target or different targets. Coefficient of variation (COV) may range from 15 to 50%.

HBV DNA

This is useful in routine monitoring on therapy to assess response to treatment every 3 months while on oral agents; and monthly for the initial 6–12 months while on interferon therapy; and also useful in the diagnosis of occult HBV infection (absence of markers but DNA positive).

HCV RNA

It is used for monitoring treatment and in some circumstances for confirmation of positive or indeterminate serology. HCV RNA is detectable 2–14 days after an exposure.

Genotyping

Genotyping of isolates for epidemiological purposes categorizes patient isolates into 8 different HBV genotypes (A to H) and 6 different HCV genotypes (1–6 with 24 subtypes) and useful in identifying treatment responders and resistance to treatment.

CONCLUSION

- Liver enzymes to a certain extent guide in the diagnosis and work-up of patients with suspected liver diseases.
- Serology still remains the cornerstone for diagnosis and screening for viral hepatitis and molecular assays are more important in the monitoring during treatment.

BIBLIOGRAPHY

1. American Gastroenterological Association. American Gastroenterological Association medical position statement: evaluation of liver chemistry tests. Gastroenterology. 2002; 123:1364-6.
2. Centers for Disease Control and Prevention. Surveillance for viral hepatitis-United States, 2012. *http://www.cdc.gov/hepatitis/Statistics/2012Surveillance/Commentary.htm.* Updated January 5, 2015. Accessed July 15, 2015.
3. Friedman SF, Martin P, Munoz JS. Laboratory evaluation of the patient with liver disease. Hepatology, A Textbook Of Liver Disease. Philadelphia; Saunders. 2003;1:661-709.
4. Government of British Columbia, Ministry of Health Services. (2005, May). Guidelines and Protocols Advisory Committee. Viral Hepatitis Testing. Retrieved from *http://www.bcguidelines.ca/gpac/pdf/vihep.pdf*
5. Green RM, Flamm S. AGA technical review of evaluation of liver chemistry tests. Gastroenterology. 2002;123:1367-84.
6. Reichling JJ, Kaplan MM. Clinical use of serum enzymes in liver disease. Dig Dis Sci. 1988;33:1601-14.

8.2 Stool Examination and Cracking Malabsorption Syndromes

Sumathi Bavanandam, P Thirumal

Reviewers: *PSN Menon, Alok Gupta, R Remesh Kumar*

INTRODUCTION

Malabsorption is a condition where there is defective absorption of nutrients which can be due to small bowel, pancreatic, hepatobiliary or gastric disorders. The tests for malabsorption depend upon on signs and symptoms, as well as epidemiological and ethnic background of the affected children. The panel of diagnostic tests to be ordered rests on the clinical suspicion of the underlying cause. Initial evaluation should be done with noninvasive, inexpensive tests called *screening* tests and then proved by *confirmatory* tests.

HISTORY AND CLINICAL EXAMINATION

A good history with thorough physical examination remains the first and essential step in tackling malabsorption. Carbohydrate malabsorption is suspected in children with history of abdominal bloat, discomfort and borborygmi (a rumbling sound heard along with passage of loose watery and frothy stools). Fat malabsorption is suspected when there is sticky oily stool with liquidity in small bowel disease or frank oily bulky stool in pancreatic disease. Protein-losing enteropathy is suspected if there is pedal edema, facial puffiness or anasarca along with anemia and multivitamin deficiencies. The common causes of malabsorption are listed in **Table 8.2.1**.

STOOL EXAMINATION

Stool should be examined macroscopically and microscopically along with chemical and microbiological tests (**Table 8.2.2**).

Freshly passed stool should be examined for pH, fat globules, and microbiological tests. Special stains are needed to look for organisms. Laxatives, antimotility agents and cholestyramine are to be avoided.

Table 8.2.1: Common causes of malabsorption in children

Age group	*Common etiologies*
Infants and children below 3 years	Lactose intolerance Giardiasis Cow's milk protein allergy Celiac disease Immunodeficiency states Hepatobiliary diseases
Older children	Giardiasis Cryptosporidiosis Strongyloidiasis Intestinal tuberculosis Celiac disease Pancreatic disorders Inflammatory bowel disorders HIV enteropathy Hepatobiliary disorders Short gut syndrome

Table 8.2.2: Stool tests in malabsorption

Macroscopy	Should look for blood; appearance (oily, frothy, or bulky); and foul smell
Microscopy	Should look for trophozoites of *Giardia lamblia,* oocysts of *Cryptosporidium parvum*, larvae of *Strongyloides stercoralis,* sheets of pus cells, exudates and fungal hyphae
Chemistry	Should test for pH, reducing substances, occult blood, fat globules, calprotectin Alpha-1 antitrypsin (A1AT) clearance for protein-losing enteropathy

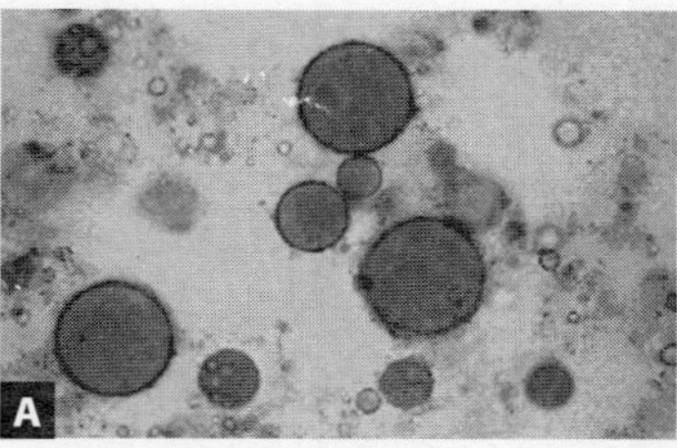
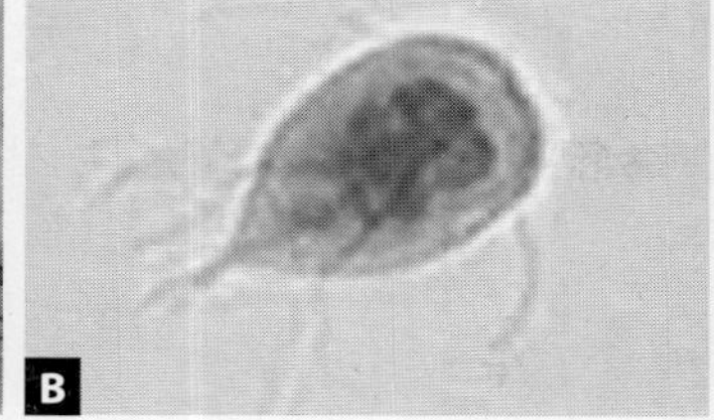
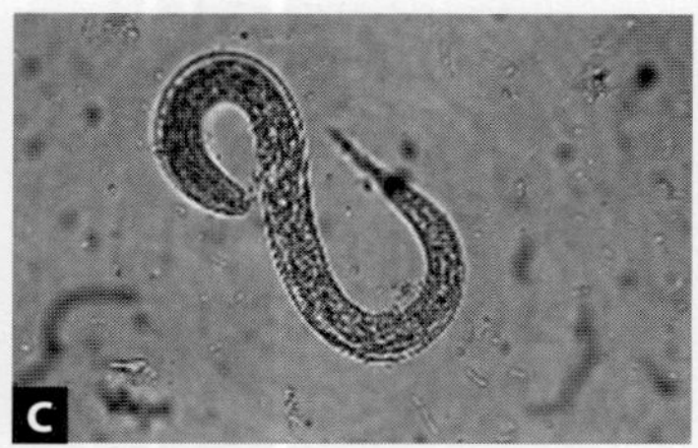

Figs 8.2.1A to C: Stool examination. (A) Stool fat globules; (B) *Giardia lamblia* trophozoite in stool; (C) Strongyloides stercoralis larva (*For color version, see Plate 6*)

Blood and mucus in stool occur in Crohn's colitis, intestinal tuberculosis, eosinophilic enterocolitis and lymphoma involving the intestines. Positive fecal occult blood indicates mucosal ulcerations of gut due to various causes. Stool should be examined for giardia trophozoites, strongyloides larva, Cryptococcus oocyst and isosporiasis, one of which can be the cause of malabsorption (**Figs 8.2.1A to C**). Acidic pH and presence of reducing substances indicate carbohydrate malabsorption such as lactose intolerance. Elevated fecal calprotectin indicates mucosal inflammation and is used in follow-up of patients with inflammatory bowel disease. Stool alpha-1 antitrypsin clearance is used for diagnosing protein-losing enteropathy.

Stool Fat Tests

Stool fat tests can be qualitative or quantitative. Fecal fat excretion of less than 7 g/day with a fat intake of 100 g/day is usually considered normal in a normal individual whereas in children with diarrhea up to 14 g/day is taken as normal. Qualitative tests are generally used more in clinical practice. More than 100 fat globules with less than 4 mm diameter per high power field is abnormal indicating fat malabsorption with a sensitivity of 78% and a specificity of 70% for the detection of steatorrhea. Acid steatocrit is another semi-quantitative test. Van de Kamer method of fat analysis is considered the gold standard. Fatty acid equivalents are expressed as fecal output of fat in grams per 24 hours, i.e. quantitative fat analysis; but they are cumbersome requiring 48–72 hours of stool collection with 80–100 g of fat intake. It cannot, however, differentiate among biliary, pancreatic and enteric causes of malabsorption.

BLOOD TESTS

Complete Blood Counts

Complete blood counts (CBC) are useful to look for anemia and type of anemia.

- Presence of microcytic hypochromic anemia (**Fig. 8.2.2A**) is suggestive of iron deficiency which can be due to reduced absorption in small bowel disease or due to chronic blood loss from the gut.
- Macrocytic anemia (**Fig. 8.2.2B**) indicates deficiency of vitamin B_{12} or folate which can occur due to terminal ileal disease or folate deficiency.
- Presence of acanthocytes (**Fig. 8.2.2C**) indicates abetalipoproteinemia, excess eosinophils suggest food allergy.
- Lymphopenia is common in intestinal lymphangiectasia.

ESR and CRP

Elevated erythrocyte sedimentation rate (ESR) and C-reactive protein (CRP) indicates disease activity in Crohn's disease which can result in malabsorption.

Blood Biochemistry

- *Blood sugar* in children with diabetes mellitus and diarrhea, malabsorption and in celiac disease.
- *Liver function tests (LFTs):* Increased levels of serum bilirubin, transaminases, and alkaline phosphatase indicate hepatobiliary cause of malabsorption.

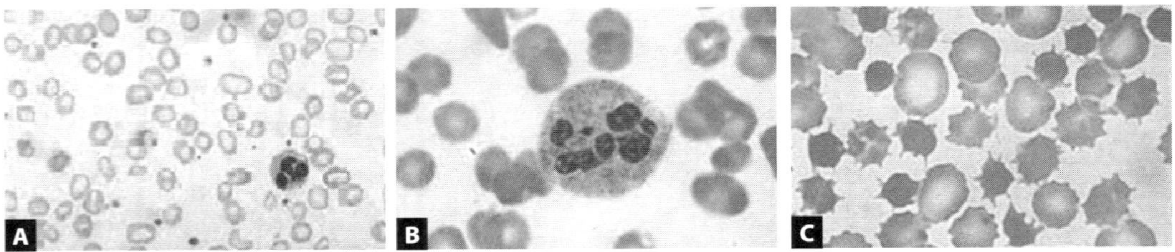

Figs 8.2.2A to C: Peripheral blood smear study. (A) Hypochromic microcytic anemia; (B) Macrocytic anemia; (C) Acanthocytes (*For color version, see Plate 6*)

Table 8.2.3: The interpretation of Schilling test

Abnormality	*Stage 1 (B_{12})*	*Stage 2 (Supplementation of intrinsic factor, IF)*	*Stage 3 (Supplementation of pancreatic enzymes)*	*Stage 4 (Administration of antibiotics)*
Vitamin B_{12} malabsorption	Decreased			
Pernicious anemia	Decreased	Normal		
Chronic pancreatitis	Decreased	Decreased	Normal	
Small intestinal bacterial overgrowth (SIBO)	Decreased	Decreased	Decreased	Normal
Terminal ileal resection	Decreased	Decreased	Decreased	Decreased

- Reduced zinc level and alkaline phosphatase indicate zinc deficiency.
- Reduced serum albumin indicates protein-losing enteropathy.
- Low serum levels of vitamin D_3, calcium, triglycerides and cholesterol indicate fat malabsorption whereas low levels of folate, iron and albumin indicate malabsorption of water soluble vitamins due to small bowel mucosal diseases.
- *Serological studies:* Serum tissue trans-glutaminase assay of IgG and IgA— serum IgA levels are useful screening tests for celiac disease.
- *Immunoglobulin profile* is used in suspected primary immune deficiency disorders involving small bowel.
- *Retroviral screening* is advisable in children with opportunistic infections of the gut.

SCHILLING TEST

Schilling test (urine) is used to distinguish between gastric, pancreatic and ileal causes of vitamin B_{12} deficiency. The test is performed by administering small oral dose of radiolabeled vitamin B_{12}. Simultaneously or within 1–2 hours, intramuscular dose of nonradiolabeled vitamin B_{12} is given. If urine has less than 7–10% of orally administered dose of radiolabeled B_{12}, it is indicative of vitamin B_{12} malabsorption. To identify the site of malabsorption, second phase of the study is done with oral administration of intrinsic factor. If the levels are normalized, it suggests intrinsic factor deficiency as in pernicious anemia whereas normalization after pancreatic enzyme supplementation indicates a pancreatic cause. Correction after administration of antibiotics indicates small intestinal bacterial overgrowth (SIBO) as the cause of malabsorption as detailed in **Table 8.2.3**.

RADIOLOGICAL TESTS

- *X-ray chest:* It can indirectly give a clue for tuberculosis.
- *X-ray abdomen:* Calcification on abdominal X-ray indicates chronic pancreatitis.
- *Barium contrast studies:* Flocculation of barium, mucosal edema and intestinal hurry indicate malabsorption. Apart from

strictures, dilated bowel loops and diverticula can be identified (See Chapter 8.5 for more details).

ENDOSCOPY

- *Gross appearance:* Gross inspection of the duodenal mucosa can provide clues to some causes of malabsorption such as:
  - Presence of aphthae suggests Crohn's disease
  - Small, diffuse, white, punctate lesions suggest lymphangiectasia.
  - Reduced folds with scalloping of duodenal folds are highly suggestive of villous atrophy in celiac disease, although not specific (**Fig. 8.2.3**).
- *Small bowel biopsy* has diagnostic value in intestinal lymphangiectasia, abetalipoproteinemia, agammaglobulinemia, eosinophilic enteritis and Whipple's disease. Other diseases where biopsy is useful include celiac disease (**Figs 8.2.4A and B**), intestinal tuberculosis, Crohn's disease, immunoproliferative small intestinal disease, tropical sprue and lymphoma.
- *Aspiration:* Microscopy of the fluid aspirated from the descending part of the duodenum can locate presence of *Giardia lamblia.* The aspirated fluid can also be cultured to detect bacterial overgrowth in patients with suspected small intestinal bacterial overgrowth (SIBO).

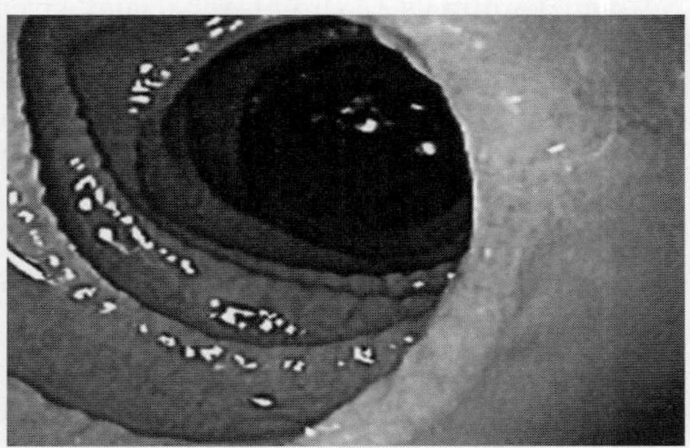

Fig. 8.2.3: Upper endoscopic view showing scalloping of duodenal folds (*For color version, see Plate 7*)

COLONOSCOPY WITH TERMINAL ILEOSCOPY WITH MUCOSAL BIOPSY

Colonoscopy with terminal ileoscopy with mucosal biopsy is useful in diagnosis of Crohn's disease, intestinal tuberculosis, lymphoma, eosinophilic enteritis (**Fig. 8.2.5**).

IMAGING STUDIES

- *Ultrasonography (USG) of abdomen and Doppler studies:* Altered liver echoes, dilated portal vein, dilated splenoportal axis and collaterals indicate portal hypertension as a cause of protein-losing enteropathy. Hepatosplenomegaly, ascites, nodal mass and bowel thickening can occur in tuberculosis and lymphoma. Pancreatic ductal dilatation with or without calcification is suggestive of chronic pancreatitis.

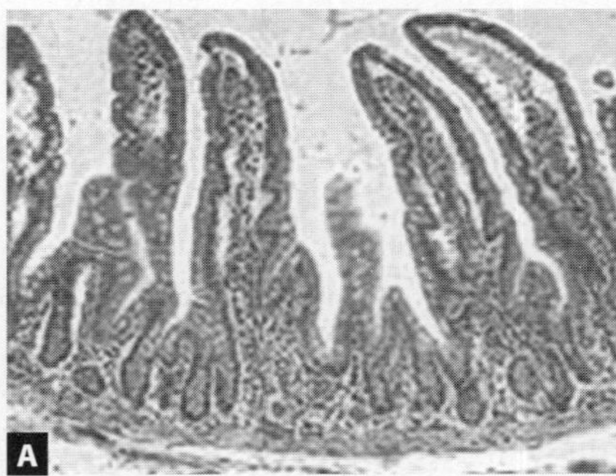

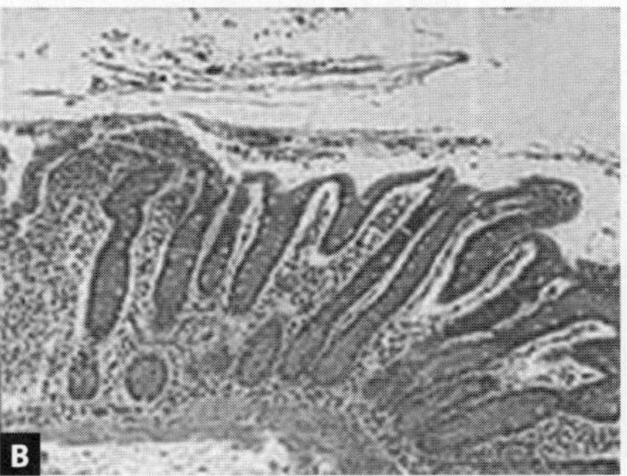

Figs 8.2.4A and B: Small bowel histology showing normal and mucosal changes in celiac disease. (A) Normal mucosa; (B) Celiac disease (*For color version, see Plate 7*)

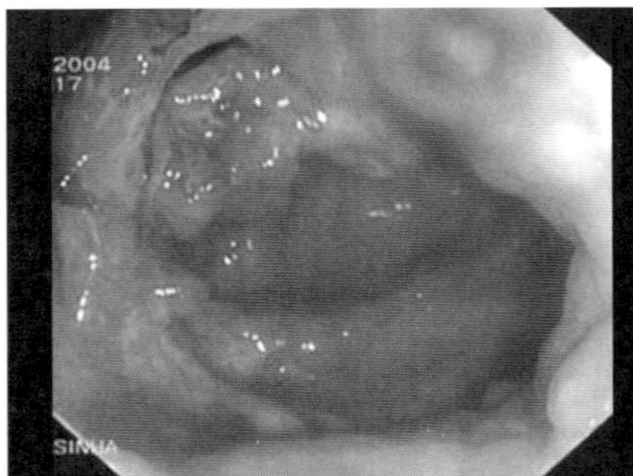

Fig. 8.2.5: Colonoscopy showing ulcer and nodularity of ileum (*For color version, see Plate 7*)

- *Computed tomographic (CT) enterography or magnetic resonance (MR) enterography* can identify mucosal changes earlier in Crohn's disease as well pick-up complications like fistulae. They are also useful in the diagnosis of tuberculosis and lymphoma.

SPECIALIZED TESTS

Hydrogen breath tests and capsule endoscopy are beyond the scope of this chapter as they are to be done in specialized pediatric gastroenterology centers with technical expertise.

CONCLUSION

Malabsorption is not uncommon in children. A good clinical history and thorough physical examination are essential to tailor the investigations towards a diagnosis of the etiology of malabsorption. Baseline tests like stool examination and complete hemogram offer valuable information. Endoscopy with intestinal biopsy is useful and diagnostic in certain diseases and should be planned accordingly. Imaging studies and highly specialized tests may be required in some situations.

BIBLIOGRAPHY

1. Bhatnagar B, Gautam R, Srivastava G, Khan KA, Thakur S. Chronic diarrhea in North Indian children: a widening etiological spectrum. Int J Contemp Pediatr. 2014;1(1):37-41.
2. Hogenauer C, Hammer HF. Maldigestion and Malabsorption, Chapter 89. In: Feldman M, Friedman LS, Sleisenger MH, (eds). Sleisenger and Fordtran's Gastrointestinal and Liver Disease, 7th edn. Philadelphia; Saunders Publishers. 2002.pp.1751-82.
3. Yachha SK, Mishra S, Malik AK, Nagi B, Mehta S. Spectrum of malabsorption syndrome in North Indian children. Indian J Gastroenterol. 1993;12(4):120-5.

8.3 Constipation

Sumathi Bavanandam

***Reviewers:** K Nedunchelian, Jaydeep Choudhury, RV Dhakshayani*

INTRODUCTION

Constipation is a common problem in toddlers and preschool children with equal frequency in boys and girls. Most common cause of constipation is functional (97%). Good history, thorough physical examination and a rectal examination are adequate for diagnosis of functional constipation. When the presentation is atypical and there is a failure of response to treatment, one has to rule out organic causes of constipation. Treatment of functional constipation consists of laxatives, dietary modification and bowel training.

DEFINITION

Constipation has been defined as "delay or difficulty in defecation, present for two or more weeks, sufficient enough to cause significant distress to the patient". It is also defined by the occurrence of any of the following characteristics, independent of stool frequency- passage of hard, scybalous, pebble like, or cylindrical cracked stools; straining or painful defecation; passage of large stools that may clog the toilet; or stool frequency less than thrice per week except in breastfed infants.

EPIDEMIOLOGY

Twenty five percent of the pediatric gastroenterology consultations are for children with constipation requiring further evaluation. Worldwide, 0.3–28% of children are constipated. Up to a third of children aged 6–12 years report constipation during any given year.

CAUSES OF CONSTIPATION (Table 8.3.1)

"*Functional constipation*" is the one, where no anatomical, physiological or pathological causes could be identified, and it is the most common cause of constipation. Some of the organic causes of constipation include Hirschsprung's disease, pseudo-obstruction, spinal cord abnormality, hypothyroidism, congenital anorectal malformations diabetes insipidus, cystic fibrosis, gluten enteropathy, etc. **Table 8.3.2** illustrates the differences between functional and organic constipation.

PATHOGENESIS OF FUNCTIONAL CONSTIPATION

Normal bowel continence is maintained by internal anal sphincter (under involuntary control), which relaxes on rectal distension, external anal sphincter (under voluntary control), which maintains the tonic state of contraction and puborectalis muscle which maintains anorectal angle of 85–100°.

Idiopathic/Functional constipation often starts as a painful bowel movement due to any reason which makes the child withhold stools in fear of pain during bowel movement, making this vicious cycle, since withholding stools makes the stool even harder and more painful subsequent bowel movement resulting in incomplete evacuation and chronic constipation. Other factors like genetic, dietary habits, especially low intake of fiber in the diet and disturbances of intestinal motility may play a role in causation and perpetuation of functional constipation. A change from human milk to cow's milk or cow's milk to soya-based formula may lead to firmer stools and hence painful bowel movements in infantile constipation. In functional constipation, the child responds to the urge to defecate by voluntarily contracting the external anal sphincter and gluteal muscles to withhold stools and avoid pain of defecation. Child often adopts various postures including standing with legs crossed and straining, to hold stools- referred to as 'fecal withholding', or 'functional fecal retention'. In due course, this will lead to inhibition of reflex defecation and reduced rectal movement and the rectum will be filled with hard stool and fecal soiling follows. One-third of children with functional constipation present with encoperesis. This leads to frustration, decreased self-esteem, depression, loss of coping skills, anxiety and other affective disturbances.

Table 8.3.1: Causes of constipation

Causes	*Conditions*
Idiopathic	Functional (95–97%)
Anal lesions and congenital anorectal malformations	Anal fissure, anteriorly placed anus, anal stenosis
Neurological disorders	Hirschsprung disease Spinal cord abnormalities: myelomeningocele, spina bifida, cerebral palsy, tethered cord
Endocrine/metabolic	Hypothyroidism, hypercalcemia, hypokalemia, diabetes insipidus, diabetes mellitus
Drugs	Anticonvulsants, heavy-metal (lead) poisoning, antidiarrheals, antipsychotic agents
Miscellaneous	Prune belly syndrome, Down syndrome, cystic fibrosis, CMP allergy, connective tissue disorders, tumors

Table 8.3.2: Comparison of functional fecal retention and Hirschsprung's disease

Symptom	*Functional fecal retention*	*Hirschsprung's disease*
Delayed meconium passage	Rarely	60%
Constipation in newborn	Rarely	Almost always
Failure to thrive	Uncommon	Possible
Enterocolitis	None	Possible
Onset after age 2 years	Common	Sometimes
Abdominal distension	Rare	Common
Fecal incontinence	Common	Almost never
Difficult bowel training	Common	Rare
Avoidance of toilet	Common	Rare
Withholding behavior	Common	Rare
Stool in rectal ampulla	Common	Rare
Fissure	Common	Rare
Obstructive symptoms	Rare	Common
Transition zone on X-ray view	Absent	Present
Aganglionosis on biopsy	Absent	Present

Red Flag Signs and Symptoms

Fever, abdominal distension, anorexia, nausea, vomiting, weight loss, blood in the stools, poor weight gain, anemia, hypotonia, anal dimple, pilonidal sinus, areflexia, absent anal reflux.

When to Suspect Functional Constipation?

Functional constipation to be suspected in preschool children with history of infrequent stools, prolonged defecation, abnormal posturing, painful act of defecation, withholding of stools, soiling of undergarments and fecal impaction, especially in older children.

Laboratory Tests

Laboratory investigations are not required to diagnose functional constipation and are rarely required. Plain X-ray skiagram of abdomen may pick-up fecal impaction in those children where per-rectal examination is not possible. 30% of childhood constipation is associated with urinary tract infection and a urine culture may be required.

Role of Barium Contrast Study

A barium enema in an unprepared colon will demonstrate a transition zone in a case of Hirschsprung disease and is also useful when other anatomic abnormalities such as a colonic or rectal stricture are suspected.

SPECIALIZED INVESTIGATIONS

Specialized investigations are not needed to diagnose functional constipation. In those children where there is no or poor response, despite good compliance with adequate dose and duration of laxative therapy, before ordering further tests, pediatric gastrointestinal consult is required. Radiopaque marker study is useful in children with refractory constipation and segmental colonic transit evaluation, especially in refractory constipation. Anal manometry, full thickness rectal biopsies are useful in Hirschsprung's disease. Endorectal USG, MRI spine and pelvis are some of the investigations that may be rarely required in some children with refractory constipation.

Table 8.3.3: Laxatives

S. No.	Drug	Dosage	Side effects
1.	Lactulose	1–3 mL/kg/day, 1–2 doses. Adjust dosage to response seen	Abdominal cramps, flatulance
2.	Milk of magnesia	1–3 mL/kg/day,1–2 doses. Adjust dose to response seen	Over dose—hypermagnesemia, hypophosphatemia, hypocalcemia
3.	Sorbitol	1–3 mL/kg/day,1–2 doses	Abdominal cramps, flatulance
4.	Mineral oil (Liquid Paraffin)	Disimpaction 15–30 mL/year of age. (max 240 mL) Maintenance— 1–3 mL/kg/day	Lipoid pneumonia
5.	PEG (Poly Ethylene Glycol)	Disimpaction—25 mL/kg/hour Maintenance—5–10 mL/kg/day or 0.5–1 g/kg/day	Nausea, bloating, cramps, vomiting, anal irritation
6.	Senna syrup	8.8 g sennoside/5 mL 2–5 years: 2.5–7.5 mL/day in two divided dosages. 6–12 years 5–15 mL/day in two divided dosages (Tablets and granules available)	Idiosyncratic hepatitis, melanosis coli, hypertrophic osteoarthropathy, analgesic nephropathy, abdominal cramping. Melanosis coli improves after medication is stopped
7.	Bisacodyl	5 mg tablets, 1–3 tablets/dosage 1–2 times daily 10 mg suppositories, 0.5–1 suppository, 1–2 times daily	Abdominal cramping, diarrhea, hypokalemia

MANAGEMENT

Constipation due to functional etiology is the most common type seen is clinical practice. Treatment consist of stool disimpaction, prevention of further stool retention, promotion of regular bowel habits, dietary advice, psychosocial support and close follow-up.

Disimpaction

Whenever child has a loaded rectum, disimpaction is indicated which can be achieved via oral or by rectal route. Usually oral administration of medication is better than the rectal route as this is noninvasive and is not associated with discomfort or pain. Rectal administration of drug usually causes discomfort to children, making stool retention worse. Polyethelene glycol (PEG) is ideal for oral disimpaction. The dose is 20 mL/kg/hr for four hours and can be repeated the next day if necessary which can be given orally or by nasogastric tube (25 mL/kg/hr) or at a dose of 1-1.5 g/kg/day for 3-6 days. Phosphate enema, glycerin suppositories may be used rectally.

Maintenance Therapy

Once the impacted feces is disimpacted and evacuated, further treatment should aim to prevent fecal reimpaction by maintenance therapy with laxatives **(Table 8.3.3)**, dietary modifications, bowel training and close follow-up. In general, the dosage of drugs used depend on the response and need to be modified constantly based upon the nature of the stools with adequate duration of therapy.

Dietary Modification

Children with functional constipation should be advised to consume diet rich in fiber and the recommended amount of daily dietary fiber for all children is equal to 5 g plus the child's age in years. Fruits like apple, pear and prune juices that contain nonabsorbable carbohydrates like sorbitol are helpful. Fluid intake should be encouraged. The diet should contain whole grains, fresh fruits and vegetables rich in fiber.

Toilet Training

This is possible after 2–3 years of age. Child should be encouraged to sit in the toilet for

Flow chart 8.3.1: Algorithm approach for management of childhood constipation

Constipation

No red flag signs (functional)

- Fecal impaction present
- Adequate disimpaction followed by maintenance laxatives, diet, training

- No fecal impaction Maintenance laxative, diet, toilet training

Red flag signs present (Organic)

Needs GI consult for further evaluation

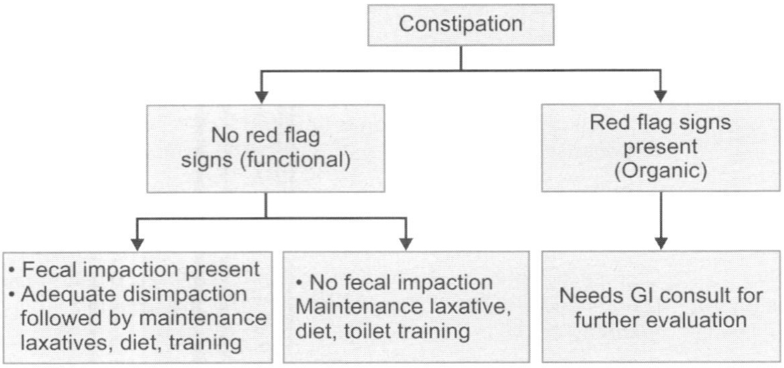

Abbreviation: GI, gastrointestinal

5–10 minutes, 3–4 times per day immediately after meals for initial few months, regularly. The gastrocolic reflex that occurs after meals can be made use of, to ease the bowel movement. Child should be rewarded whenever there is no fecal soiling as this will act as a positive reinforcement and provide psychological support to these children. Re-education is an important part of bowel training. Child should be advised not to strain excessively and never to ignore/suppress the urge to defecate.

OUTCOME

In studies on functional constipation, recovery is defined as greater than three stools per week with no soiling. However, the response depends on age of onset and associated encoperesis. Approximately two-thirds of cases of functional constipation need laxative therapy for months to years and the rest require even longer term treatment. Significant number may continue to have constipation into adulthood. In one study, 52% of children with constipation and encopresis, the symptoms persisted even after five years of treatment. Clayden has shown that 22% of children required laxatives for less than 6 months, 44% for less than 12 months, and the rest for more than 12 months.

FOLLOW-UP

The successful management of functional constipation in childhood depends on close follow-up, till normal bowel movement is achieved, followed by review every two to three months for the next 2 years and then yearly thereafter.

SUMMARY

Functional constipation is the most common cause of constipation in children. Good history and thorough physical examination including per rectal (PR) are all that is needed for a diagnosis of functional constipation. Laxative therapy is usually needed for several months and early withdrawal of therapy leads to relapse. Effective treatment depends on (a) child and family education, (b) adequate disimpaction and (c) maintenance phase which includes behavioral therapy, medication and dietary modification. Summary of approach to the management of childhood constipation is given in **Flow chart 8.3.1**.

BIBLIOGRAPHY

1. Baker SS, Liptak GS, Colletti RB, et al. Constipation in infants and children: evaluation and treatment. A medical position statement of the North American Society for Pediatric Gastroenterology and Nutrition. J Pediatr Gastroenterol Nutr. 1999;29:612-26.
2. Benninga MA, Voskuijl WP, Taminiau JA. Childhood constipation: Is there new light in the tunnel. J Pediatr Gastroenterol Nutr. 2004;39:448-64.

3. Biggs Ws, Dery WH. Evaluation and treatment of constipation in infants and children. Am Fam Phys. 2006;73:469-77.
4. Candy DCA, Edwards D. The management of chronic constipation. Current Paediatr. 2003;13: 101-6.
5. Clayden GS. Management of chronic constipation. Arch Dis Child. 1992;67:340-4.
6. Clinical Practice Guideline. Evaluation and treatment of constipation in infants and children: Recommendations of the North American Society for Pediatric Gastroenterology, Hepatology and Nutrition. J Pediatr Gastroenterol Nutr. 2006;43(3):e1-e13.
7. Croffie MJ. Constipation in children. Indian J Pediatr. 2006;73:697-701.
8. Di Lorenzo C. Pediatric anorectal disorders. Gastroenterol Clin North Am. 2001;30: 269-87.
9. Hyams J, Colletti R, Faure C, Gabriel-Martinez E, Maffei HV, Morais MB, et al. Functional gastrointestinal disorders J Pediatr Gastroenterol Nutr. 2002;35(suppl):110-7.
10. Loening-Baucke V. Prevalence, symptoms and outcome of constipation in infants and toddlers. J Pediatr. 2005;146:359-63.
11. Morais MB, Vítolo MR, Aguirre AN, Fagundes-Neto U. Measurement of low dietary fiber intake as a risk factor for chronic constipation in children, J Pediatr Gastroenterol Nutr. 1999;29:132-5.
12. Partin JC, Hamill SK, Fischel JE, Partin JS. Painful defecation and fecal soiling in children. Pediatrics. 1992;89(6 Pt 1):1007-9.
13. Position of the American Dietetic Association. Health implications of dietary fiber. J Am Diet Assoc. 1997;97(10):1157-9.
14. Soares AC, Lederman HM, Fagundes-Neto U, de Morais MB. Breath methane associated with slow colonic transit time in children with chronic constipation. J Clin Gastroenterol. 2005;39(6):512-5.
15. Staiano A, Andreotti MR, Greco L, Basile P, Auricchio S. Long-term follow-up of children with chronic idiopathic constipation. Dig Dis Sci. 1994;39:561-4.
16. Van den Berg, Maartje M, Benninga, Di Lorenzo C. Epidemiology of childhood constipation: a systematic review. Am J Gastroenterol. 2006; 101(10):2401-9.
17. Youssef NN, Di Lorenzo C. Childhood constipation: evaluation and treatment. J Clin Gastroenterol. 2001;33(3):199-205.

8.4 Neonatal Cholestasis Syndrome

B Bhaskar Raju

***Reviewers:** K Nedunchelian, Jaydeep Choudhury, RV Dhakshayani*

Neonatal cholestasis syndrome (NCS) is a heterogeneous disorder characterized clinically by jaundice, high colored urine staining the diapers, with or without pale stools, beyond 14 days of life. "Prolonged cholestasis of infancy" is the preferred terminology in infants who develop cholestasis within 90 days of life (serum direct bilirubin greater than 2 mg/dL or > 20% of total fraction).

Cholestasis can occur either due to hepatocellular or obstructive causes. In general cholestasis results from impairment in bile formation, impairment in bile secretion or impediment to bile flow. Cholestasis results in retention of substances that are normally excreted in bile, production of abnormal lipoproteins, defective absorption of fat and fat soluble vitamins, with resultant clinical manifestations. If left untreated, this eventually leads to end stage liver disease requiring liver transplantation. Treatment aims at alleviating the signs and symptoms of cholestasis by improving bile excretion and by prevention of malnutrition. Malnutrition, a common consequence of cholestasis, significantly increases morbidity and mortality and also transplant outcomes.

For some conditions, curative therapy may be available.

The treatment of cholestasis is broadly classified as *medical* and *surgical*.

MEDICAL THERAPY

Consists of:
- Definitive treatment
- Supportive treatment with choleretics
- Nutritional therapy
- Treatment of complications.

Definitive Therapy

Definite and possible curative therapy is available only for a few conditions presenting with cholestasis in infancy. They include:
- Cholestasis secondary to neonatal sepsis is often reversible and requires treatment with appropriate antibiotics for adequate duration.
- TPN-related cholestasis in the newborn can be prevented by using lipid solutions containing omega 3 fatty acids.
- Some forms of intrauterine infections are treatable, though not curable. They include intravenous ganciclovir for proven CMV infections (by blood/tissue PCR or by histological proof) and IV acyclovir for Herpes infection related cholestasis. Spiramycin/sulfadiazine/pyrimethamine combination is indicated for proven Toxoplasmosis (diagnosed by four-fold rise in antibody titer.)
- Thyroid replacement therapy for hypothyroidism-related cholestasis.
- NTBC (Nitisinone) long-term, may help in neonatal cholestasis due to tyrosinosis.
- Soy-based lactose-free milk will clear jaundice due to galactosemia.

Choleretic Therapy

Drugs can be used to improve bile flow in situations where there is intracellular cholestasis without physical blockage of bile pathways. Two drugs that are commonly used are:
- Ursodeoxycholic acid
- Phenobarbitone.

The reasons for necessitating treatment in cholestasis is summarized in **Flow chart 8.4.1**.

Ursodeoxycholic Acid

Ursodeoxycholic acid (UDCA) is a tertiary bile acid-not present in humans. It is a nontoxic, benign bile acid which, when consumed, is absorbed into portal circulation and excreted by hepatocytes into bile. In the process, it drags some water too along, improving bile volume and bile's capacity to excrete other substances. In other words, it enhances "bile acid dependent" bile flow. It also has inhibitory effect on cholesterol micelle formation and absorption, and hence used for treatment of cholesterol gallbladder stones.

Liver synthesizes bile acids, cholic acid and chenodeoxycholic acid through cytochrome P450 mediated oxidation of cholesterol. They are called primary bile acids. They are essential for micelle formation in the intestines and digestion of fats. In the raw form, they are mildly toxic to liver cells. Hence, they are rapidly conjugated and excreted through bile. In the intestine, bacterial action on primary bile acids produces deoxycholic and lithocholic acids both of which are very toxic to liver. In normal conditions, they are reabsorbed, re-enter hepatocytes, rapidly conjugated and excreted again, thereby preventing any damage to hepatocytes. In cholestasis however, delay

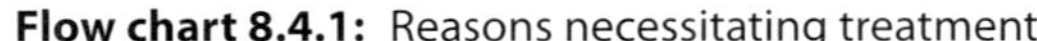
Flow chart 8.4.1: Reasons necessitating treatment

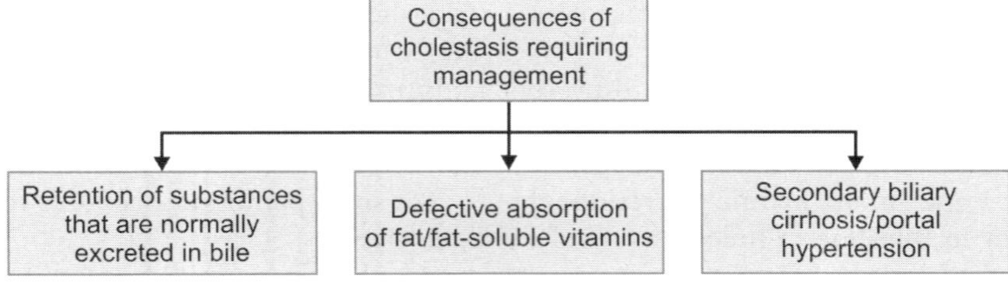

in excretion of these toxic bile acids and their accumulation in liver is the primary reason for severe hepatocellular damage that is seen in cholestasis of any etiology.

- UDCA, besides enhancing bile acid dependent bile flow, also reduces toxicity of secondary bile acids by suppressing their absorption through competitive inhibition in the ileum.
- Since UDCA is preferentially absorbed, the toxic bile acids levels are reduced in blood and in hepatocytes.
- UDCA is also known to be cyto-protective for hepatocytes. It reduces cell membrane damage and apoptosis.

UDCA is given in doses of 15–20 mg/kg/day in divided doses. It is available as 150 mg and 300 mg tablets and 125 mg/5 mL syrup.

Phenobarbitone

Phenobarbitone is a powerful cytochrome P450 stimulator and a multiple enzyme inducer. When given long-term, it results in upregulation of cytochrome 450 (CYP8B1) activity which in turn leads to increased excretion of electrolytes (Cl and HCO_3) and consequently water as well. This results in general increase in bile volume due to increase in "bile salt independent" bile flow, and opens up closed bile ducts.

Phenobarbitone is given in doses of 5 mg/kg/day. It is available as 30 mg tablets and 20 mg/5 mL syrup.

Nutritional Supplementation

Nutritional therapy is a vital part of management of NCS, since failure to thrive and nutritional deficiencies are extremely common in NCS. Failure to thrive negatively impacts success of Kasai/liver transplant in NCS, besides increasing general morbidity and mortality. Hence, this needs to be addressed at all costs.

Breast milk (directly suckled) is the best milk for babies with NCS. Since fat in breast milk (BM) is pre-emulsified, lack of bile salts will not affect fat absorption, when the baby is fed exclusively on BM. Hence, every attempt must be made to encourage exclusive breastfeeds in babies with NCS.

If child has no access to BM, he/she will need to be fed alternative milk, rich in medium chain triglycerides (MCT). Commercial infant formulas are available in the market with bulk of the fat provided as MCT (Simyl MCT) which may be used. Where the buying capacity is poor, the following high MCT milk may be used:

Skimmed milk	100 mL
Coconut oil	2 mL
Ground nut oil	1 mL

This has to be boiled for a few minutes and used. Coconut oil provides MCT and ground nut oil provides essential fatty acids which coconut oil lacks.

The nutritional aim in NCS is to provide 125% of daily requirement of calories, proteins, minerals (Fe, Ca, Mg, P) and water-soluble vitamins. Fat-soluble vitamins will need to be given in doses much higher than the recommended doses for children, in view of poor fat digestion in cholestasis.

The recommended oral doses of fat-soluble vitamins in NCS are:

- Vitamin A 2000–5000 IU/day
- Vitamin D_3 2000 IU/day
- Vitamin K 5 mg/weekly
- Vitamin E (TPGS) 15–25 IU/day

Oral preparations of the above may not always available everywhere and all may not be able to afford it. In such instances, all of the above vitamins (except Vit E) can be given parenterally at periodic intervals.

Other minerals requirement in NCS:

- Calcium 50–100 mg/kg/day
- Phosphorus 25–50 mg/kg/day
- Zinc 1 mg/kg/day
- Magnesium 1–2 mEq/kg/day
- Elemental iron 5–6 mg/kg/day.

Management of Hypercholesterolemia

Bile is the sole pathway of excretion of cholesterol and hence, any reduction or block in bile flow will result in accumulation of cholesterol in the body. While the type of cholesterol that accumulates, does not predispose to heart or vascular disease, children with persistent hypercholesterolemia do develop ugly xanthomas and xanthelasmas. Such children will need long-term drugs to reduce synthesis of cholesterol. Atorvastatin at 0.5 mg/day will help.

Treatment of Complications

Management of Pruritus

Pruritus is believed to be due to increase in levels of bile acids and related substances in blood. It becomes obvious once baby develops hand control. Management has to be multifaceted since it is an extremely difficult complication of NCS to treat.

Management of Pruritus Includes:

↓Levels of bile acids and related substances in blood by

↓Reabsorption of bile acids

↑Excretion of bile acids

Enterohepatic reabsorption of bile acids is a major factor in causation of both pruritus and liver damage.

Reabsorption of excreted bile acids can be reduced by cholestyramine 250 mg/kg/day or colestipol 200 mg/kg/day. They both are binding resins that bind bile acids excreted through bile and prevent reabsorption. UDCA too helps reduce reabsorption by competitively inhibiting their absorption. Receptors absorb UDCA preferentially.

Bile salt excretion can be increased by choleretics (already discussed) in intrahepatic cholestasis. In the presence of pruritus, rifampicin can be added since it is an enzyme inducer like phenobarbitone and works synergistically with it to increase bile salt independent bile flow.

↓Local inflammation and irritation at the level of nerve endings

This can be achieved with antihistamines, especially sedative antihistamines and emollients. Some studies have shown reduction in itching with steroids, but they are not recommended because of serious side effects on long-term use.

Suppress Transmission of ITCH Impulses through Nerves

Serotonin and opioids transmit itch impulses across nerves to CNS and drugs designed to reduce their activity will help in pruritus.

Opioid Antagonists

- Naloxone (IV/IM/Nasal spray)
- Naltrexone 2 mg/kg/day
- Nalmefene 0.5 mg/kg/day.

Antiserotonin Drugs

Ondansetron 2 mg/QID.

Nonspecific Nerve Conduction Suppressants

Carbamazepine15 mg/kg/day.

Pruritus secondary to cholestasis is very difficult to treat. Babies with NCS often require a cocktail of drugs, long-term, to reduce pruritus. Some severe cases may not respond to any medication. In such situations, small doses of propofol, given as continuous subcutaneous infusion through infusion pump may help. The dose required to suppress inching does not cause significant sedation. The drugs used in pruritus is summarized in **Table 8.4.1**.

Liver transplant is curative in severe pruritus secondary to NCS. Biliary diversion surgery which reduces reabsorption of bile acids also help ameliorate itching besides improving cholestasis. Cold water baths, closely cut nails and avoidance of sweating also help. The management of pruritus is summarized in **Flow chart 8.4.2**.

Coagulopathy

Vitamin K malabsorption secondary to cholestasis leads to coagulopathy. Many cases are often diagnosed following postvaccination bleeds. While subcutaneous bleed may be harmless, bleed into internal organs especially brain can be life-threatening. Vitamin K orally or parenterally can prevent bleeds. Active bleeds will need fresh frozen plasma, and intensive care. Factor VII can arrest bleeds fast, but it is exorbitantly expensive.

SURGICAL THERAPY IN NCS

The surgical options possible in various conditions are shown in **Flow chart 8.4.3** and the entire management is summarized in **Flow chart 8.4.4**.

Flow chart 8.4.2: Summary of management of pruritus in cholestasis in NCS

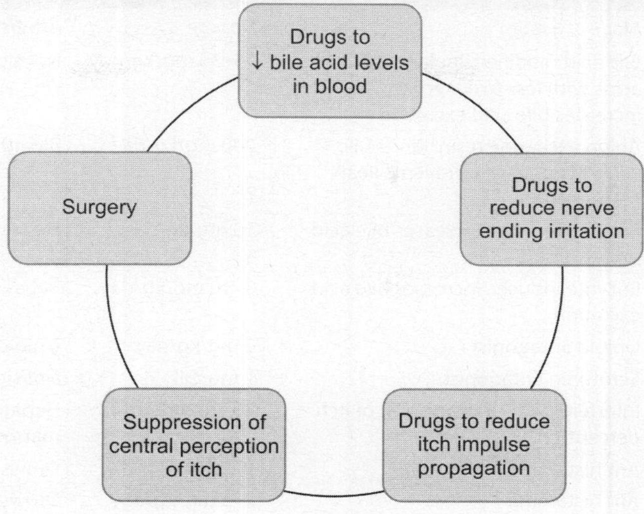

Flow chart 8.4.3: Surgical options in NCS

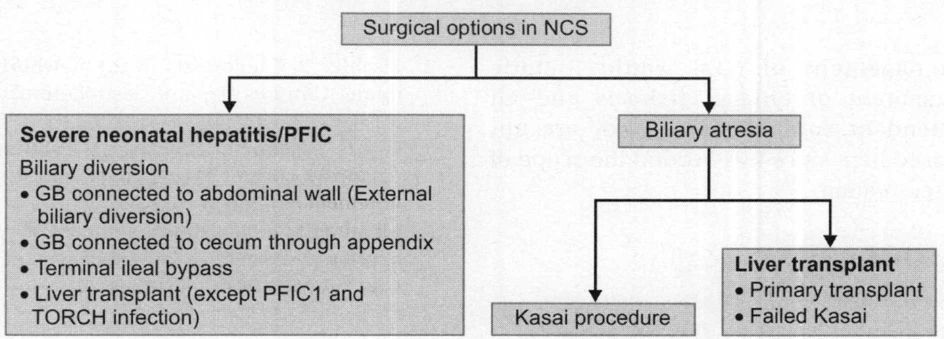

Abbreviations: NCS, neonatal cholestasis syndrome; PFIC, progressive familial intrahepatic cholestasis; GB, gallbladder; TORCH, toxoplasmosis, other (syphilis, varicella-zoster, parvovirus B11), Rubella, cytomegalovirus and herpes

Flow chart 8.4.4: Summary of management

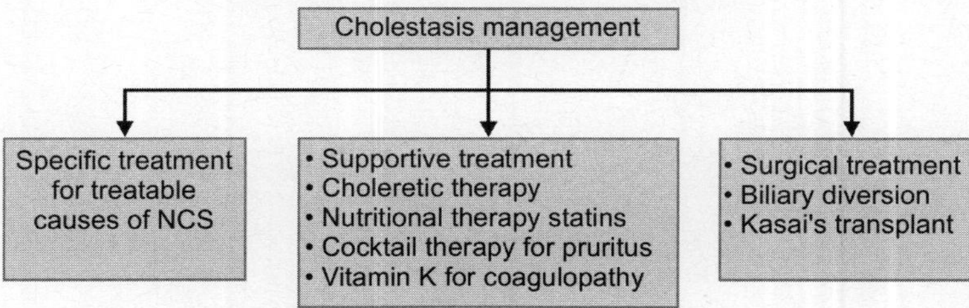

Abbreviation: NCS, neonatal cholestasis syndrome

Table 8.4.1: Drugs used in pruritus

Drugs	*Mode of action*	*Dosage*	*Adverse effects*
UDCA	Bile acid modifier. Replaces toxic bile acids with less toxic tertiary bile acids, increases bile acid excretion	15–30 mg/kg/day	Not significant
Cholestyramine Colestipol	Anion exchange resin. Binds bile acids in intestines. Prevents ileal reabsorption	200 mg/kg/day	Bloating, constipation
Rifampicin	Enzyme inducer, increases bile acid excretion	10 mg/kg/day	Hepatotoxicity
Phenobarbital	Enzyme inducer, increases bile acid excretion	3–10 mg/kg/day	Behavioral changes
Naltrexone	Opioid antagonist	2 mg/kg/day	Opioid withdrawal effect
Ondansetron	Serotonin antagonist	2 mg/QID	Not significant
Carbamazepine	Interferes with transmission of itch perception	10–20 mg/kg/day	Hepatotoxicity, bone marrow depression
Diphenhydramine	Antihistamine	5–10 mg/kg/day	Drowsiness
Hydroxyzine	Antihistamine	2–5 mg/kg/day	Drowsiness
Steroids	Immunosuppressive/anti-inflammatory	10 mg/day	Hypertension, Cushing's etc

Management of NCS would include management of biliary cirrhosis and all its attendant complications. They are not discussed here since it is beyond the scope of this presentation.

BIBLIOGRAPHY

1. Brumbaugh D. Conjugated hyperbilirubinaemia in children. Pediatr Rev. 2012;33(7):291-302.
2. Fischler B. Cholestasis in the newborn and infant. Clin Res Hepatol Gastroenterol. 2014; 38(3):263-7.
3. Gotze T. Neonatal choelastasis—Differential diagnosis, current diagnostic procedures, and treatment. Front Pediatr. 2015;3:43.
4. Moreira RK. Biliary atresia-a multi-disciplinary approach to diagnosis and management. Arch Path Lab Med. 2012;136:746-60.

8.5 Contrast Studies in Pediatric Gastroenterology

Ganga Devi Rajapandian, Balakrishnan Natarajan
Reviewers: *PSN Menon, Alok Gupta, R Remesh Kumar*

INTRODUCTION

Conventional contrast imaging studies are a useful tool in the diagnostic armamentarium of the pediatric gastroenterologist and pediatric radiologist. A detailed description of contrast imaging in pediatric gastrointestinal (GI) disorders is beyond the scope of this chapter and the discussion will be limited to the following aspects:

- Contrast media
- Study methodology
- Barium swallow and meal follow through studies
- Barium enema examination.

CONTRAST MEDIA USED IN PEDIATRIC IMAGING

Water-insoluble Contrast Media

Barium sulfate is the preferred contrast medium to study pediatric gastrointestinal tract. It is administered orally or rectally in a finely divided aqueous suspension. Barium sulfate is a white crystalline powder with atomic number of 56. It is highly radiopaque. In suspension, it has a pH of 5.3 and is stable in gastric acid. It is non-absorbable, nontoxic and insoluble in water and lipids. Advantages of barium sulfate include its low cost and good mucosal coating.

For barium swallow, barium is given as a paste or in semisolid consistency, mixed with water in a proportion of 1:1. For barium meal and follow through, barium is given as thick suspension in a milk shake consistency mixed with water in a proportion of 1:2. The quantity required is about 30–75 mL for infants and 480 mL for older children. For barium enema, barium is used as a thin suspension mixed with water in a dilution of 1:4. The quantity varies from 30 mL to 50 mL to 1 liter depending on the age of the child and indication of the study.

If a contrast enhanced computed tomography (CECT) scan of abdomen is indicated, it must be scheduled before a barium study because it takes at least 2–4 weeks for the barium to be cleared from the bowel and a subsequent CT in the next 2 weeks will be rendered difficult for interpretation.

Rarely complications may be encountered with barium studies. These are due to the entry of barium into peritoneal cavity or mediastinum (due to bowel perforation). Extravasation of barium into the urinary tract may produce inflammation if entry occurs due to an abnormal communication, e.g. a fistula. Aspiration of barium may occur into the bronchial tree as well. Rarely barium inspissation in the bowel may occur in cases of colonic obstruction.

Water-soluble Contrast Media

Iohexol and gastrografin are the commonly used water soluble contrast media in children. They contain iodine which is radiopaque. Iohexol is a nonionic and low osmolar contrast agent and is used for oral and rectal administration. Gastrografin is an ionic and high osmolar contrast agent with high incidence of complications. Gastrografin is *never* given orally and is used only for rectal examination. The water soluble contrasts are used in a dilution of 1:1.

Oral iohexol is indicated in children with suspected bowel perforation especially in corrosive poisoning or in case of recent biopsy. Oral iohexol is used in immediate postoperative states to assess an anastomotic leak. It is also used for the diagnosis of enteric fistula. In a sick child with duodenal obstruction or intestinal malrotation, oral iohexol is used. Iohexol is used to do distal loopogram in a child with anorectal malformation to evaluate for rectourethral and rectovesical fistulae.

Gastrografin enema is used only in neonates for the evaluation and treatment of meconium ileus and unused colon. Iohexol enema is used nowadays with equal efficacy in the treatment of meconium ileus.

STUDY METHODOLOGY

Request

A detailed written request from the referring pediatrician should include provisional diagnosis, past history (including known diagnoses if any), signs and symptoms and the specific reason for the examination. This is helpful for the proper performance and interpretation of the examination.

Consent

Written consent is obtained from the child's parent or guardian.

Patient Preparation

This depends on the type of barium study:

- Barium swallow/oral contrast esophagogram -fasting for a minimum of 2 hours.
- Barium meal/oral contrast upper gastro-intestinal (GI) examination—fasting for 2–3 hours for neonates and young infants, 4 hours for older infants and children and 6–8 hours for adolescents.
- Single contrast barium enema—no specific preparation required.
- Double contrast barium enema—dietary restriction, hydration and laxatives previous night.

Equipment

Contrast GIT procedures are performed using standard fluoroscopy and radiographic equipment with pediatric settings. It should be capable of producing kilovoltages greater than 100 kilovoltage peak (kVp). Other dose-reduction procedures, such as last image-hold, image-capture and video recording are also recommended.

Scout Radiograph

A scout radiograph of the abdomen is always taken before contrast medium is given. Plain radiograph of the abdomen with chest in anteroposterior (AP) projection with the child supine is taken particularly in the presence of acute abdominal symptoms. Horizontal beam decubitus and lateral radiograph of the abdomen should be performed if there is any suspicion of pneumoperitoneum or if the patient has an underlying condition that predisposes to bowel perforation.

In the frontal radiograph of the abdomen with chest, one needs to look for the following:

- Anomalies of situs—liver in the right upper quadrant, spleen in the left and levocardia indicate situs solitus
- Organomegaly, mass or mass effect
- Bowel gas pattern—dilated loops with no rectal air is suggestive of intestinal obstruction
- Pneumoperitoneum—if present, barium is contraindicated
- Abnormal calcifications
- Skeletal abnormalities
- Evidence of prior surgery
- Position of the catheters and monitoring electrodes in a sick child.

In a neonate with bilious vomiting, presence of few dilated proximal bowel loops without any distal air is suggestive of complete high intestinal obstruction (atresia) and no further imaging is needed before surgery. If the radiograph shows multiple dilated loops, it is suggestive of a low intestinal obstruction (distal to mid-ileum); barium/contrast enema is indicated. If any other plain radiographic finding is present, then barium meal study is performed.

Some examples of pneumoperitoneum, pica and tracheoesophageal fistula seen in scout films are demonstrated in **Figures 8.5.1A to C**.

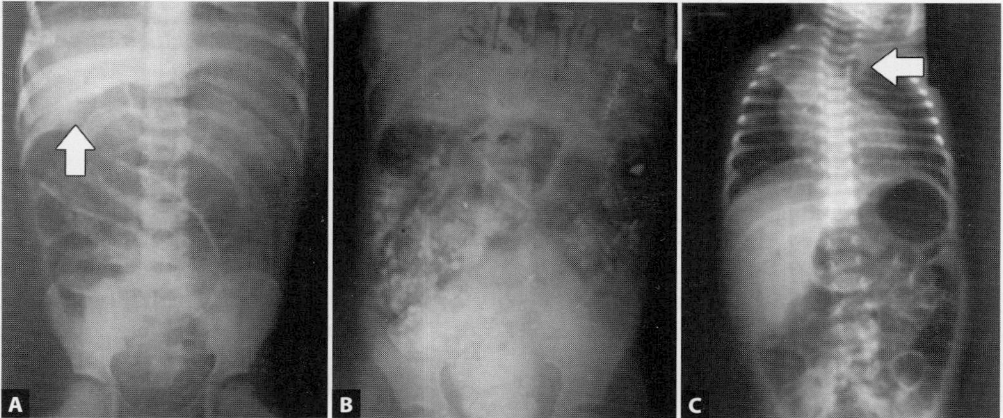

Figs 8.5.1A to C: Scout radiograph of the abdomen supine and AP views. (A) Extraluminal air (white arrow)—Pneumoperitoneum; (B) Multiple abnormal radiopacity seen in the colonic lumen and rectum—pica; (C) Normal bowel gas pattern with coiling of nasogastric tube (white arrow) in the upper esophagus—esophageal atresia with tracheoesophageal fistula

BARIUM SWALLOW EXAMINATION

Barium swallow is the radiographic procedure to study the anatomy and function of pharynx and esophagus. The study is useful in children with the following history and symptoms:

- Dysphagia
- Odynophagia (painful swallowing)
- Noncardiac chest pain
- Recurrent pneumonia
- Chronic tracheobronchial inflammation.

The conditions that can be diagnosed include:

- Esophageal obstruction, strictures and radiolucent foreign bodies
- Extrinsic compression including great vessel anomalies
- Postsurgical leak or stricture
- H-type tracheoesophageal fistula
- Suspected or known motility disorders
- Esophagitis
- Unexplained pneumomediastinum or suspected esophageal perforation
- Neoplasm and varices.

Technique

Single Contrast Barium Swallow

Neonates and infants may be fed barium from a native milk dispenser or small tumblers. Older children are asked to swallow a mouthful of barium. Lateral and frontal anteroposterior (AP) projections of pharynx and esophagus are taken, with visualization from the nasopharynx to the gastric fundus.

Barium Swallow in Infants with Suspected Tracheoesophageal Fistula

In infants and small children, the contrast can be administered in small amounts initially through a small feeding tube placed in the upper esophagus near the thoracic inlet, with the infant in a right anterior oblique (RAO) or lateral position. Fluoroscopic monitoring of the contrast injected from the tube is done (from the level of hypopharynx to carina) in the lateral position. This helps to differentiate contrast in the trachea due to aspiration or from a fistula. If no fistula is identified, the study may be completed with standard oral administration of contrast.

Double Contrast Barium Swallow

The child is asked to swallow an effervescent agent (Eno) followed by barium. It is seldom performed in pediatric patients, but it may help to evaluate mucosal integrity in adolescents.

Barium Swallow in Infants with Suspected Gastroesophageal Reflux

The child is made to drink barium so as to fill the stomach. Sips of water are given to the child to clear the esophagus of barium. AP and lateral projections of the barium filled stomach and esophagus are taken in supine and Trendelenburg positions. Images of gastroesophageal reflux should be recorded by last image hold, if reflux occurs during the fluoroscopic examination.

BARIUM MEAL STUDY AND FOLLOW THROUGH EXAMINATION

Barium meal study is a radiographic procedure to examine stomach and duodenum up to the duodenojejunal junction. The study is useful in children with the following history and symptoms:

- Abdominal pain, epigastric distress or discomfort
- Bilious or nonbilious vomiting
- Unexplained fever, weight loss and failure to thrive
- Chronic or recurrent respiratory disease including cough and acute life-threatening event
- Abdominal masses
- Signs and/or symptoms of upper GI bleeding
- Chronic diarrhea.

The conditions that can be diagnosed include:

- Intestinal malrotation anomalies
- Hernia including hiatus hernia and recurrent diaphragmatic hernia
- Hypertrophic pyloric stenosis when ultrasound is equivocal
- Gastric outlet or suspected small bowel obstruction
- Peptic ulcer disease
- Duodenal laceration or intramural hematoma
- Neoplasms
- Unexplained gastrointestinal bleeding or anemia
- Malabsorption
- Suspected enteric fistula
- Small bowel trauma
- Congenital anomaly such as an omphalo-mesenteric duct remnant
- Polyposis syndromes such as Cowden or Peutz-Jeghers syndromes
- Evaluation of postoperative anatomy.

Procedure

Flavoring agents may be added in older patients. Neonates and infants may be fed contrast from a native milk dispenser or small tumblers. The contrast may be given by straw or taken directly from a cup by an older child. A nasogastric tube, gastrostomy tube, or jejunostomy tube may be used as appropriate.

In neonates or young infants with a history of bilious emesis, a nasogastric tube can be placed with tip in the distal stomach to empty the stomach. A controlled upper GI study with a small amount of contrast and air can effectively evaluate malrotation and/or volvulus using the least amount of contrast and fluoroscopic time.

The films taken include the following:

- *Immediate:* Anteroposterior (AP), postero-anterior (PA), right anterior oblique (RAO), and right lateral views.
- *Follow-up:* AP views at 10 minutes, 30 minutes, 1 hour, 3 hours, and at 6 hours.

Initial passage of contrast through the duodenum should be observed directly with fluoroscopy to confirm the position of the duodeno jejunal junction (DJJ). The lateral view is important to assure the retroperitoneal position of the normally rotated duodenum and the normal height of the DJJ at the level of the duodenal bulb. The normal position of the DJJ is at or to the left of the left pedicle of the L2 vertebra and at a height approximately at the level of the duodenal bulb. A final image must document ileocecal junction and barium entry into the large bowel.

Figures 8.5.2 to **8.5.5** illustrate the barium swallow images of some common disorders in children such as gastroesophageal reflux disease, congenital esophageal stenosis, and barium meal images of hypertrophic pyloric stenosis, and malrotation of midgut.

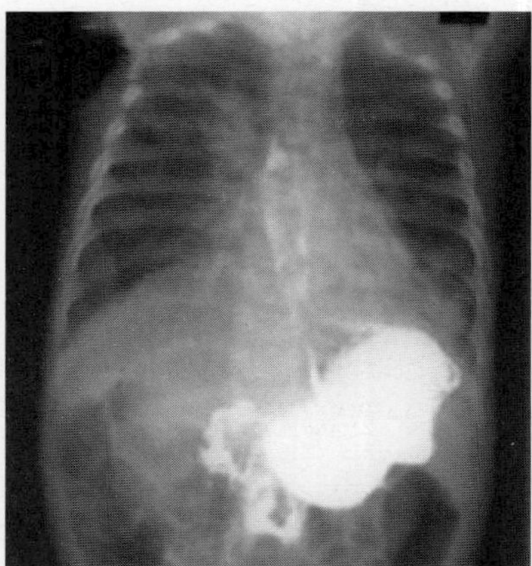

Fig. 8.5.2: Neonate with respiratory distress and vomiting—gastroesophageal reflux disease with bilateral lower lobe consolidation

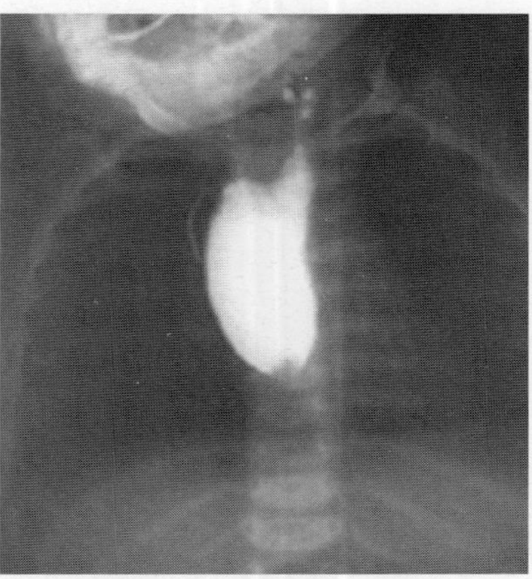

Fig. 8.5.3: Child with difficulty in swallowing—concentric narrowing of the lower thoracic esophagus suggestive of congenital esophageal stenosis

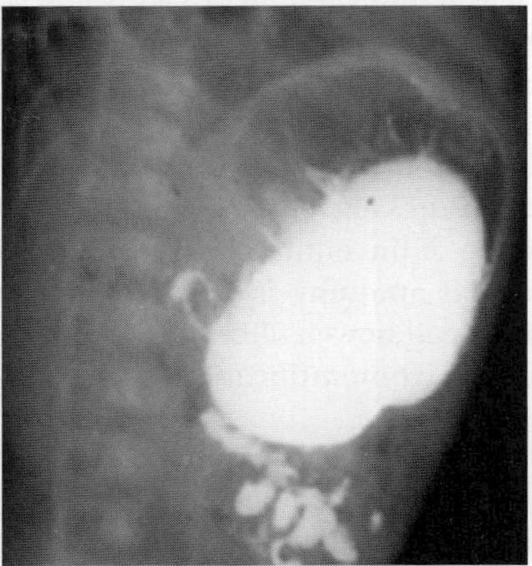

Fig. 8.5.4: Infant with vomiting/barium meal-narrow pyloric canal with a thin tract of barium called string sign which is diagnostic of hypertrophic pyloric stenosis

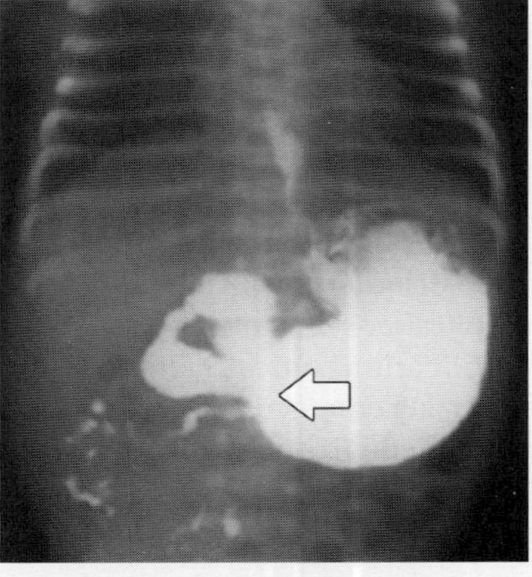

Fig. 8.5.5: Neonate with bilious vomiting/barium meal—duodenojejunal junction (white arrow) is overlying the spine with proximal jejunal loops in the right upper quadrant-diagnostic of malrotation of midgut

Figure 8.5.6 demonstrates the utility of contrast study in the diagnosis of Trichobezoar and **Figure 8.5.7** in intestinal ascariasis.

BARIUM ENEMA EXAMINATION

The radiographic study of large intestine by retrograde rectal administration of barium is called barium enema. The study is useful in children with the following history and symptoms:

- Chronic constipation
- Chronic diarrhea
- Bleeding per rectum
- Weight loss
- Abdominal pain.

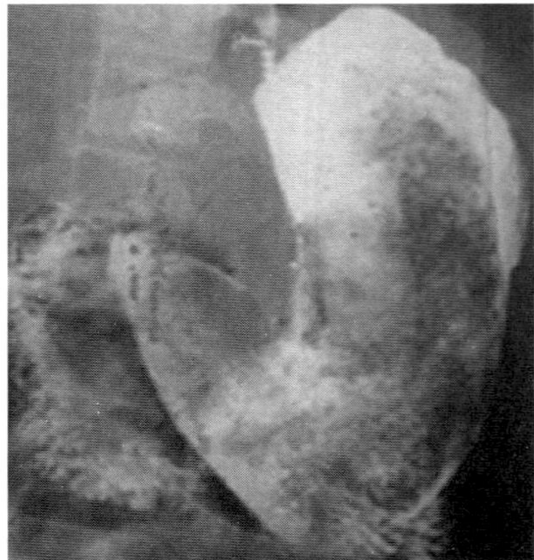

Fig. 8.5.6: Intraluminal filling defect is seen in the stomach with a speckled appearance—diagnostic of Trichobezoar

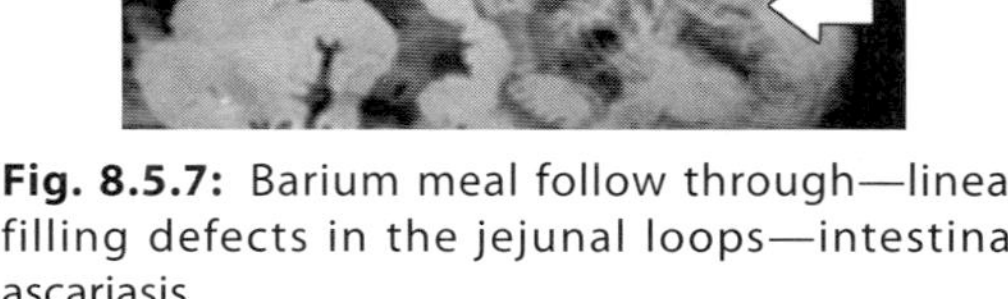

Fig. 8.5.7: Barium meal follow through—linear filling defects in the jejunal loops—intestinal ascariasis

The disorders that can be diagnosed include:

- Distal intestinal obstruction in the neonate (such as Hirschsprung disease, meconium ileus, ileal atresia, meconium plug, small left colon syndrome or colonic atresia), infant, child, or adolescent
- Familial polyposis syndromes or multi-system disorders involving the colon
- Complications due to surgery
- Complications due to diseases such as necrotizing enterocolitis (NEC)
- Intussusception (including reduction).

Contraindications for barium enema in children include the following:

- Evidence of colonic perforation—pneumoperitoneum
- Ischemic colon
- Toxic megacolon
- Hypovolemic shock
- Peritonitis.

Procedure

Single Contrast Barium Enema

- *Preparation:* No specific patient preparation is required.
- *Technique:* The smallest possible catheter permitting adequate contrast flow is used.
- Rectal administration of a sufficient volume of contrast agent (air, barium, and/or water soluble contrast) is used to provide colonic distension.
- The patient is then positioned to visualize the flexures and entire colon.
- Filling of the entire colon in children with normal anatomy is confirmed by reflux into small bowel, filling of the appendix or conclusive identification of the ileocecal valve.
- Images should be obtained of the rectum in the lateral projection.
- Images of the cecum should be obtained to document its position.
- Frontal views (AP, PA), oblique views (RAO, LAO) and lateral views including the rectum are obtained.

Hirschsprung's Disease

- *Examination preparation:* No bowel preparation prior to the enema including oral or rectal cleansing medications is necessary. Avoid recent digital rectal examination.
- *Examination technique:* Barium or water soluble contrasts are the routine contrast media used for evaluating childhood

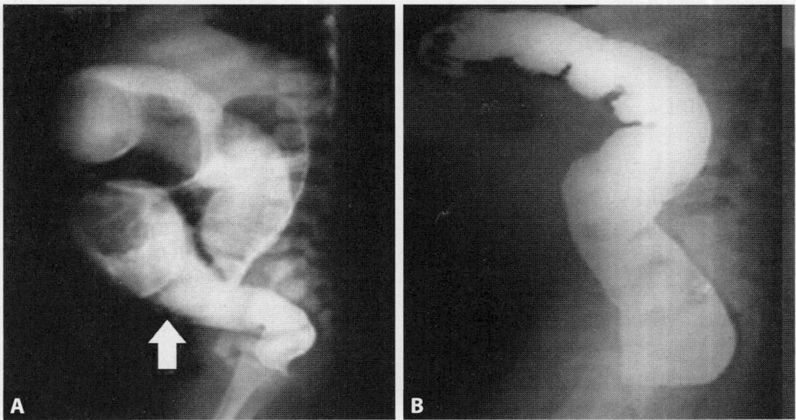

Figs 8.5.8A and B: Child with constipation/Barium enema/lateral radiograph. (A) Transition zone in the proximal sigmoid—Hirschsprung's disease; (B) Uniform dilatation of the colon up to anorectal junction—habit constipation

Hirschsprung's disease. In the neonate or infant, water soluble media diluted to near isotonic or iso-osmolar concentration are preferred. Barium is mixed in normal saline.

- The child is imaged initially in the lateral position when the rectum and sigmoid colon first fill with contrast. Images are obtained immediately upon early filling and during distension.
- The colon should be gravity filled with contrast. Once a transition zone is demonstrated, colonic filling is stopped.
- AP, PA, RAO, LAO and left lateral radiographs of the abdomen are taken.
- 24-hour film is taken to assess barium retention.

Figures 8.5.8A and **B** show the barium enema study in children with constipation. The transition zone in the proximal sigmoid junction is diagnostic of Hirschsprung disease. The uniform dilatation of the colon upto anorectal junction is diagnostic of habit constipation.

Meconium Ileus of the Neonate

A diagnostic contrast enema usually employs a near isotonic or iso-osmolar water soluble agent. If the diagnosis of meconium ileus is made by the contrast enema, the examination

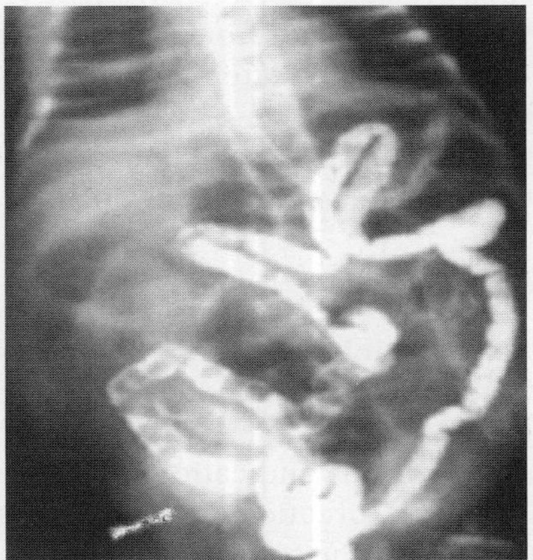

Fig. 8.5.9: Neonate with abdominal distension/contrast enema–small caliber of colon and terminal ileum with filling defects in the terminal ileum–meconium ileus

may proceed to a therapeutic contrast enema using contrast in a moderately hyperosmolar concentration. **Figure 8.5.9** illustrates the utility of contrast enema study in meconium ileus.

Double Contrast Barium Enema

- *Colon preparation:* Dietary restriction of solid food is done. Adequate hydration is maintained. Laxatives (in a dose appropriate for body weight) are given previous night and cleansing enemas is given in the morning.

- *Examination technique:*
  - High density (100% w/v) barium suspension should be used.
  - High kVp technique which produces lesser doses to the patient is preferred.
- Barium is instilled per rectum upto the splenic flexure under fluoroscopic guidance.
- The patient is turned on the right side to promote barium coating of the right colon.
- The patient is then elevated to empty the rectum and coat the cecum.
- Air is instilled slowly using Higginson syringe. If good coating is not initially achieved, the patient should be rotated as needed to coat the mucosa throughout the colon.
- Images may include frontal anteroposterior, posteroanterior, lateral view and both oblique views.
- Supplemental views such as upright and both decubitus views may be obtained.

CONCLUSION

Contrast imaging is advised by a pediatric gastroenterologist or pediatric surgeon to arrive at a diagnosis in various disorders. There are specific indications for their use and standard practice guidelines for the performance of the tests in children. Barium swallow, barium meal with follow through and enema are the commonly performed contrast imaging modalities in children. With careful monitoring, complications are rare. Scout film of the abdomen should be reviewed for possible emergencies before a contrast is administered. Iohexol is useful in the evaluation of post-operative leak and stricture. Gastrografin should never be given orally due to the risk of complications.

BIBLIOGRAPHY

1. Adam A, Dixon AK, Gillard J, Schaefer-Prokop C, Grainger RG, Allison DJ (eds). Grainger and Allison's Diagnostic Radiology, 6th edn. Elsevier Health Sciences, Edinburgh, 2015.
2. Aitchison F (Ed). Chapman & Nakielny's Guide to Radiological Procedures, 5th edn. Edinburgh, Saunders Elsevier; 2009.
3. American College of Radiology. ACR-SPR practice guideline for the performance of pediatric contrast examinations of the small bowel-Revised; 2008.
4. American College of Radiology. ACR-SPR practice parameter for the performance of contrast esophagograms and upper gastro-intestinal examinations in infants and children-2010/revised 2015 (resolution 36).
5. American College of Radiology. ACR-SPR practice parameter for the performance of pediatric fluoroscopic contrast enema examinations-Amended 2014 (Resolution 39)/ revised 2011 (resolution 51)
6. Berrocal T, Lamas M, Gutierrez J, Torres I, Pieto C, del Hoyo ML. Congenital anomalies of the small intestine, colon and rectum. Radiographics. 1999;19:1219-36.
7. Berrocal T, Torres I, Gutierrez J, Pieto C, del Hoyo ML, Lamas M. Congenital anomalies of upper gastrointestinal tract. Radiographics. 1999;19:855-72.
8. Cohen M. Choosing contrast media for the evaluation of gastrointestinal tract of neonates and infants. Radiology. 1987;162:447-56.
9. Coley BD (Ed). Caffey's Pediatric Diagnostic Imaging, 12th edn. Saunders Elsevier; 2014
10. Lee NK, Kim S, Jeon TY, Kim HS, Kim DH, Seo HI. Complications of congenital and developmental abnormalities of the gastro-intestinal tract in adolescents and adults: Evaluation with multimodality imaging. Radiographics. 2010;30:1489-507.
11. Narla LD, Hingsbergen EA. Case 22: Total Colonic Aganglionosis—Long-Segment Hirschsprung Disease. Radiology. 2000;215:391-4.
12. Timpone VM, Lattin GE, Lewis RB, Azuar K, Tubay M, Jesinger RA. Abdominal twists and turns: Part I, gastrointestinal tract torsions with pathologic correlation. Am J Radiol. 2011; 197:86-96.

Nephrology

Reviewers: *K Nedunchelian, Jaydeep Choudhury, RV Dhakshayani, MKC Nair, S Thangavelu, S Narmada*

9.1 Nephritic and Nephrotic Syndrome: An Investigatory Approach

Sangeetha

Reviewers: *K Nedunchelian, Jaydeep Choudhury, RV Dhakshayani*

Human kidney can be injured by various mechanisms. To know the degree of injury, impact on the kidney, progression and prognosis, we need laboratory evaluation and occasionally, a renal biopsy.

ACUTE NEPHRITIC SYNDROME

Acute nephritic syndrome (ANS) is characterized by sudden onset of variable degrees of hematuria, edema and hypertension. Acute nephritic syndrome following post-streptococcal infection is the most common type in children, accounting for 80% of cases. It can present acutely with any infection which is termed as "*infection related glomerulonephritis*".

First Line Investigations

- *Urinalysis:* To look for proteinuria, red blood cells (RBC) and casts. Usually proteinuria is mild, in non-nephrotic range. Dysmorphic RBCs favor glomerular etiology. A fresh uncentrifuged urine sample is necessary to look for the cast which may get lysed on standing and centrifugation. During the acute phase, urine may show significant white blood cells which is often mistaken for an urinary tract infection. But, ANS is one of the common conditions presenting with sterile pyuria.
- *Renal function test:* Blood urea and serum creatinine levels are elevated. In children presenting with acute kidney injury, hyponatremia, hyperkalemia and metabolic acidosis can occur.
- *Complete blood count:* Mild dilutional anemia can occur in ANS. Blood counts will show evidence of infection. Thrombocytopenia in a child with ANS picture favors systemic lupus erythematosus (SLE) and hemolytic uremic syndrome (HUS). They should be ruled out with other corroborative investigations.
- *Evidence of preceding streptococcal infection:* Rise in anti-streptolysin O (ASO) titer > 200 IU/mL is considered as positive. Eighty percent of children with ANS following streptococcal pharyngitis will have positive titers whereas only 20% of pyoderma patients will show elevated titers. They may also have elevated anti-hyaluronidase and anti-DNase B titers. The streptozyme test and anti zymogen antibodies are helpful in detecting the infection, but are not available everywhere.
- *Serum complement C3 levels:* Hypocomplementemia will be seen in 90% of children which becomes normal in 6–8 weeks.
- *Imaging:* X-ray chest will reveal signs of volume overload like cardiomegaly and pulmonary congestion.

  Ultrasound abdomen may show alteration in corticomedullary differentiation, ascites and pleural effusion.

Second Line Investigations

- Serum complement *C4* level in case of suspected SLE.
- Genetic mutation analysis of CH 50, factor H, factor B, factor I, CD 46, membrane cofactor protein (MCP), thrombomodulin and antifactor-H antibodies in case of suspected atypical HUS.
- *Renal biopsy:* Acute nephritic syndrome is not an indication for renal biopsy as

majority of the children recover well. ANS presentation following acute respiratory illness favors IgA nephropathy rather than post-infectious glomerulonephritis. IgA nephropathy needs renal biopsy to prove the diagnosis.

Renal biopsy is indicated in children with atypical presentations like:
- Nephritic onset of nephrotic syndrome
- Secondary causes like Henoch-Schönlein purpura, SLE and HUS
- Rapidly progressing renal failure
- Hypocomplementemia beyond 12 weeks
- Persistent microscopic hematuria for more than 12–18 months.

NEPHROTIC SYNDROME

Nephrotic syndrome (NS) is characterized by massive proteinuria, hypoalbuminemia, hyperlipidemia and edema. Idiopathic nephrotic syndrome is one of the common renal ailments in children and the various blood as well as urine investigations to support the diagnosis of the same are outlined here.

First Line Investigations

- *Urinalysis:* Urine examination by heat coagulation/dipstick showing 3+ or more proteinuria on three consecutive days sample proves nephrotic range proteinuria (massive proteinuria). Spot urine protein creatinine (PCR) ratio of >2 mg/mg or 24 hours urine protein >40 mg/m^2/hour or >3 g/1.73m^2/day denotes nephrotic range proteinuria. Since 24 hours urine collection is a very cumbersome procedure in children, spot PCR can be taken as an investigatory tool, especially in infants and young children.

  Microscopic examination of urine to look for red blood cells (5–10% can have microscopic hematuria) and casts (lipid cast in nephritic syndrome which supports nephrotic syndrome. RBC casts in nephritic onset of nephrotic and secondary NS like SLE, HSP). When there is persistence of microscopic hematuria (>5 RBCs/HPF), nonminimal change disease is more likely.
- *Complete blood count:* To look for any evidence of infection. The infection should be treated before starting steroids.
- *Kidney function tests:* Blood urea, serum creatinine and serum electrolytes as a baseline is necessary. Usually in minimal change disease, renal function will be normal. Altered renal functions in the form of elevated creatinine at presentation again favors significant renal pathology other than minimal change disease.
- *Serum albumin and cholesterol:* Serum albumin <2.5 g/dL and serum cholesterol >200 mg/dL are the classical biochemical features of nephrotic syndrome. Severity of these values is related to duration of proteinuria.
- Tuberculin test and X-ray chest are done prior to starting corticosteroid therapy.
- Ultrasound abdomen is done to look for kidney size, site, echogenecity. It may also show ascites and pleural effusion.

Second Line Investigations

- Serum complement C3 levels and anti streptolysin O titers in children presenting with acute nephritic onset nephrotic syndrome.
- Hepatitis B surface antigen will be useful in children with the history of recent jaundice and raised levels of transaminases.
- *Anti-nuclear antibody (ANA) and anti-double stranded DNA (anti-dsDNA):* In case of suspected systemic lupus erythematosus causing secondary nephrotic syndrome, they may be needed.
- *Screening for intrauterine infections and genetic mutation analysis:* May be required in congenital and infantile nephrotic syndrome patients. Nephrotic syndrome caused by genetic mutations is resistant to steroids and other immunosuppressive therapy. Hence, proper diagnosis is mandatory to discuss the prognosis, therapy and genetic counseling. Genetic mutation analysis should also be offered to children

with steroid resistance and family history of nephrotic syndrome.

- *Renal biopsy—indications*
  - Age of presentation—less than one year and more than eight years
  - Nephrotic syndrome with acute kidney injury after ruling out diuretic usage and hypovolemia
  - Steroid resistant nephrotic syndrome
  - Suspected secondary causes like systemic lupus erythematosus and Henoch-Schönlein purpura
  - Before starting calcineurin inhibitor therapy
  - Biopsy after 2 years of starting the therapy in children on calcineurin inhibitors.

Light microscopy and immunofluorescence methods: The biopsy specimen should be examined by light microscopy and immunofluorescence.

Electron microscopy study will be useful in hereditary nephropathies like Alport syndrome and thin basement membrane disease.

FOLLOW-UP INVESTIGATIONS

After the initiation of alternative therapy like cyclophosphamide, total and differential counts should be monitored fortnightly. In case of Levamisole and Mycophenolate mofetil (MMF), counts should be checked once in 2–3 months. Counts <4000/cu mm mandate discontinuation of the drug. Also, transaminase levels should be monitored with Levamisole and MMF therapy.

Children on Tacrolimus and Cyclosporine should undergo renal function test, blood sugar testing every 2–3 months and lipid profile annually. Blood levels of Cyclosporine or Tacrolimus should be measured 2–4 weeks after initiation of therapy. Subsequent drug level monitoring is needed in case of suspected noncompliance, unsatisfactory response and renal toxicity which are proven by elevated serum creatinine level of 30% or more from the baseline value. Trough (12-hour) blood levels of Cyclosporine should be maintained at 80–120 ng/mL and Tacrolimus at 5–8 ng/mL.

BIBLIOGRAPHY

1. Bagga A, Srivastava RN. Diagnostic Evaluation. Pediatric Nephrology, 5th edn. New Delhi: Jaypee Brothers Medical Publishers (P) Ltd; 2011.pp.20-47.
2. Indian Pediatric Nephrology Group, Indian Academy of Pediatrics. Consensus Statement on Evaluation of Hematuria. Indian Pediatr. 2006;43:965-73.
3. Indian Pediatric Nephrology Group, Indian Academy of Pediatrics. Management of Steroid Sensitive Nephrotic Syndrome: Revised guidelines. Indian Pediatr. 2008;45: 203-14.
4. Van der Watt G, Omar F, Brink A, McCulloch M. Laboratory investigation of the child with suspected renal disease. In: Avner ED, Harmon WE, Niaudet P, Yoshikawa N, Emma F, Goldstein SL (Eds). Pediatric Nephrology, 7th edn. Verlag Berlin Heidelberg: Springer; 2016. pp. 613-36.
5. Vijayakumar M, Prahlad N, Nammalwar BR. Evaluation of renal functions. In: Vijayakumar M, Nammalwar BR (Eds). Principles and Practice of Pediatric Nephrology, 2nd edn. New Delhi: Jaypee Brothers Medical Publishers (P) Ltd. 2013.pp.110-23.

9.2 Urinalysis and More in Urinary Tract Infection

A Somasundaram, S Kirupa

***Reviewers:** MKC Nair, S Thangavelu, S Narmada*

INTRODUCTION

Urinary tract infection (UTI) is one of the most common pediatric infections. It distresses the child, concerns the parents, and may cause permanent kidney damage. Occurrences of a first-time symptomatic UTI are highest in boys and girls during the first year of life and markedly decrease after that. The need for accurate diagnosis of UTI is emphasized due to important implications concerning evaluation and follow-up. UTI is diagnosed on a positive culture in a symptomatic child, and not merely by the presence of leukocyturia. Patients with asymptomatic bacteriuria do not require treatment. Infants with the first UTI should be evaluated with micturating cystourethrography. Children with vesicoureteral reflux (VUR) should be followed up with serial ultrasonography and direct radionuclide cystograms every 2 years, while awaiting resolution. The diagnosis of UTI is often missed in infants and young children, as urinary symptoms are minimal and often non-specific. This chapter discusses in detail the urine testing strategies, the urine microscopy interpretation and the recommended imaging schedule for the diagnosis of UTI in infants and children.

When to Suspect Urinary Tract Infection?

The history and clinical course of a UTI vary with the patient's age. No one specific sign or symptom can be used to identify UTI in infants and children. **Table 9.2.1** shows the symptoms to suspect UTI in the various age groups.

SAMPLING OF URINE

Urine collection must occur before starting antibiotics because a single dose of an effective antibiotic rapidly sterilizes the urine.

The methods to obtain urine are:

- Midstream clean catch urine
- Urethral catherization
- Urine bag collection
- Suprapubic aspiration (SPA).

For toilet-trained children, a midstream urine sample should be collected. Asking little girls to sit backward on the toilet seat spreads the labia and may prevent contamination. It appears that perineal cleansing may not be necessary before collection of midstream urine, presumably because the first drops of urine wash away contaminants.

For children who are not toilet trained, only urethral catheterization and SPA are considered to be reliable methods for specimen collection for the purpose of culture. Although collecting urine using a bag for urinalysis is simple and noninvasive, bag samples have a high a rate of contamination (up to 63%), making culture

Table 9.2.1: Signs and symptoms of UTI in various age groups

0–2 months	*2 months to 2 years*
• Jaundice • Fever • Failure to thrive • Poor feeding • Vomiting • Irritability	• Poor feeding • Fever • Vomiting • Strong-smelling urine • Abdominal pain • Irritability
2–6 years	*Older than 6 years and adolescents*
• Vomiting • Abdominal pain • Fever • Strong-smelling urine • Enuresis • Urinary symptoms (dysuria, urgency, frequency)	• Fever • Vomiting, abdominal pain • Flank/back pain • Strong-smelling urine • Urinary symptoms (dysuria, urgency, frequency) • Enuresis • Incontinence

results unreliable for diagnosis of UTI. In some hospital and clinic settings, a bag specimen is used as an initial screen and a subsequent specimen is obtained by catheterization or SPA if the urinalysis is abnormal.

Suprapubic aspiration is the method of choice for obtaining urine from:

- Uncircumcised boys with a redundant or tight foreskin
- From girls with tight labial adhesions
- From children of either sex with clinically significant periurethral irritation.

PRESERVATION OF URINE

Urine must be refrigerated if it cannot be examined promptly. Delay of more than two hours between collection and examination often cause unreliable results. If delay is anticipated, the sample can be stored in a refrigerator at 4°C for up to 12–24 hours. Boric acid is a well established preservative for urine.

URINALYSIS

Urinalysis (UA) is vital in the confirmation of diagnosis of UTI, because it indicates the presence of bacteriuria and pyuria.

Macroscopic analysis by dipstick methods (rapid tests) and microscopic analysis of urine is supportive in the confirmation of UTI.

Macroscopic Urinalysis (Dipstick)

Leukocyte Esterase Test

Leukocyte esterase is produced by neutrophils and may signal pyuria associated with UTI. To detect significant pyuria accurately, five minutes should be allowed for the dipstick reagent strip to change color. It may be falsely negative when leukocytes are present in low concentration.

Nitrite Test

Nitrites normally are not found in urine, but occur when bacteria reduce urinary nitrates to nitrites. Many gram-negative and some gram-positive organisms are capable of this conversion, and a positive dipstick nitrite test indicates that these organisms are present in significant numbers. This test is specific but not highly sensitive. Thus, a positive result is helpful, but a negative result does not rule out UTI. **Figure 9.2.1** shows a positive urine dipstick for nitrite and leukocyte esterase.

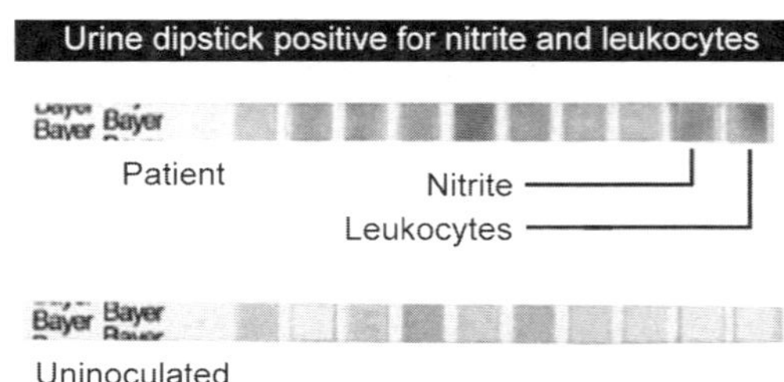

Fig. 9.2.1: Urine dipstick (*For color version see Plate 7*)

Microscopic Urinalysis

Microscopic examination of spun urine can evaluate for the presence of white blood cells (WBCs), red blood cells (RBCs), bacteria, casts and skin contamination (e.g. epithelial cells). Presence of WBCs in the urine is a sensitive indicator of inflammation associated with infection.

Significant pyuria is defined as the presence of the following:

In fresh uncentrifuged sample >10 leukocytes/mm^3 (or)

In centrifuged sample >5 leukocytes per high power field

It is now recognized that pyuria is a hallmark of true UTI and helps distinguish UTI from asymptomatic bacteriuria. It is the host's inflammatory response that results in scarring.

Sterile pyuria (positive leukocytes, negative culture) may occur in the conditions listed in the **Table 9.2.2**.

Asymptomatic bacteriuria is the demonstration of bacteria in Gram stained specimen of fresh uncentrifuged urine. The presence of bacteria without manifestation of infection and pyuria denotes asymptomatic bacteriuria. It is most common in girls and is rare in boys with an incidence of <1% in preschool children and school going girls. This condition is benign and does not cause renal damage.

Table 9.2.2: Causes of sterile pyuria

- Partially treated bacterial UTI
- Viral infections
- Renal tuberculosis
- Renal abscess
- UTI in the presence of urinary obstruction
- Urethritis because of STDs
- Inflammation near bladder or ureter (Crohn's disease)
- Interstitial nephritis

Table 9.2.3: Sensitivity and specificity of components of urinalysis, alone and in combination

	Test	*Sensitivity*	*Specificity*
1.	LE	83	78
2.	NT	53	98
3.	Either LE or NT positive	93	72
4.	Microscopy, WBCs	73	81
5.	Microscopy, bacteria	81	83
6.	LE, NT or microscopy positive	99.8	70

Data presented as %.
Abbreviations: LE, leukocyte esterase; NT, nitrite; WBCs, white blood cells
Source: Pediatrics. American Academy of Pediatrics. 2011;128:595-610.

Thus, the combination of dipstick tests and microscopy will help in predicting the presence of UTI and the sensitivity and specificity of various components of urinalysis is given in **Table 9.2.3.**

The *enhanced urinalysis* (EA) technique developed to predict UTI in low-risk infants and children. It utilizes uncentrifuged urine and a neubauer hemocytometer to evaluate the number of WBC/mm^3 (cell count). This method is far superior to the standard urinalysis in successfully distinguishing between colonization, contamination, and asymptomatic bacteriuria, thus providing health care providers with the ability to detect a true UTI, especially in the febrile infants. A positive enhanced UA is defined as ≥ 10 white blood cells per cubic millimeter and presence of any bacteria per 10 oil immersion fields on a Gram-stained smear.

A positive *automated urinalysis* is defined as ≥ 2 white blood cells per high-powered field and presence of any bacteria using the IRIS iQ200 ELITE.

URINE CULTURE

Urine collection must occur before starting antibiotics because a single dose of an effective antibiotic rapidly sterilizes the urine. Urine culture should be repeated, in case, contamination is suspected, e.g. mixed growth of two or more pathogens, or growth of organisms that normally constitute the periurethral flora (lacto-bacilli in healthy girls; enterococci in infants and toddlers). The culture should also be repeated in situations where UTI is strongly suspected but colony counts are equivocal.

The number of bacteria required for defining UTI depends on the method of urine collection is given in **Table 9.2.4**.

In the past, frequent follow-up cultures were recommended to identify asymptomatic recurrences. However, it is now understood that this practice will mistake girls with asymptomatic bacteriuria as having recurrent or chronic UTI. Because it is the host response that causes scarring, and the host response includes both fever and inflammation (pyuria), it is more appropriate to detect and treat febrile recurrences than to perform periodic cultures.

BLOOD TESTS

Hematologic studies do not tend to help in the diagnosis of UTIs, although they should be obtained in patients who appear ill. Complete blood counts, serum BUN, creatinine and a blood culture should be done in infants and children with complicated UTI to document bacteremia and to assess renal function.

IMAGING STUDIES

There is limited evidence that intensive imaging and subsequent management alters the long-term outcome of children with reflux nephropathy diagnosed following a

Table 9.2.4: Criteria for the diagnosis of UTI

Method	*Finding*
Suprapubic aspiration	If a UTI is present, bacteria are likely to be proliferating in bladder urine with growth of any number of organism
Urethral catherization	Febrile infants and children with UTI usually have >50,000 CFU/mL of a single urinary pathogen; however, UTI may be present with 10,000–50,000 CFU/mL of a single organism.*
Midstream, clean-void collection	UTI is diagnosed when >100,000 CFU/mL of a single urinary pathogen is present in a symptomatic patient. Pyuria usually present. A UTI may be present with 10,000–50,000 CFU/mL of a single bacterium.*
Any method in a girl or boy	If the patient is asymptomatic and bacterial growth is usually >100,000 CFU/mL of the same organism on different days and if pyuria is absent, this result probably indicates colonization rather than infection.

* Patients with urinary frequency (i.e. decreased bladder incubation time) are those most likely to have bacteria proliferating in the urinary bladder in the presence of low colony counts.

Source: E medicine medscape article on Pediatric Urinary Tract Infection Work-up

Table 9.2.5: Recommended imaging schedule for children with urinary tract infection

Test	*Responds well to treatment within 48 hours*	*Atypical UTI**	*Recurrent UTI**
For infants younger than 6 months			
Ultrasound during the acute infection	No	Yes	Yes
Ultrasound within 6 weeks	Yes	No	No
DMSA 4–6 months following the acute infection	No	Yes	Yes
VCUG	No	Yes	Yes
For infants and children 6 months or older but younger than 3 years			
Ultrasound during the acute infection	No	Yes	No
Ultrasound within 6 weeks	No	No	Yes
DMSA 4–6 months following the acute infection	No	Yes	Yes
VCUG	No	No	No
For children 3 years or older			
Ultrasound during the acute infection	No	Yes	No
Ultrasound within 6 weeks	No	No	Yes
DMSA 4–6 months following the acute infection	No	No	Yes
VCUG	No	No#	No#

Source: NICE Guidelines for Pediatric UTI

Abbreviations: UTI, urinary tract infection; VCUG, voiding cystouretrogram

+ Consider if USG abnormal

Not routine, consider if dilatation on USG, poor urine flow, non-*E. coli* infection

Atypical UTI includes:
- Seriously ill
- Poor urine flow
- Abdominal or bladder mass
- Raised creatinine
- Septicemia
- Failure to respond to treatment with suitable antibiotics within 48 hours
- Infection with non-*E. coli* organisms

Recurrent UTI:
- Two or more episodes of UTI with acute pyelonephritis/upper urinary tract infection, or
- One episode of UTI with acute pyelonephritis/upper urinary tract infection plus one or more episode of UTI with cystitis/lower urinary tract infection, or
- Three or more episodes of UTI with cystitis/lower urinary tract infection.

UTI. With availability of antenatal screening, most important anomalies have already been detected and managed after birth. Therefore, there is considerable debate regarding the need and intensity of radiologic evaluation in children with UTI.

The goal of imaging studies in children with a UTI is identify the following:

- Anatomic abnormalities that predispose to infection
- Determine whether there is active renal involvement
- To assess whether renal function is normal or at risk.

Current common imaging options for children with UTI include:

- Renal/bladder ultrasound (RBUS),
- Radiographic (e.g. Voiding cystourethrogram [VCUG])
- Radioisotope (e.g. Dimercaptosuccinic acid [DMSA]) techniques.

The recommended imaging schedule in Pediatric UTI as per NICE Guidelines is given in **Table 9.2.5**.

An ultrasonogram provides information on kidney size, number and location, presence of hydronephrosis, urinary bladder anomalies and post-void residual urine. DMSA scintigraphy is a sensitive technique for detecting renal parenchymal infection and cortical scarring. VCUG detects VUR and provides anatomical details regarding the bladder and the urethra.

At the time of the first acute infection, clinicians will be concerned as to whether the child is predisposed to recurrent urinary infection, because of kidney stones or anatomical anomalies of the kidney, ureter or bladder, which may cause VUR or urinary stasis. Antibiotic prophylaxis, pending results of imaging, is no longer advised routinely.

Because recurrence is more common in infants and young children with high grade VUR, whether they have received prophylaxis or not, postponing VCUG until after a recurrence accomplishes two things: it avoids the radiation, cost, and discomfort of VCUG in 90% of these patients with a first febrile UTI, and it identifies those with high-grade VUR, albeit after a recurrence.

A DMSA scan can be used to diagnose acute pyelonephritis (when performed during acute illness) and to identify renal scars (when performed months following the acute illness).

POINTS TO REMEMBER

- Diagnosis of UTI requires evidence of infection from both abnormal urinalysis results and positive urine culture results
- Voiding cystourethrography is not recommended routinely after the first febrile UTI; ultrasonography should include the bladder and the kidneys.
- On follow-up, emphasis is on urine testing with subsequent febrile illnesses, rather than on regularly repeated urine cultures after treatment.

BIBLIOGRAPHY

1. Diagnosis and management of urinary tract infection in children: summary of NICE guidance. BMJ. 2007;335(7616):395-7.
2. Elder JS. Urinary tract infections. In: Kliegman RM, Stanton BMD, Geme J, et al. (Eds.) *Nelson Textbook of Pediatrics,* 20th ed. Philadelphia, PA: Elsevier; 2016. pp. 2556-62.
3. Robinson JL, Finlay JC, Lang ME, Bortolussi R. Urinary tract infection in infants and children: Diagnosis and management, Canadian Paediatric Society, Paediatr Child Health. 2014; 19(6):315-19.
4. Urinary Tract Infection: Clinical Practice Guideline for the Diagnosis and Management of the Initial UTI in Febrile Infants and Children 2 to 24 Months, Subcommittee on Urinary Tract Infection, Steering Committee on Quality Improvement and Management. Pediatrics. 2011;128(3):595-610.
5. Vijayakumar M, Kanitkar M, Nammalwar BR, Bagga A. Indian Society of Pediatric Nephrology, Revised Statement on Management of Urinary Tract Infections. Indian Pediatr 2011;48: 709-17.

Hematology

Reviewers: *PSN Menon, Alok Gupta, R Remesh Kumar, MKC Nair, S Thangavelu, S Narmada, K Nedunchelian, Jaydeep Choudhury, RV Dhakshayani*

10.1 ABC of CBC

Ramamurthi Palaniraman
Reviewers: *PSN Menon, Alok Gupta, R Remesh Kumar*

INTRODUCTION

Complete blood count (CBC) is the most common test done in a day-to-day practice. But it is often given cursory appraisal with incomplete interpretation. Ideally, CBC should be accompanied by a peripheral blood smear study.

WHAT DOES CBC ACTUALLY MEAN?

CBC includes the following tests:

- Hemoglobin (Hb)
- Hematocrit (Hct): Measures the percentage of the volume of whole blood that is made up of red blood cells
- Red blood cell (RBC) count
- White blood cell (WBC) total count (TC)
- WBC differential count (DC)
- Platelet count
- *Red blood cell indices:*
  - *Mean corpuscular volume (MCV):* Average volume of red cells.
  - *Mean corpuscular hemoglobin (MCH):* Calculation of the average amount of hemoglobin inside a single red blood cell.
  - *Mean corpuscular hemoglobin concentration (MCHC):* Calculation of the average concentration of hemoglobin inside a single red blood cell.
  - *Red cell distribution width (RDW):* A parameter that measures variation in red blood cell size or red blood cell volume.
- *Platelet indices:*
  - *Mean platelet volume (MPV):* Reflects the average size of platelets present in a person's sample of blood.
  - *Platelet distribution width (PDW):* Reflects how uniform the platelets are in size.

CBC IN CHILDREN

The normal ranges for values are not static; CBC values change with age and one should be aware of this before interpretation. **Table 10.1.1** provides the age-related changes in RBCs. **Table 10.1.2** demonstrates the age-related changes in WBCs.

Indications

In Whom to Do?

- Primary hematological complaints—pallor, bleeding, etc.
- In day-to-day infections.

Table 10.1.1: Age-related RBC changes

Age	*Hb (G/dL)*	*RBC (Million cells/μL)*	*MCV (fL)*
Birth	16.5	4.7	108
Day 3	18.5	5.3	108
6 months	11.5	3.8	91
12 years	13.5	4.6	86
18 years (Female)	14.0	4.6	90
18 years (Male)	14.5	5.9	88

Table 10.1.2: Age-related WBC changes

Age	*Polymorphs (%)*	*Lymphocytes (%)*
Birth	61	31
2 weeks	40	48
1 month	35	56
1 year	31	61
6 years	51	42
16 years	57	35

- Monitoring the progress of the illness and response to treatment—in the hospital.

When to Do?

- *Timing of CBC:* In a well-baby, it has less relevance on day 1 of fever, cold, cough or loose stools, as stress of day 1 illness itself may induce erroneous results.
- In the diagnosis of infection it gives valuable guidance from day 3 onwards.
- In a malarial endemic zone, it is useful on day 1 itself along with blood smear study.

How to Do?

- Manual CBC with differential counts is outdated now.
- Three-part and five-part differential cell counters are commonly used now.
- Electrical impedance method or light refraction method is preferred.
- Standardized equipment (Beckman Coulter, Sysmex, Celldyne, etc.) should preferably be used.
- Standardization (QC or Quality Control) is essential to ensure consistent results.

Limitations of Coulter Counter

- Ethylenediaminetetra-acetic acid (EDTA) may cause clumping of platelets giving rise to pseudo-thrombocytopenia whereas direct peripheral smear may show normal platelet count.
- In case of severe neutropenia, the immature monocytes are picked up by the Coulter counter as neutrophils giving rise to erroneous results.
- In case of thalassemia, normoblasts are picked up as lymphocytes.
- For any test result especially the platelet count to be absolutely sure, it is always necessary to cross-check manually on direct peripheral smear.

How to Interpret Results

Having ensured that there are no technical errors and standardization-related errors, interpretation of the results is an interesting exercise. It is just an extension of clinical examination. So it should be interpreted only in the context of clinical picture and not in isolation.

Often in office practice, CBC is used to diagnose bacterial infection and to decide about starting antibiotics. But the evidence says that CBC is a weak screening test to diagnose bacterial infection with less than 50% sensitivity and specificity.

COMMON SCENARIOS IN PEDIATRIC PRACTICE

Common scenarios that we come across in pediatric clinical practice are:

- *Leukocytosis:* Neutrophilic or lymphocytic
- Leukopenia

Please do not forget to watch what happens in the other cell lines (RBC and platelets) in all examinations.

Leukocytosis

Neutrophilic leukocytosis (neutrophilia) is considered when absolute neutrophil count (ANC) >10,000 cells/mm^{3}and total WBC count (TC) >15,000 cells/mm^3 of blood. It may occur in the following situations:

- Stress response
- Serious bacterial infections
- Invasive viral infections
- Inflammatory disorders (e.g. systemic onset juvenile rheumatoid arthritis (SoJRA) and Kawasaki disease).

Depending on the day of performing the test and clinical picture, the interpretation will vary.

Lymphocytosis in Childhood

Lymphocytosis is diagnosed when TC >15,000 cells/mm^3 of blood and lymphocytes are predominant (absolute lymphocytosis) or when TC <10,000 cells/mm^3 of blood and lymphocytes are predominant (relative lymphocytosis secondary to neutropenia). Conditions causing absolute lymphocytosis include the following:

- Pertussis
- Common viral infections: e.g. Echovirus, Coxsackie virus

- Infectious mononucleosis like conditions, e.g. infections due to Epstein-Barr virus (EBV), cytomegalovirus (CMV), toxoplasma
- Leukemia (when ANC is low, Hb is low, and platelets are low)

Leukopenia

Viral infections are the commonest cause of transient neutropenia with leukopenia which recovers within 3–5 days, but may persist for weeks at times. Shigella produces leukopenia with marked increase in band cells. Overwhelming acute sepsis caused by *Meningococcus, Pneumococcus* and *Staphylococcus* as well as conditions like typhoid and paratyphoid fevers cause leukopenia. Rickettsial infections (e.g. scrub typhus) also, at times, behave like typhoid with leukopenia and thrombocytopenia in the second week of fever.

INFECTIONS AND PLATELETS IN CBC

Most infections whether viral, bacterial or protozoal, cause thrombocytopenia. It should be confirmed by peripheral blood smear that it is not pseudo-thrombocytopenia. Depending on the day of thrombocytopenia along with other parameters, you may get a clue to which infection you are dealing with as shown below:.

- Week 1 – Malaria, dengue fever
- Week 2 – Malaria, scrub typhus, typhoid, leptospirosis
- Week 3 – Infections due to EBV, CMV, human immunodeficiency virus (HIV), leukemia, collagen vascular diseases (e.g. systemic lupus erythematosus [SLE])

Considering the fact noted above, practical interpretation of CBC with respect to infectious diseases is as follows **(Table 10.1.3)**:

Short Duration Fever

- Day 1: Avoid doing CBC as far as possible.
- Day 3: *Neutrophilic leukocytosis*—always rule out occult pneumonia and urinary tract infection (UTI).
- Day 5–7: *Neutrophilic leukocytosis*—infections (occult abscess), inflammatory conditions (SoJRA, Kawasaki disease, etc.)
- CBC: *Lymphocytosis* (4–7 days)—viral, rarely bacterial; always keep malignancy as a possibility.
- CBC: *Leukopenia* (4–7 days)—suggests dengue fever, typhoid or malaria; needs interpretation along with RBC and platelet indices. This gives a valuable clue for diagnosis.

Eosinophilia

Eosinophilia is often associated with rashes, wheezes and helminthic (tissue invading-visceral larva migrans) infections. Eosinophilia is also associated with drug hypersensitivity, asthma, cow's milk allergy, hay fever, urticaria, eczema, other skin disorders, Job's syndrome, and malignancy.

Eosinopenia

In the clinical setting of typhoid fever if absolute eosinopenia is present, it is an excellent clue that we are dealing with typhoid fever. Studies have shown that in typhoid, absolute eosinopenia is present in 70–75% of cases.

Table10.1.3: Hematological profile on day 4–5 of fever

Parameter	*Enteric fever*	*Malaria*	*Dengue fever*	*Other viral infections*
Hb/Hct	Normal	Low	Normal/High	Normal
TC	Normal/Low	Normal/Low	Low	Normal/Low
DC	Eosinopenia	Monocytosis	Lymphocytosis	Lymphocytosis
Platelets	Normal /Low	Low	Low	Normal/Low

CBC INTERPRETATION TIPS IN HEMATOLOGY FOR AN OFFICE PRACTITIONER

Anemia

- Low Hb, low RBC count, decreased MCV, high RDW, and increased platelets—*Iron deficiency anemia*
- Low Hb, high RBC count, decreased MCV, normal RDW, normal platelets—*Thalassemia minor and intermedia*
- Low Hb, low RBC count, increased MCV, high RDW, decreased platelets—*Megaloblastic anemia (B_{12} or folate deficiency)*
- Low Hb, low RBC count, increased MCV, normal RDW, decreased platelets—*Aplastic anemia*

Bleeding

- Platelet count low, mean platelet volume (MPV) increased and rest of the cell lines (RBC and WBC) normal—*Immune thrombocytopenic purpura (ITP)*
- Whenever more than two cell lines are affected (e.g. RBC and platelets or WBC and platelets), always check the absolute neutrophil count (ANC)—calculated as ANC [= % of (Neutrophils + Band cells) in DC × TC ÷ 100]. If ANC is less than 1000/μL, it is a red flag and sinister sign in CBC. Malignancy has to be ruled out. If it is an infection-related illness, it may indicate hemophagocytosis.
- In the same way in a family with sibling deaths and early infantile deaths, calculating absolute lymphocyte count (ALC) in cord blood is useful—calculated as ALC (=% of lymphocytes in DC × TC ÷ 100). If ALC is less than 1000/μL, it is a red flag sign and gives a clue for severe combined immunodeficiency (SCID).

CONCLUSION

- Utility value of CBC is very high for primary hematological problems such as anemia, and thrombocytopenia—along with smear study.
- CBC a useful tool in diagnosis and management of dengue fever.
- With respect to day-to-day infections, CBC needs cautious interpretation. Utilize CBC as a starting point for further evaluation. CBC gives direction for further definitive investigations.

BIBLIOGRAPHY

1. Carry J, Rosmarin AG. Why does my patient have leukocytosis? Hematol Oncol Clin North Am. 2012;26(2):303-19.
2. Indian Academy of Pediatrics (IAP). Problem-solving in pediatric infectious diseases (PSPID module under IAP Vision). 2007.
3. Walters MC, Ableson HT. Interpretation of the complete blood count. Pediatr Clin North Am. 1996;43(3):599-622.
4. Witmer CM. Hematologic manifestations of systemic disease (Including iron deficiency, anemia of inflammation and DIC). Pediatr Clin North Am. 2013;60(6):1349-62.

10.2 Acute Phase Reactants: How do They Help?

P Sudhakar

Reviewers: *MKC Nair, S Thangavelu, S Narmada*

INTRODUCTION

Acute phase reactants (APRs) are a heterogeneous group of plasma proteins that increase or decrease as a response to an inflammatory stimuli following an insult. This helps to prevent ongoing tissue damage, eliminate the cause of inflammation as well as begin the repair process.

The whole process occurring in the host comprising wide variety of reactions is called as acute phase response. The causes may be infection, tissue injury, burn, trauma, surgery, cancer or immunological disorders. The acute phase response is proportional to the severity of the inflammatory stimulus. Most acute phase reactants are mainly produced by the liver, although other cell types such as macrophages, endothelial cells, fibroblasts, and adipocytes are also involved in the synthesis.

The macrophages, monocytes, and other cells participating in the inflammatory response releases proinflammatory cytokines such as interleukin (IL)-6, IL-1, tumor necrosis factor-alpha, and interferon gamma, which in turn stimulate production of acute phase proteins (APR) by the liver.

Important acute phase reactants include:

- Erythrocyte sedimentation rate (ESR)
- C-reactive protein (CRP)
- Procalcitonin (PCT)
- Ferritin
- Others including serum amyloid A (SAA) protein, alpha-1 antitrypsin, haptoglobin, alpha-1 acid glycoprotein, ceruloplasmin, complement proteins C3 and C4, transcortin, transthyretin, albumin and prealbumin and retinol binding protien, etc.

CLASSIFICATION

Acute-phase reactants can be classified as positive and negative. Acute-phase proteins whose plasma concentrations increase or decrease as a response to inflammation are called positive and negative acute phase reactants respectively.

Positive acute-phase reactants: The level of response may vary among different APRs. C-reactive protein and SAA protein can increase a few thousand-fold in response. Ceruloplasmin and complement proteins rise by approximately 25–50%, and fibrinogen levels usually increase a few fold.

Negative acute-phase reactants: Negative acute-phase proteins decrease in inflammation. Examples include transcortin, transferrin, transthyretin, albumin, prealbumin and retinol-binding protein. The decrease of such proteins may be used as markers of inflammation. The physiological role of decreased synthesis of such proteins is generally to save amino acids for producing "positive" acute-phase proteins more efficiently.

Indirect acute-phase reactants: Erythrocyte sedimentation rate is a non-protein APR that changes in response to plasma fibrinogen levels and plasma viscosity and hence is an "indirect" APR.

Functions of acute-phase reactants: They serve different physiological functions for the immune system. Some act to destroy or inhibit growth of microbes, e.g. C-reactive protein, mannose-binding protein, complement factors, ferritin, ceruloplasmin, serum amyloid A and haptoglobin **(Fig. 10.2.1)**.

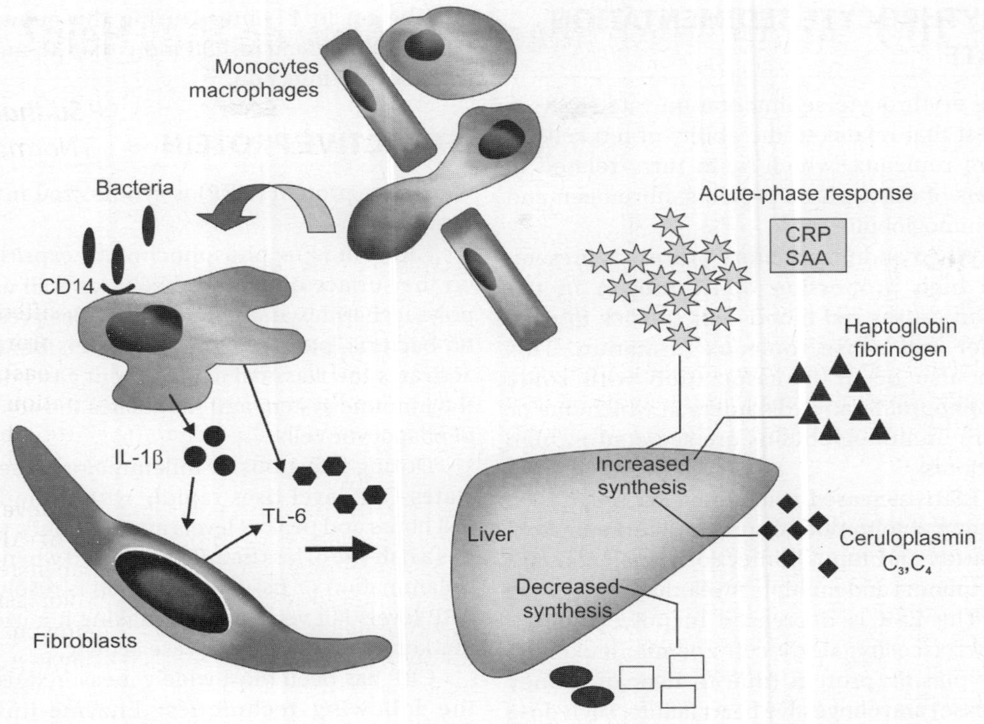

Fig. 10.2.1: Synthesis of acute-phase reactants

Source: A Brief Review. Bansal T, Pandey A, Deepa D, Asthana AK. C-reactive protein (CRP) and its association with periodontal disease: J Clin Diagn Res. 2014;8(7):ZE21–ZE24./Published online 2014 Jul 20. doi: 10.7860/JCDR/2014/8355.4646.

Others give negative feedback on the inflammatory response, e.g. serpins. Alpha 2-macroglobulin and coagulation factors affect coagulation, mainly stimulating it. This pro-coagulant effect may limit infection by trapping pathogens in local blood clots. Also, some products of the coagulation system can contribute to the innate immune system by their ability to increase vascular permeability and act as chemotactic agents for phagocytic cells.

CLINICAL USE OF ACUTE-PHASE REACTANTS

Acute-phase reactants have been used as markers for inflammation and so can be considered as "sickness index" in infectious and noninfectious conditions.

They play major role in early diagnosis, in differentiating infectious from noninfectious causes, as a prognostic marker, and in antibiotic guidance strategies. A better defined role as a supplement to clinical assessment may lead to more judicious antibiotic prescriptions, and it has the potential for a long-term favorable impact on antimicrobial stewardship and antibiotic resistance.

The ESR, CRP and procalcitonin are the most commonly used acute-phase markers in clinical practice. Other acute-phase markers are not used regularly in clinical practice for many reasons such as difficulty in measuring levels, lack of standardization and uniformity in reporting, and paucity of clinical data.

ERYTHROCYTE SEDIMENTATION RATE

The erythrocyte sedimentation rate (ESR) is a test that relates to the ability of red cells to form rouleaux, which is, in turn, related to levels of acute phase proteins, fibrinogen and immunoglobulin.

When an inflammatory process is present, the high proportion of fibrinogen in the blood causes red blood cells to stick to each other and cause rouleaux formation. This can also occur in association with some lymphoproliferative disorders in which one or more immunoglobulins are secreted in high amounts.

ESR is increased in inflammation, pregnancy, anemia, autoimmune disorders (like rheumatoid arthritis and lupus), infections, malignancies (lymphoma and multiple myeloma).

The ESR is decreased in polycythemia, hyperviscosity, sickle cell anemia, leukemia, low plasma protein (due to liver or kidney disease) and congestive heart failure. High dose of steroids and salicylates have been reported to cause lower ESR.

ESR rises within 24–48 hours of the onset of inflammation and falls back slowly with resolution.

- Normal values usually <20 mm/hr
- Extreme elevation of ESR (>100 mm/hr) seen in Infective Endocarditis, Miliary Tuberculosis, Kawasaki disease/ Malignancy/Collagen Vascular Disease such as Systemic Lupus Erythematosus and Juvenile Idiopathic Arthritis
- Abnormally low ESR value in infectious condition is a sign of DIC reflecting low plasma fibrinogen concentration

Elevated ESR has poor discriminating power as a single test to differentiate an inflammation due to infectious or noninfectious reason

Micro-ESR is a simple marker used in neonatal infection. It is not a very reliable marker. Its normal value is 6 mm during the first 3 days of life. By the end of first month, maximum value may be up to 11 mm. During the neonatal period value of micro-ESR more than 15 mm is suggestive of infection.

C-REACTIVE PROTEIN

C-reactive protein (CRP) is synthesized in the liver.

CRP binds to phosphocholine expressed on the surface of damaged cells, as well as to polysaccharides and peptosaccharides present on bacteria, parasites and fungi. This binding activates the classical complement cascade of the immune system and modulates the activity of phagocytic cells.

During infectious or inflammatory disease states CRP level rises rapidly within the first 6–8 hours and peak at levels after 48 hours. CRP has a half-life of less than 24 hours and when the inflammation or tissue destruction is resolved, CRP levels fall very quickly, making it a useful marker for monitoring disease activity.

CRP has been most widely measured using the following techniques: Enzyme-linked immunosorbent assays (ELISA), immuno-turbidimetry, or antibody-based nephelometric assays.

C-Reactive protein used for:

- Detecting systemic inflammatory processes.
- Detecting infection and assessing response to antibiotic treatment of bacterial infections.
- Differentiating between active and inactive disease forms with concurrent infection.
- Serum high sensitivity C-reactive protein (HSCRP) is the appropriate C-reactive protein test to order to assess risk of cardiovascular disease or events.

The main advantage of CRP levels is its earlier rise and earlier fall. It is unaffected by anemia, protein levels, red blood cell shape or patient age or sex.

False positive CRP: It occurs in intrauterine infections, birth asphyxia, respiratory distress syndrome, intracerebral hemorrhage and meconium aspiration.

Interpretation

In normal healthy individuals, C-reactive protein (CRP) is a trace protein (<8 mg/L).

Elevated values are consistent with an acute inflammatory process but nonspecific and should not be interpreted without a complete clinical history.

Concentrations above 100 mg/L are associated with severe stimuli such as major trauma and severe infection (sepsis).

Serial CRP values provide useful diagnostic information about the level of activity and severity of a disease. Persistence of a high serum CRP concentration is usually a grave prognostic sign that generally indicates the presence of an uncontrolled infection.

Serial CRP values are better with negative predictive value of up to 99% indicating that if CRP determinations remain persistently normal, it is strong evidence that bacterial sepsis is unlikely and antibiotics can be safely discontinued. Usually, it returns to normal within 2–7 days of successful treatment.

Persistent elevation of CRP may indicate persistent bacterial infection or development of some complication. Persistent elevation of CRP has been found with persistent bacterial meningitis and abscess formation in necrotizing enterocolitis.

A systematic review on diagnostic value of CRP in identifying serious infections in febrile children by Van den Bruel A et al. showed the relation between risk of serious bacterial and CRP level **(Table 10.2.1)**.

Table 10.2.1: Relation between risk of serious bacterial and CRP level

CRP mg/L	*Risk of serious bacterial infection*
< 20	5%
20–80	15%
> 80	72%

Source: Diagnostic value of laboratory tests in identifying serious infections in febrile children: systematic review BMJ 2011;342 doi: http://dx.doi.org/10.1136/bmj.d3082 (Published 08 June 2011). Cite this as: BMJ 2011;342:d3082

PROCALCITONIN

Procalcitonin (PCT) is a propeptide of calcitonin.

PCT levels increase rapidly by 2 hours of an infection, peak by 12 hours, and normalize by 2–3 days. PCT has high sensitivity and specificity.

After birth, the PCT values of the newborn increase over the first 24 hours and stay elevated during the first 2 days of life. The adult reference range applies from day 3 after birth and the mean normal serum PCT level is around 2 ng/mL.

The *optimal cut-off values ranges of* procalcitonin (PCT) are variable and depends upon the clinical condition and comorbidities.

PCT is used for:

- Diagnosis of bacteremia and septicemia in children (including neonates)
- Diagnosis of renal involvement in urinary tract infection in children
- Diagnosis of bacterial infection in neutropenic patients
- Diagnosis, risk stratification, and monitoring of septic shock
- Monitoring of therapeutic response to antibacterial therapy
- Diagnosis of systemic secondary infection post-surgery, and in severe trauma, burns, and multiorgan failure
- Differential diagnosis of bacterial versus viral meningitis/pneumonia.

Sepsis: One major advantage of PCT compared to other parameters is its early and highly specific increase in response to bacterial infections and sepsis. Elevated levels usually not seen in other noninfectious inflammatory conditions. Thus, in septic conditions increased PCT levels can be observed 3–6 hours after infectious challenge.

Low PCT values (<0.25 μg/L) in patients with clinical signs of infection (CAP, UTI) indicate a low probability for blood culture proof of bacterial infection, whereas elevated PCT values (>0.25 μg/L) seem to correlate with the bacterial load and positive blood culture result.

PCT levels in sepsis are generally greater than 1–2 μg/L and often reach values between 10 and 100 μg/L, or considerably higher in individual cases, thus enabling the diagnostic differentiation

Table 10.2.2: Possibility of bacterial infection and recommendation of antibiotics with reference to procalcitonin level

Procalcitonin concentration (μg /L)	*Possibility of bacterial infection*	*Recommendation for starting antibiotics*
< 0.1	Very unlikely	No antibiotics
0.1–0.25	Unlikely	No antibiotics
0.25–0.5	Likely	Start antibiotics
> 0.5	Very likely	Strongly recommended

between various clinical conditions and a severe bacterial infection (sepsis).

Lower respiratory infection: The possibility of bacterial infection and recommendation of antibiotics with reference to serum procalcitonin level can be predicted as shown in **Table 10.2.2**.

Neonates: Early and reliable differentiation of infected and non-infected newborns is possible with PCT determination directly after birth from cord blood when neonatal infection is suspected. A value <0.5 μg/L practically excludes the presence of infection. PCT has been found to be a reliable marker of late onset sepsis in newborn babies with a sensitivity and specificity of nearly 100%.

Meningitis: Serum and cerebrospinal PCT levels are likely to have a high diagnostic accuracy in bacterial meningitis.

Post-neurosurgical procedures: Serum PCT levels of >0.15 have a high diagnostic value for bacterial infections.

Infective endocarditis: An initial value of PCT > 0.5 is predictor for poor outcome.

Pyelonephritis in children: PCT level >0.5 is associated with high likelihood of pyelonephritis and renal scars in pediatric patients with urinary tract infection.

There are few noninfectious conditions and non-bacterial etiology which show elevated PCT:

- Neonates < 48 hours of life (physiological elevation).
- The first days after a major trauma, major surgical intervention, severe burns, treatment with drugs stimulating the release of pro-inflammatory cytokines.
- Patients with invasive fungal infections, acute attacks of *Plasmodium falciparum* malaria.
- Patients with prolonged or severe cardiogenic shock, prolonged severe organ perfusion anomalies, small cell lung cancer, medullary C-cell carcinoma of the thyroid.

Low PCT level does not always indicate absence of bacterial infection.

Falsely low PCT levels in the presence of bacterial infection may occur in:

- Early course of infections
- Localized infections
- Subacute infectious endocarditis.

FERRITIN

Ferritin as an acute-phase reactant is elevated in inflammation, autoimmune disorders, chronic infection and liver disease.

Normal Serum Ferritin Level

- Children up to 6 months: 50–200 ng/mL
- Children 6 months to 15 years: 7–140 ng/mL.

Very high levels of ferritin (>500) are seen in inflammatory conditions.

Elevated levels of ferritin are well-established in macrophage activation syndrome, adult onset Still's disease, multiple sclerosis, and in both synovial fluid and synovial cells of rheumatoid arthritis patients. High concentrations of serum ferritin levels have been reported in patients with active SLE as compared to inactive SLE. Elevated levels of urinary ferritin have also been reported in lupus nephritis (LN) patients.

CONCLUSION

In conclusion, serial values of acute phase reactants are more important adjunct to comprehensive clinical assessment than as single value. During infections, procalcitonin has an advantage over CRP and ESR due to its better specificity but the high cost is a limiting factor in using PCT as a marker of infection.

The inflammatory proteins CRP and PCT do not appear to be adequate markers of invasive bacterial infections in children with severe acute malnutrition and, therefore, cannot be much helpful in reducing antibiotic use. However, these markers could be helpful in identifying children most at risk for dying, which could potentially be useful for triage purposes.

BIBLIOGRAPHY

1. Anne-Laure Diagnostic and Prognostic Value of Procalcitonin and C-reactive Protein in Malnourished children/Pediatrics. 2014; 133:2.
2. Bansal T, Pandey A, Deepa D, Asthana AK. C-reative protein (CRP) and its association with periodontal disease: A brief review. J Clin Diagn Res. 2014;8(7):ZE21-ZE4.
3. Diagnostic value of laboratory tests in identifying serious infections in febrile children: systematic review, BMJ. 2011;342 doi: http://dx.doi.org/10.1136/bmj.d3082 (Published 08 June 2011), Cite this as: BMJ. 2011;342:d3082.
4. Dowton SB, Colten HR. Acute phase reactants in inflammation and infection. Semin Hematol. 1988;25:84-90.
5. Gabay C, Kushner I. Acute-phase proteins and other systemic responses to inflammation. N Engl J Med. 1999;340:448-54.
6. Patel PS. Markers of infection. Indian Pract Pediatr. 2009;11(3).
7. The hyperferritinemic syndrome: macrophage activation syndrome, Still's disease, septic shock and catastrophic antiphospholipid syndrome/ BMC Medicine. 2013:11:185.

10.3 Interpretation of Coagulation Tests in Office Practice

M Deenadayalan

***Reviewers:** K Nedunchelian, Jaydeep Choudhury, RV Dhakshayani*

INTRODUCTION

Hemostasis is a complex process that leads to the formation of a blood clot at the site of vessel injury. Abnormalities in hemostasis can result in bleeding/hemorrhage and or clotting/thrombosis.

Hemostasis is divided into three components **(Fig. 10.3.1)**.

Primary hemostasis: Starts immediately after the endothelial damage and is characterized by vasoconstriction, platelet adhesion and aggregration resulting in the formation of platelet plug.

Secondary hemostasis or coagulation: Formation of fibrin through the coagulation pathway.

Fibrinolysis: Fibrin clot is broken down by the action of plasmin on fibrin, once vascular integrity is restored.

Primary hemostatic disorders [disorders of platelets and von Willebrand factor (VWF)]

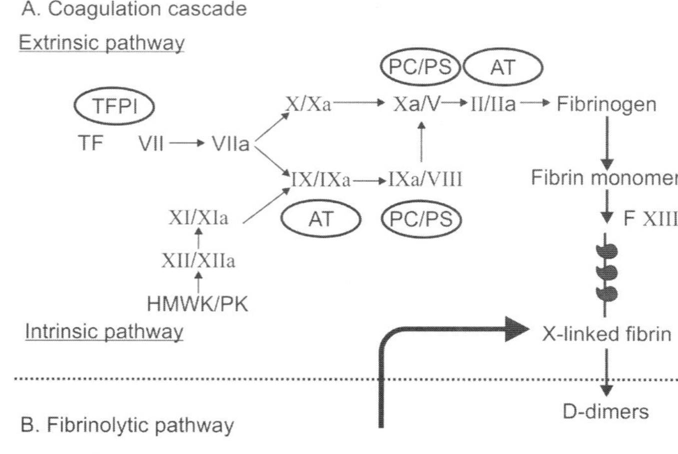

Fig. 10.3.1: Hemostasis and fibrinolysis

mainly results in mucocutaneous bleeding with symptoms such as epistaxis, menorrhagia, petechiae, easy bruising and bleeding after dental and surgical interventions. Secondary hemostatic disorders (congenital or acquired deficiencies of coagulation factors) typically manifest with delayed, deep bleeding into muscles and joints.

HOW TO INVESTIGATE A BLEEDING CHILD?

Before the interpretation of a coagulation test, the most important tool in the evaluation of a patient with a suspected bleeding disorder is a thorough history and physical examination.

HISTORY AND PHYSICAL EXAMINATION

General condition: Well child/sick child.

Age of onset: Usually inherited bleeding disorders present in infancy and are associated with family history. However, mild coagulation defects such as vWD, inherited platelet function defects and mild factor deficiency may not be diagnosed until adulthood when excessive bleeding might occur after trauma or surgery.

History of umbilical bleeding and delayed wound healing should be sought.

Type of bleeding: Mucocutaneous bleeding or joint/muscle bleeding.

History of medication: Antiplatelet medications, anticoagulants, prolonged use of antibiotics causing vitamin K deficiency.

Underlying medical conditions: Liver disease, renal failure, malabsorption.

History of Child Abuse

History of prolonged bleeding after trauma/surgery including dental extraction, circumcision, immunization/intramuscular injection, etc.

Unexplained menorrhagia and post-partum bleeds, family history of bleeding and history of consanguinity will be useful. However, a negative family history does not exclude an inherited coagulation disorder as up to one-third of patients with hemophilia have a negative family history.

Complete physical examination includes looking for petechiae, pathological bruising, hematomas, echymoses, joint effusion, evidence of joint laxity or hyperextensibility.

Clinically significant bleeds are defined as:

- Spontaneous or provoked bleeding from 2 or more distinct mucocutaneous sites
- Bleeding from a single site warranting blood transfusion
- Bleeding from a single site on 3 or more occasions
- Epistaxis for more than 10 minutes or requiring interventions
- Clinical menorrhagia (>7 days/>80 mL/day)

How do We Investigate for These Conditions in the Laboratory?

Once a clinical history and physical examination are suggestive of a bleeding disorder, we have to proceed with coagulation tests. It should be emphasized that, at present, no single test reliably screens the overall process of hemostasis particularly for abnormalities of platelet function or the fibrinolytic pathway.

The baseline investigations **(Table 10.3.1)** should include complete blood counts, examination of the peripheral blood smear for platelet morphology prothrombin time/ international normalized ratio (PT/ INR), activated partial thromboplastin time (aPTT) and the fibrinogen activity level. Normal values may vary with age and among different laboratories. In particular, normal prothrombin and activated partial thromboplastin times should be based upon an individual clinical laboratory's reference ranges.

Approach to a child with prolonged PT and aPTT is shown in **Flow chart 10.3.1**.

Abnormal prolongation of PT or APTT occurs only when coagulation factors are less than 40%. Depending upon the initial screening

Table 10.3.1: Initial screening test

- Complete blood count and blood smear
- Bleeding time
- Prothrombin time
- Activated partial thromboplastin time
- PT and aPTT mixing studies
- Fibrinogen level
- Thrombin time
- Clot stability test

Flow chart 10.3.1: Approach to a child with prolonged PT and aPTT

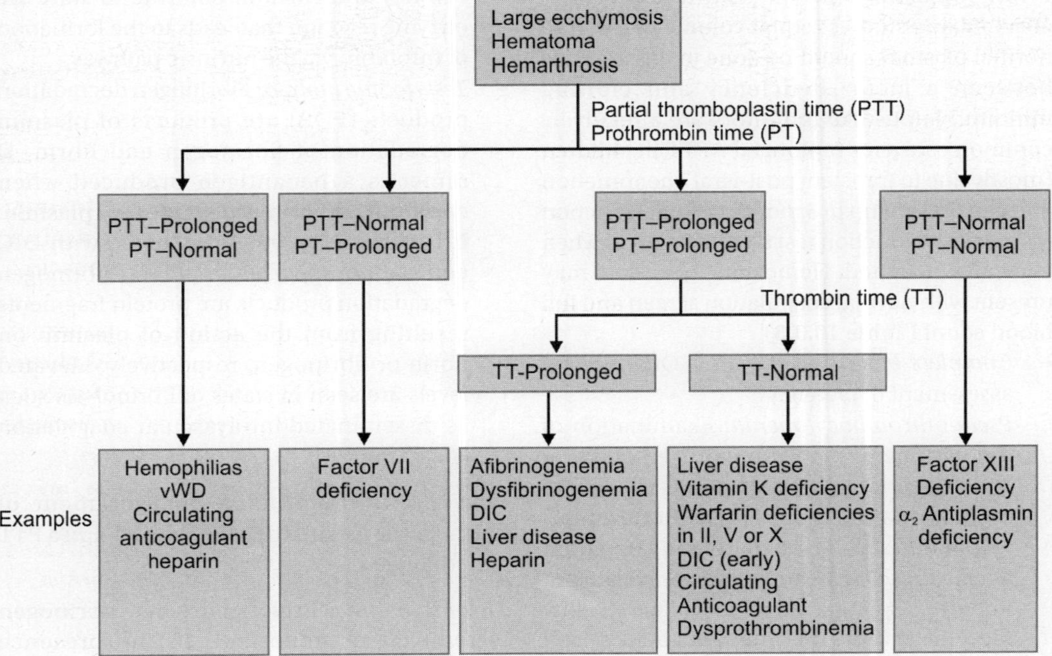

Table 10.3.2: Second-stage investigations

- von Willebrand disease panel, multimer assay
- Platelet aggregation studies
- Specific factor levels
- Euglobulin lysis time
- Lupus anticoagulant
- Plasminogen activator inhibitor level

Table 10.3.3: Hemostatic disorders with normal coagulation screen and full blood count

- Mild von Willebrand disease
- Mild hemophilia A or B
- Mild factor XI or other single factor deficiency
- Factor XIII deficiency
- α_2-antiplasmin deficiency
- Plasminogen activation inhibitor-1 deficiency
- Glanzmann thrombasthenia
- Platelet storage pool disease
- Platelet release defect
- Collagen disorders
- Vitamin C deficiency

test, *second line investigations* should be done **(Table 10.3.2)** so that investigative approach becomes cost-effective and patient-friendly. If there is prolongation of activated partial thromboplastin time or prothrombin time, 50:50 mixing studies (equal volume of test and normal plasma) should be done to differentiate between a factor deficiency and clotting inhibitor. Lupus like inhibitors are a relatively common cause for prolonged APTT in children (mostly due to transient post-viral phenomenon and can present up to 3 months). Renal function test and liver function test should be done when clinically indicated. Hemostatic disorders may present with normal coagulation screen and full blood count **(Table 10.3.3)**.

- *Complete blood count (CBC):* Quantitative assessment of platelets
  Pseudothrombocytopenia: Examination of the peripheral blood smear is essential in patients with low platelet counts in order to exclude the presence of pseudothrombocytopenia caused by platelet aggregation after using EDTA as an in vitro anticoagulant. Platelet aggregation causes falsely low platelet counts by the automated cell counter, but the platelet clumps are obvious on examination of the smear. Alternative anticoagulants (e.g. trisodium citrate or heparin) may circumvent in vitro EDTA-associated platelet aggregation.
- *Bleeding time:* Prolonged with impaired platelet function, platelet counts below 80,000–100,000/mm^3 or impaired vascular integrity. This test is no longer used because of difficulties in standardization and interpretation.
- *Platelet function analyzer (PFA 100):* Assesses flow through a membrane, membrane closure time is measured in response to ADP and to epinephrine. This is often prolonged with impaired platelet function.
- *Prothrombin time (PT) assay* (assesses the extrinsic system): This test utilizes tissue thromboplastin and calcium chloride, to initiate the formation of thrombin via the extrinsic pathway.
- *Partial thromboplastin time (PTT) assay* (assesses the intrinsic system): This test utilizes a phospholipid reagent, a particulate activator (e.g. ellagic acid, kaolin, silica, soy extract) and calcium chloride to start the enzyme reaction that leads to the formation of thrombin via the intrinsic pathway.
- *Tests for fibrinolysis:* Fibrinogen degradation products (FDP) are products of plasmin degradation of fibrinogen and fibrin. D dimer is a neoantigen produced when cross-linked fibrin is degraded by plasmin. It is elevated in 90% of patients with DIC and is more specific than FDPs. Fibrinogen degradation products are protein fragments resulting from the action of plasmin on fibrin or fibrinogen, respectively. Elevated levels are seen in states of fibrinolysis such as disseminated intravascular coagulation specifically.

Fibrinogen: Quantitative measurement of fibrinogen is useful when both the PT and a PTT are prolonged.

Thrombin time: Prolonged when fibrinogen is reduced or abnormal, in the presence

Table 10.3.4: Laboratory causes for prolongation of test results

- Patient's hematocrit (HCT >55 or <30%)
- Citrate concentration (3.2% sodium citrate)
- Under-fill or overfill of tube
- Collection from heparin line
- Clotted or hemolyzed sample
- Time between collection and assay (within 6 hrs)
- Medications
- Time of collection of sample
- Preparation of platelet poor sample
- Prolongation incubation at 37°C
- Wrong label and clinical error

of inhibitors (fibrin degradation products, D-dimers) and in the presence of thrombin inhibiting drugs. Useful test to diagnose dysfibrinogenemas (qualitatively abnormal fibrinogen). Useful when both the PT and a PTT are prolonged.

Clotting factor activity assays: Performed to identify clotting factor deficiencies if mixing studies normalize the PT and aPTT. FXII, FXI, FIX and FVIII assays are useful if aPTT normalizes in mixing studies. The FVII assay is useful if the PT normalizes in mixing studies. FX, FV, FII and fibrinogen assays are useful if both PT and aPTT normalize in mixing studies.

von Willebrand antigen: Quantitative assay for von Willebrand factor: useful when bleeding time or PFA-100 closure time is prolonged or when von Willebrand disease is suspected:

- *von Willebrand factor (ristocetin cofactor activity):* functional/qualitative assay for von Willebrand factor; useful when the bleeding time or PFA-100 closure time is prolonged or when von Willebrand disease is suspected.
- *Platelet aggregation studies:* A qualitative assessment of platelet function; useful when the bleeding time or PFA-100 closure time is prolonged.
- *Urea clot lysis assay:* Useful screen for FXIII deficiency beyond the newborn period. In the absence of fibrin cross-linkage by FXIII, a clot will degrade with incubation in 5 M urea. Prolongation of test results can sometimes be due to laboratory, sample and technique dependent errors. In case of patients with a negative bleeding history, it is, therefore, important to rule out an artefactual prolongation of the hemostatic test before further testing or treatment **(Table 10.3.4)**.

BIBLIOGRAPHY

1. Khair K. Bruising and bleeding in infants and children: a practical approach. Br J Haematol. 133:221-31.
2. Kumar R. Inherited abnormalities of coagulation. Pediatr Clin N Am. 2013;60:1419-41.
3. Lanzkowsky P (Ed). Manual of Pediatric Hematology and Oncology, 5th edn. 2016.
4. van Herrewegen F, Meijers JC, Peters M, van Ommen. Clinical practice: the bleeding child. Part II: disorders of secondary hemostasis and fibrinolysis. Eur J Pediatr. 2012;171(2):207-14. *doi: 10.1007/s00431-011-1571-x.*
5. van Ommen CH, Peters M. The bleeding child. Part I: primary hemostatic disorders. Clinical practice Eur J Pediatr. 2012;171(1):1-10. *doi: 10.1007/s00431-011-1532-4.*

Endocrinology

Reviewers: *K Nedunchelian, Jaydeep Choudhury, RV Dhakshayani*

11.1 Hypothyroidism and Hypocalcemia: How to Diagnose Early?

Hemchand K Prasad, Umamaheshwari B

Reviewers: *K Nedunchelian, Jaydeep Choudhury, RV Dhakshayani*

Hypothyroidism and hypocalcemia are the two most common endocrine conditions encountered by a pediatrician in office practice.

HYPOTHYROIDISM

Universal screening of congenital hypothyroidism is mandatory for an optimal neurological outcome in neonates. Presented below are simple algorithmic approaches to the three common endocrine issues in office practice:

1. Congenital hypothyroidism
2. Juvenile hypothyroidism
3. Hypocalcemia.

Congenital Hypothyroidism

Congenital hypothyroidism (CH) is the most common preventable cause of mental retardation. The incidence of congenital hypothyroidism reported in the western world is 1 in 3500. The incidence reported in our country is much higher. A two-stepped approach to a positive thyroid screening should be followed:

- *Step 1:* Confirmation of a positive screen
- *Step 2:* Establishing the cause of congenital hypothyroidism.

Step 1: Establish Hypothyroidism

All babies must be screened for congenital hypothyroidism by a day 3 heel prick TSH screening. A heel prick TSH ≥6 mIU/mL is considered as positive. As per the latest 2014 European guidelines **(Flow chart 11.1.1)**, the way to proceed with a positive screen is as follows:

- Heel prick TSH ≥40 mIU/mL – Start therapy after taking venous sample, do not wait for reports
- Heel prick TSH <40 mIU/mL and ≥6 mIU/mL – Take a venous sample
- Venous TSH ≥20 mIU/mL – Start therapy irrespective of Free T_4
- Venous TSH 6–20 mIU/mL – Treat only if free T_4 is low, otherwise retest in 1–2 weeks
- Venous TSH <6 mIU/mL – Interpret as a negative screen.

Step 2: Establish Cause for Hypothyroidism

After establishing a diagnosis of hypothyroidism, further evaluation with ultrasound and technetium scan of thyroid gland, done at diagnosis or at 3 years of age (after 6 weeks of stoppage of therapy), helps finding the cause of hypothyroidism. While ultrasound aids in identifying the presence and size of the gland, technetium scan helps in functional assessment of thyroid.

A technetium scan is done by injecting Tc-99m pertechnetate in the arm and images of thyroid gland are obtained with a scintillation camera after 20 minutes. Images are obtained from anterior, left and right anterior oblique projections with a sternal notch marker to detect substernal extension of thyroid. Fasting is not required and TSH must be high for a technetium scan. The cause for hypothyroidism is established as per **Flow chart 11.1.2**.

Special issues in a preterm baby **(Table 11.1.1)**: A pediatrician dealing with a preterm baby may encounter false reports in a preterm baby. Preterm babies may give a picture like central hypothyroidism (transient hypothyroxinemia of prematurity) or a false-positive elevation of TSH (transient hyperthyrotropinemia). Conversely, preterm babies with hypothyroidism may not be able to

Flow chart 11.1.1: Approach to positive thyroid screening

Capillary TSH

≥40 mU/L
Take venous FT_4 and TSH
Do not wait for reports–Treat

<40 mU/L
Take venous FT_4 and TSH
>20 mU/L
Even if FT_4 N–Treat
6–20 mU/L FT_4
Low FT_4
Treat
N FT_4
Treat or Evaluate or Repeat in 2 weeks

<6 mU/L
Reassure

Flow chart 11.1.2: Evaluation of a hypothyroid neonate

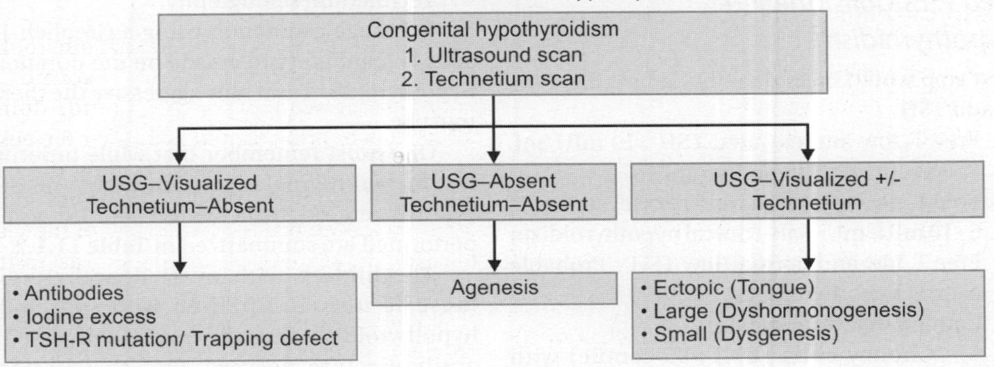

mount a TSH surge (because of axis immaturity) and hence need to be retested at term (or prior to discharge). Also preterm babies are prone for transient hypothyroidism because of conditions like maternal thyroid disease and iodine exposure.

Hence, thyroid function must be interpreted very carefully in a preterm baby and must be repeated at term, irrespective of the initial screening results.

Juvenile Hypothyroidism

Juvenile hypothyroidism (JH) may be primary hypothyroidism due to defect in thyroid gland or central hypothyroidism as part of pan hypopituitarism while most common cause for JH is autoimmune thyroiditis. Hypothyroidism is a great mimic and presentation is highly variable. The common applicable dictum is—it is better to suspect it and not find it, rather than not suspect it and find it.

Table 11.1.1: Important thyroid function test abnormalities seen in a preterm baby

	T_3	T_4	TSH	Free T_4	Causes	Action to be taken
Transient hypothyroxinemia of prematurity	Low	Low	Low	Normal	Immature HP axis <30 weeks	Retest at term/ discharge
Delayed elevation of TSH	Low	Low/ N	Normal	Normal	Immature HPT axis	Retest at term/ discharge
Transient hyperthyrotropinemia	Normal	Normal	Mildly elevated	Normal	Erroneous assay, iodine deficiency or excess, idiopathic	Retest at term/ discharge
Transient primary	Low	Low	Mildly elevated to normal	Low normal	Maternal thyroid therapy, iodine deficiency, maternal antibodies, idiopathic	Thyroxine replacement till 3 years

- *Step 1:* Establishment of hypothyroidism (primary or secondary)
- *Step 2:* Establishing the cause of hypothyroidism and further evaluation.

Step 1: Establishment of Hypothyroidism

First step would be to do a thyroid profile: Free T_4 and TSH

- Free T_4 low and elevated TSH >10 mIU/mL—overt primary hypothyroidism
- Free T_4 normal and marginally elevated TSH 6-10 mIU/mL - sub-clinical hypothyroidism
- Free T_4 low and normal/low TSH - Probable central hypothyroidism
  Caution in interpretation
  - Chubby child (BMI >95 centile) with TSH 6–10 and normal FT_4 is not hypothyroidism
  - Sick child with low TSH and low total T_4 is not central hypothyroidism
  - Micropenis with normal testes, high TSH may be related to BMI not thyroid disease.

Step 2: Establishing the Cause of Hypothyroidism and Further Evaluation

Primary hypothyroidism: Establishment of Hashimotos thyroiditis is done by estimation of antithyroid peroxidase and antithyroglobulin antibody. Significant titers of antibody proves the diagnosis of Hashimotos thyroiditis. Presence of abnormal thyroid echoes and increased vascularity and increased gland size supports the diagnosis. If antibodies are negative, further evaluation to establish the etiology include:

- FNAC (if goiter is present)
- Technetium scintigraphy.

Bone age estimation using a Greulich-Pyle atlas is mandatory to decide on the duration of hypothyroidism and how aggressive the therapy must be.

One must remember that while ordering a test for antithyroglobulin antibody, the other thyroid-related tests which should not be performed are summarized in **Table 11.1.2**.

All children with overt hypothyroidism must be treated. Children with sub-clinical hypothyroidism must be treated only if: either antibodies are positive, growth faltering is present or ultrasound thyroid abnormalities are present.

Secondary hypothyroidism: If a diagnosis of central hypothyroidism is suspected, one must estimate serum cortisol immediately to look for concomitant central adrenal insufficiency. An MRI brain to look at the morphology of pituitary gland or intracranial tumors is a necessary part of the evaluation.

Hypocalcemia

Hypocalcemia is a common metabolic abnormality seen by pediatricians in practice. Hypocalcemia may be symptomatic

Table 11.1.2: Laboratory investigations related to thyroid related to antithyroglobulin antibody

Investigations	*Normal*	*Indication*
Thyroglobulin	3–40 ng/mL	Post-thyroidectomy status in thyroid cancer Dyshormonogenesis
Thyroid binding globulin	14–30 μ/mL	Genetic condition
Anti-thyroglobulin antibodies	<100 IU/mL	Autoimmune thyroid disease

Flow chart 11.1.3: Evaluation of child with hypocalcemia

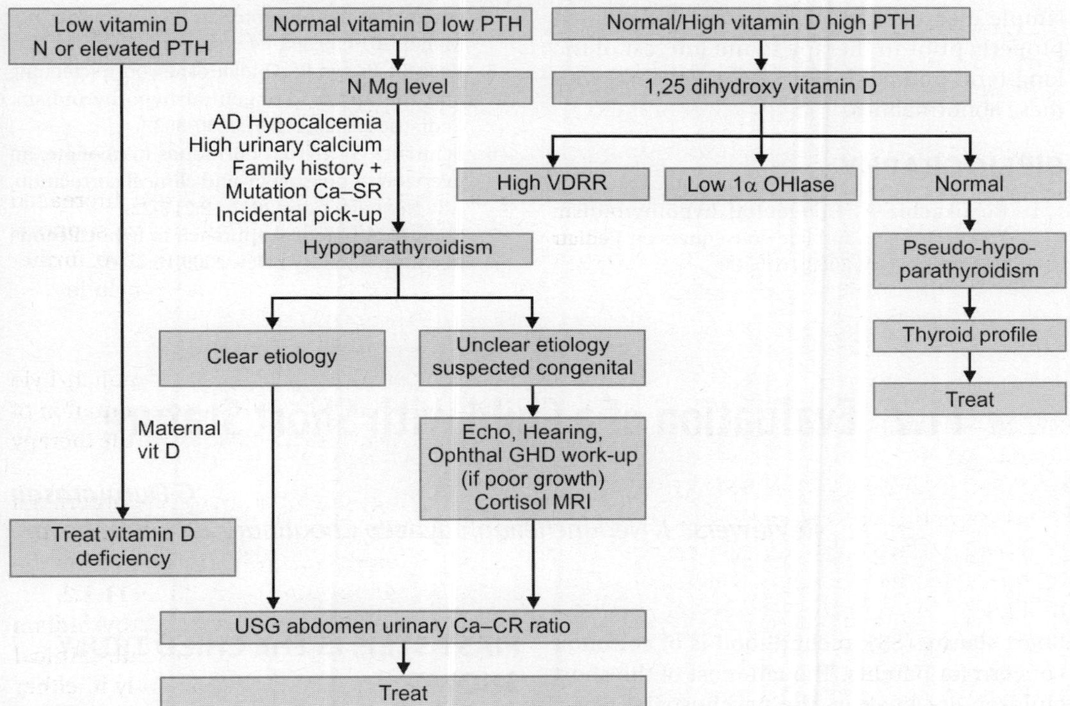

or asymptomatic. Also, hypocalcemia may be related to an acute illness, transient metabolic abnormality or a permanent underlying condition. A stepwise approach to hypocalcemia includes:

- *Step 1:* Establishment of hypocalcemia
- *Step 2:* Establishment of the cause of hypocalcemia.

Step 1: Establishment of Hypocalcemia

Hypocalcemia is considered when serum calcium is <8.5 mg/dL or ionized calcium is <4.4 mg/dL. A serum calcium estimation must always be coupled with estimation of serum creatinine and serum phosphorus estimation.

Step 2: Establishment of Cause of Hypocalcemia

Once hypocalcemia is established, prior to therapy, sample must be taken for estimation of parathormone, 25-hydroxy vitamin D and 1,25 dihydroxy vitamin D (if clinically warranted). The algorithm for interpretation and further evaluation in summarized in **Flow chart 11.1.3**.

- When vitamin D levels are low with normal or elevated PTH, treat as vitamin D deficiency.
- If PTH is low or inappropriately normal for the degree of hypocalcemia with normal vitamin D levels—suspect hypoparathyroidism.

- If vitamin D is normal or high with high PTH proceed with active vitamin D (1,25 OH Vit D)—Look for rare causes of hypocalcemia like vitamin D-dependent rickets.

If hypoparathyroidism is suspected, baseline documentation of urine calcium creatinine ratio and ultrasound for nephrocalcinosis is mandatory.

Hypothyroidism and hypocalcemia are simple disorders which need to be evaluated properly prior to therapy in the interest of the long-term optimal health of a given child with these abnormalities.

BIBLIOGRAPHY

1. Buyukgebiz A. Congenital hypothyroidism clinical aspects and late consequences. Pediatr Endocrinol Rev. 2003;1:185-90.
2. Cho WI, Yu HW, Chung HR, Shin CH, Yang SW, Choi CW, et al. Clinical and biochemical characteristics of neonatal hypocalcemia. Pediatr Endocrinol Metab. 2015;20(2):86-91.
3. Davies JH, Shaw NJ. Investigation and management of hypercalcaemia in children. Arch Dis Child. 2012;97:533-8.
4. Léger J, Olivieri A, Donaldson M, Torresani T, Krude H, Guy van Vliet, et al. ESPE Guidelines on screening, diagnosis and management of congenital hypothyroidism. J Clin Endocrinol Metab. 2014;99:363-84.
5. Rose SR, Brown RS. Update of newborn screening and therapy for congenital hypothyroidism. Pediatrics. 2006;117(6):2290-303.
6. Schmaltz C. Thyroid hormones in neonate, an overview of physiology and clinical correlation. Adv Neonatal Care. 2011;12:217-22.
7. Shaw N. A practical approach to hypocalcemia in children. Endocr Dev. 2009;16:73-92.

11.2 Evaluation of a Child with Short Stature

G Duraiarasan

Reviewers: *K Nedunchelian, Jaydeep Choudhury, RV Dhakshayani*

Short stature (SS) in childhood is of common concern for parents. Though most of the short children are healthy, the psychosocial stress associated with shortness is more distressing, depending upon height deficit and child's coping skills.

Normal variation accounts for the majority of cases of suspected short stature. Pathologic causes are numerous but rare. A stepwise approach, with a careful history, physical examination and targeted laboratory and radiological evaluation is recommended in order to determine the etiology and guide treatment. Meticulous measurements, accurate plotting, growth velocity derivations and pubertal status assessments help the physician elucidate the cause.

FIRST STEP: IS THE CHILD TRULY SHORT?

"Short stature"is defined as height below 3rd centile or less than two standard deviations (SDs) below the mean height for that age and sex according to the population standard; or even if the height is within the normal percentiles the growth velocity being consistently below 25th percentile over a period of 6–12 months of observation.

SECOND STEP: WHETHER THE CHILD'S HEIGHT IS APPROPRIATE FOR THE FAMILY?

To determine whether a child's height is consistent with his or her genetic potential, a target height (mid-parental height) can be calculated using the formulas **(Box 11.2.1)**. Most of the children's expected adult height will fall within their target height range. Clinicians should be more concerned only when a child's height percentile differs from the target range percentiles.

After calculating the target height, the target range is calculated by plotting two points, 6 cms above and below (representing the 10th and the 90th centile for that child) **(Fig. 11.2.1)**.

Box 11.2.1: Formulas for calculating target height

Target height formulas

For girls (father's height [cm] + mother's height [cm] – 13) ÷ 2

For boys (father's height [cm] + mother's height [cm] + 13) ÷ 2

For example, if the mother is 155 cm and the father is 167 cm, the target height or 50th percentile for a boy child of these parents is 167.5 cm (155 + 167 = 322/2 = 161 + 6.5) and the target range is 161.5–173.5 cm.

Thus, the 50th centile on the chart is 167.5 cm and 173.5 cm is the 90th centile for this child and the 10th centile for this child 161.5 cm

THIRD STEP: WHAT IS THE CHILD'S GROWTH RATE?

Height velocity is the most sensitive indicator in detecting growth abnormality. The growth velocity varies with age and is maximum during the first year of life and drops to 5 cm/ year after 5 years till the pubertal growth spurt **(Box 11.2.2)**. Any child more than two years

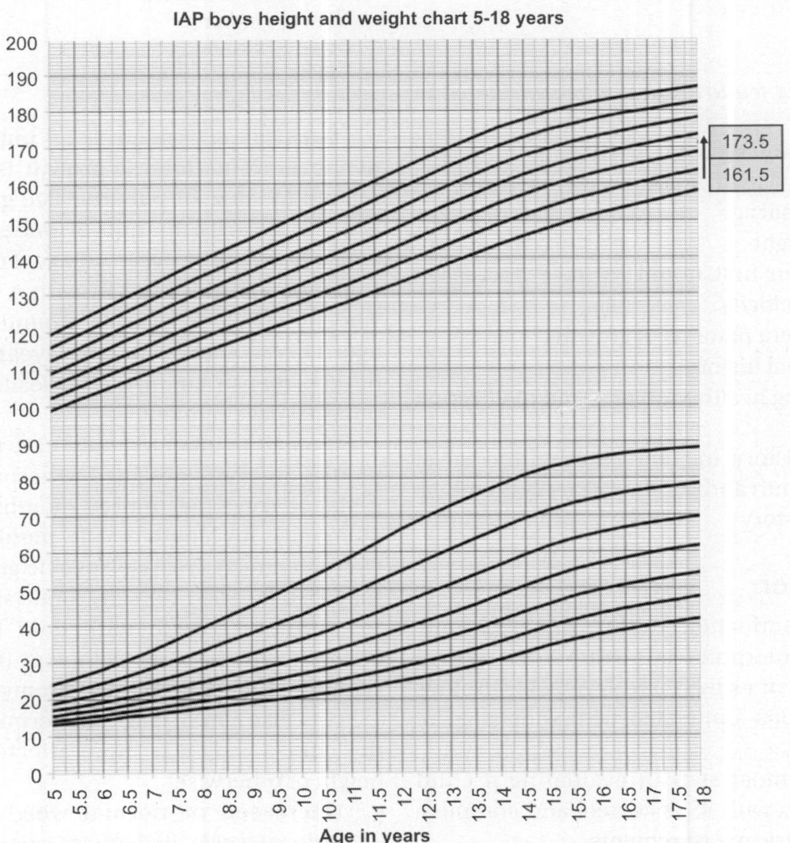

Fig. 11.2.1: 10th and 90th centile range with 50th centile for a boy with height of mother 155 cm and father 167 cm

Box 11.2.2: Growth velocity over various age groups

Age	*Growth velocity*
0–3 mo	3.5 cm/mo
3–6 mo	2 cm/mo
6–9 mo	1.5 cm/mo
9–12 mo	1.3 cm/mo
1–2 y	10–11 mm/ mo; 12 cm/y
2–3 y	8 cm/y
3–4 y	7 cm/y
4–9 y	5–6 cm/y

of age with a growth velocity of less than 4.5 cm/year has a pathological cause and needs evaluation. Children who grow at a normal rate are more likely to represent normal variations of growth.

CLINICAL APPROACH

History

The following features should be considered in the history:

- Pregnancy history, including maternal health and medications
- Gestational age
- Birth weight
- Age when first noted to have decreased growth velocity
- Subsequent patterns of growth
- Nutritional history
- Coexisting health problems and medication use
- Family history, including heights and age of growth spurt and puberty of family members
- Social history

Examination

A careful examination for the signs of chronic illness or dysmorphic features are crucial part of the assessment as there are several syndromes and conditions associated with short stature **(Box 11.2.3)**.

The foremost step in evaluating a child who presents with SS is correct and complete anthropometric measurements.

Box 11.2.3: Causes of short stature

Normal
- Constitutional growth delay
- Genetic/Familial

Pathological
- Psychosocial growth retardation
- Nutritional
- Gastrointestinal
- Cardiac
- Pulmonary—chronic lung diseases
- Renal
- Endocrine
  - GH deficiency—congenital/acquired
  - Hypothyroidism
  - Pseudohypoparathyroidism
  - Hypercortisolemia
  - Precocious puberty
  - Poorly controlled type 1 diabetes
- Skeletal dysplasias and chondrodystrophies
- Low birth weight
- Chromosomal defects
- Turner's syndrome
- Down syndrome
- Others

Pubertal assessment is an important part of the examination, as growth is intimately related to stage of puberty. The growth spurt is seen towards the end of puberty in boys, typically around 14 years of age. Puberty tends to happen earlier in girls, with a peak height velocity usually occurring around 12 years of age. This is approximately 1 year before the onset of menstruation, the last feature of female pubertal development.

Premature infants should have their growth plotted on charts designed to account for their gestational age (i.e. until 24 months for weight, 40 months for length and 18 months for head circumference). Disease-specific growth charts may also be used for syndromic short stature to compare growth with data from other children with the same pathology (e.g. Turner's syndrome, achondroplasia, trisomy 21).

It is also important to determine whether the child's weight is more affected than the height or otherwise.

- Decreased or normal weight-to-height ratio suggests inadequate caloric intake or chronic illness as the etiology for the short stature.

- A high weight-to-height ratio suggests an endocrine etiology, such as GH deficiency, GH insensitivity, hypothyroidism, or glucocorticoid excess and should be referred to a pediatric endocrinologist.

LABORATORY EVALUATION

Choice of tests should be based on the potential etiologies after a careful history and physical examination.

Skeletal Age

The most essential tool in SS work-up is estimation of bone age (BA).

When bone age is less than 2 SD or <2 years of chronological age, it is considered delayed. In familial SS, the BA matches the chronological age (CA); the height age being less than both BA and CA (HA <BA = CA).

Conversely, in pathological short stature, the BA is severely delayed as compared to HA and furthermore than the CA (BA <HA <CA).

In constitutional short stature, there is a delay in attaining normal/expected growth velocity and puberty, patients demonstrate a slower growth initially but will show peak growth later with later onset of puberty and will finish within their target height range **(Fig. 11.2.2)**. These children have delayed BA which matches their HA. Both are less for their CA (HA = BA <CA).

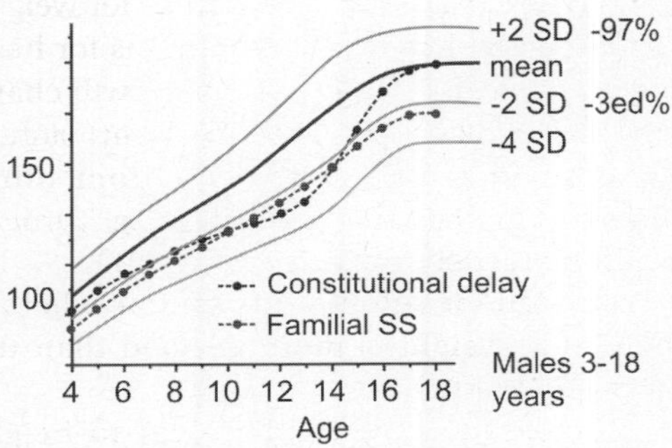

Fig. 11.2.2: Differences in growth velocity of familial short stature and constitutional short stature

A short child with delayed bone age carries a better prognosis for attainment of ultimate height than a shortchild where bone age is consistent with chronological age. Bone age of 17 years in males and 15 years in females means full maturation, i.e. no more increase in height is possible.

First-line tests include:

- CBC
- Complete metabolic profile (to screen for electrolyte abnormalities in renal and other chronic diseases) including looking for metabolic acidosis and for hypocalcemia (e.g. DiGeorge syndrome, rickets)
- ESR to rule out underlying undiagnosed chronic inflammatory illness
- Tissue transglutaminase to rule out celiac disease
- Urine analysis to rule out infection, or proteinuria (with chronic renal disease), and to detect renal tubular acidosis
- TFTs to screen for hypothyroidism
- Insulin-like growth factor 1 (IGF-1) and IGF-binding protein 3 (IGFBP-3) to screen for GH deficiency
- Karyotype in girls to rule out Turner's syndrome.

SUBSEQUENT TESTS

Depend on the diagnosis and may include:

- GH stimulation tests for GH deficiency; patients may also need an MRI brain and full pituitary evaluation to identify co-existing pathology
- Diurnal cortisol levels, urinary cortisol levels, and a dexamethasone suppression test for Cushing's syndrome.

DIAGNOSTIC ALGORITHM

A practical way to approach the differential diagnosis of pathological short stature is to divide patients into those with dysmorphic features and those without. Patients with dysmorphic features are suggestive of genetic syndromes and may be disproportionate or proportionate based on the upper-to-lower

Flow chart 11.2.1: Approach to a child with pathological short stature

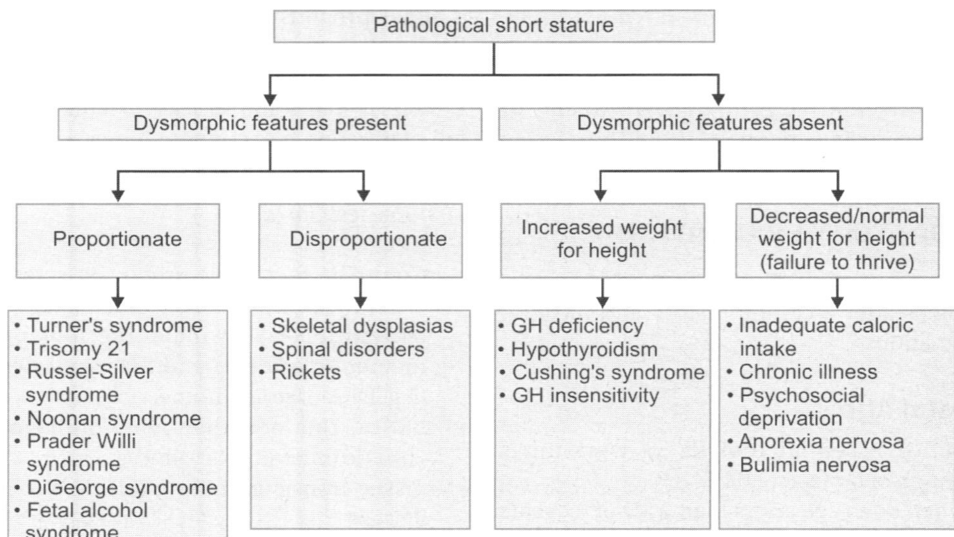

segment ratio. Those who are not dysmorphic can be further divided depending on the weight-to-height ratio.

Flow chart 11.2.1 will aid in narrowing the differential diagnosis.

MANAGEMENT

- Growth hormone subcutaneous injections (GH deficiency, Turner syndrome, SGA, CRF prior to transplant)
- Dietary advice [undernutrition, celiac disease, renal tubular acidosis (RTA)]
- Limb lengthening procedure: Skeletal dysplasia
- Levothyroxine (in hypothyroidism)
- Monitoring with regular and accurate recording of height is mandatory for a good outcome in any form of therapy.

BIBLIOGRAPHY

1. Cohen LE. Idiopathic short stature a clinical review. JAMA. 2014;311(17):1787-9.
2. Yadav S, Dabas A. Approach to short stature. Indian J Pediatr. 2015;82(5):462-70.
3. Yewale V, Khadilkar V, Yadav S, Agrawal KK, Tamboli S, Banerjee M. IAP Guidebook on growth monitoring in children. IAP Growth Chart Committee, 2014.

Critical Care

Reviewers: *P Ramachandran, NC Gowrishankar, Hemchand K Prasad*

12.1 Envenomation in Snakebite and Scorpion Sting

Janani Sankar

Reviewers: *P Ramachandran, NC Gowrishankar, Hemchand K Prasad*

SNAKEBITE ENVENOMATION

INTRODUCTION

There are 330 species of snakes found in India, of which 70 species are poisonous (40 land snakes and 30 sea snakes). The most common venomous Indian snakes are usually referred as the big four" common krait, common cobra, saw scaled viper and Russell's viper. Their toxicity is secondary to venom containing hemotoxic, neurotoxic and myotoxic components.

PATHOPHYSIOLOGY

Among the various species, though the average yield per bite in terms of dry weight of lyophilized venom is larger, the fatal doses of cobra is 12 mg, Russel's viper is 15 mg, krait is 6 mg and saw scaled viper is 8 mg. However, clinical features and outcomes are not predictable since every bite does not result in envenomation.

Snake venom is complex mixture of enzymatic and nonenzymatic compounds. Enzymes identified are phopsholipases A2, D hydrolases, proteases, hydaluronidase, nucleotidase and ATPases. The nonenzymatic components are neurotoxins and hemotoxins.

Direct cytolytic action, causes local necrosis predisposing to secondary infection. The cobra toxin of the Indian cobra and alpha-bungarotoxin of the common krait block the postsynaptic pathway and prevents depolarization. Beta-bungarotoxin of the common krait causes pre-synaptic blockage preventing release of acetylcholine. Viper bites can result in hypotension, ECG changes and acute myocardial infarction. Consumption coagulopathy results in intravascular coagulation, and qualitative and quantitative defect in platelet function causing bleeding.

Some toxins increase capillary permeability, causing loss of blood and plasma into the extravascular space resulting in edema. The resultant fall in intravascular volume, leads to shock.

SIGNS AND SYMPTOMS

Local symptoms and signs in the bitten part:

- Fang marks
- Local pain
- Local bleeding
- Bruising
- Lymphangitis
- Lymph node enlargement
- Inflammation
- Blistering
- Local infection, abscess formation
- Necrosis.

SYSTEMIC SYMPTOMS AND SIGNS

General

Nausea, vomiting, malaise, abdominal pain, weakness, drowsiness, prostration.

Cardiovascular (Viperidae)

Visual disturbances, dizziness, faintness, collapse, shock, hypotension, cardiac arrhythmias, pulmonary edema, conjunctival edema (chemosis).

Bleeding and Clotting Disorders (Viperidae)

- Traumatic bleeding—from recent wounds (including prolonged bleeding from the fang marks and from old partly-healed wounds)

Spontaneous systemic bleeding—from gums, epistaxis, bleeding into the tears, intracranial hemorrhage (meningism from subarachnoid hemorrhage, lateralizing signs and/or coma from cerebral hemorrhage), hemoptysis, hematemesis, rectal bleeding or melaena, hematuria, vaginal bleeding, antepartum hemorrhage in pregnant women, bleeding into the mucosa, skin (petechiae, purpura, discoid hemorrhages and ecchymoses) and retina.

Renal (Viperidae, Sea Snakes)

Loin pain, hematuria, hemoglobinuria, myoglobinuria, oliguria/anuria, symptoms and signs of uremia.

LONG-TERM COMPLICATIONS OF SNAKEBITE

At the site of the bite, loss of tissue may result from sloughing or surgical debridement of necrotic areas or amputation; chronic ulceration, infection, osteomyelitis, contractures, arthrodesis or arthritis may persist causing severe physical disability. Malignant transformation may occur in skin ulcers after a number of years.

MANAGEMENT

- Prehospital care (first aid)
- Supportive therapy
- Specific therapy
- Local wound management.

Prehospital Care (First Aid)

Prehospital care should focus on stabilization and rapid transport to a healthcare facility where anti-venom is available.

Aim of first aid is to attempt to retard systemic absorption of venom and prevent complications before the patient can receive specific treatment.

Immobilization

The bitten extremity is placed in a neutral position, and the patient should avoid movement. It is immobilized as for fractured limbs. Movement of even the unbitten extremities increases lymphatic absorption from the bitten site.

The following interventions are avoided: Incision or excision of the bite site, suction cryotherapy, tourniquet and electric shock therapy.

Supportive Therapy

Airway, breathing and circulation (ABCs) are stabilized and ventilatory support is provided, if needed. Vascular access should be obtained in the unbitten limb. Fluid management and inotropes may be titrated based on identification of shock. Anticonvulsants are administered for seizures. Sedation and analgesics are administered for pain but NSAIDs are usually avoided. A booster dose of tetanus toxoid may be administered. Broadspectrum antibiotics are administered in patients with an infected wound.

Specific Therapy

Antivenom Ingredients

Polyvalent snake anti-venom manufactured by Haffkine biopharmaceutical Corporation Ltd is available as a lyophilized powder. It is of equine origin and is effective against the big four (Common cobra, common krait, Russell's viper and saw-scaled viper). Each milliliter of the reconstituted snake anti-venom neutralizes 0.6 mg of venom (Indian cobra and Russell's viper) and 0.45 mg venom from krait and saw scaled viper.

Indications for Administering Antivenom

The prophylactic use of antivenom should be avoided due to the inherent risk of hypersensitivity reactions. The following are the indications for administering antivenom:

- Swelling rapidly continuing one hour after removal of tourniquet.
- *If neurotoxic:*
  - Measure single breath count, i.e. ask patient to count aloud for the duration of one breath and record the number reached. Start antivenom 10 vials.
  - 0.6 mg atropine given IV followed by 1.5 mg neostigmine given IM; Repeat single breath count every 10 minutes for 1 hour.

- If the child improves, give atropine as required followed by 0.5 mg neostigmine every 30 minutes until recovery, if no improvement, stop atropine and neostigmine.
- Monitor patient for 1–2 hours, if symptoms do not improve, or worsen repeat dose of 10 vials of ASV up to a maximum of 25 vials.

• *If hemotoxic:*
  - Monitor coagulation every 6 hours and repeat dose of 4 vials until blood becomes coagulable *up to a maximum of 8 vials.*
  - 20 minutes whole blood clotting test (20WBCT) is essential and measurement of hemoglobin concentration or hematocrit are important to detect occult bleeding and careful monitoring of urine output and measurement of blood urea/creatinine and potassium are important as renal failure is a high risk.

20 Minutes Whole Blood Clotting Test

Place a few milliliters of freshly sampled venous blood in a fresh glass test tube. Leave undisturbed for 20 minutes at ambient temperature. After that tip the test tube once. If the blood is still liquid (unclotted) and runs out, the patient has incoagulable blood. In the South-East Asian region, incoagulable blood is diagnostic of a viper bite and rules out an elapid bite.

Precautions Taken During Administration of Antisnake Venom

Antisnake venom should be administered over one hour since there is no benefit in administering it over longer periods and lengthening the period of neutralizing.

The dose is similar for adults and children.

ASV test done has been abandoned since early intervention against these reactions has shown positive outcomes. Therefore, patients should be monitored closely for the anaphylactoid reactions. At the first sign of any of the following such as urticaria, itching, fever, shaking chills, nausea, vomiting, diarrhea, abdominal cramps, tachycardia, hypotension, bronchospasm or or angioedema, ASV should be discontinued. In anti-hematostatic bites, after the initial dose has been adminstered over one hour, no further ASV is given for six hours. If whole blood clotting time exceeds 20 minutes (performed every six hours), it will be help determine whether additional ASV is required. In neurotoxic bites, once the first dose of 10 vials has been administered and the neostigmine test given, the victim is closely monitored. If after 1–2 hours the victim has not improved or has worsened, the a second or final dose should be given. The second dose also consists of 10 vials which are administered over one hour. Maximum dose of ASV is 25 vials.

Preparation and Administration of Antivenom

Antivenom is mixed with NS and rotated between the palms of the hands till the serum is fully dissolved and a clear liquid appears. Vigorous shaking is avoided since appearance of foam indicates the presence of denatured protein. Prior to the administration of anti-venom, history of previous administration of antiserum, allergy, bronchial asthma and urticaria is obtained.

Treatment of Serum Sensitive Individuals

0.01 mL/kg of 1:1000 adrenaline (maximun: 0.5 mL) is administered intramuscularly. Repeat doses may be needed. Supplemental oxygen is provided. Need for intubation is anticipated. Shock is corrected with normal saline. Chlorpheneramine maleate 0.2 mg/kg/dose IV and hydrocortisone 2 mg/kg/dose IV are administered. If the child is found to be sensitive to equine ASV, de-sensitivization may be necessary by administering graded doses of anti-venom at regular and adequate intervals.

Once the patient recovers, ASV may be restarted over 10–15 minutes while monitoring closely. The normal rates may then be resumed.

Timing of Antivenom

Beneficial effects are observed within 4 hours if bite, but it is never too late to start ASV in viperine bites. Venom requiring neutralization may be present even 3 weeks after the bite.

Local Wound Management

The wound is cleaned and left open. If the proximal edge of the swelling or tenderness is apparent, it is marked with ink, such that progression with time may be easily monitored.

The circumference of the injured extremity is measured at level, if the edema and hourly progression of edema is recorded. Wound debridement may be required on the 3rd of 5th day after hemodynamic stabilization.

Fasciotomy should be performed for massive edema secondary to compartment system.

BIBLIOGRAPHY

1. WHO Guidelines 2010. Management of Snake Envenomation.

SCORPION STING

INTRODUCTION

Scorpion stings are not uncommon. In India, 86 species of scorpions have been identified; two types of poisonous species are important namely the small red *Buthus tamulus* and the large black *Palamneus gravimanus*; of the two *Buthus tamulus* is more toxic. *Mesobuthus tamulus* (the Indian red scorpion) is the most lethal amongst all poisonous species of scorpions in India with fatalities in adults and children.

PATHOPHYSIOLOGY

The scorpion does not always inject the venom when it stings, since it can control its ejaculation to total, partial or nonexistent (dry sting). The scorpion venom is a mixture of various active substances namely polypeptides and enzymes. Venom consists of: (1) Neurotoxin, which acts on the respiratory, vasomotor centers, nerve terminals and end plates of both striped and unstripped muscles, (2) hemolysins, agglutinins, hemorrhagins, leukocytolysins, coagulins, lecithin, cholesterin, cardiotoxins, nephrotoxins, hyaluronidases, phosphodiesterases, phopholipases, glycosaminoglycans, histamine, tryptophan and cytokine releasers. The main molecular targets of scorpion neurotoxins are the voltage-gated sodium channels and potassium channels including calcium-activated potassium channels resulting in an autonomic storm where both the sympathetic and parasympathetic systems are activated. The toxin induces a predominantly alpha-receptor stimulatory effect, resulting in pulmonary edema, myocardial dysfunction, tachycardia, shock, hypertension and excessive sweating. Scorpion venom also suppresses secretion of insulin which in turns leads to hyperglycemia, lipolysis and increased free fatty acid concentrations. Increased free fatty acids is considered an important contributory factor to the occurrence of arrhythmias and heart failure in scorpion-sting victims.

CLINICAL FEATURES

Venom is deposited deep to subcutaneous tissue after sting; almost complete absorption of the venom from sting site would occur in 7–8 hours (70% of maximum concentration of venom in the blood reached within 15 minutes of sting). The severity of envenoming is related to age (high fatality is seen in children and 50% mortality in less than 4 years old in the past), size of scorpion and the season of sting (April to early June and September to October).

Clinical manifestations may be local or systemic. The symptoms may progress to maximal severity in 3–5 hours and subside within 1–2 days. The local manifestations include intense pain at the site of sting, swelling and ecchymosis. It has also been observed that if the pain is severe, there is less propensity for progression to severe manifestation.

The "autonomic storm", is the most important manifestation of scorpion envenomation. The initial cholinergic stimulation leads to vomiting, salivation, sweating, and cold extremities, priapism and bradycardia. Sweating and salivation may persist for 6–12 hours. Occurrence of priapism, a poor prognostic sign, seems to be associated with myocardial dysfunction.

Stimulation of the sympathetic system, leads to tachypnea, pulmonary edema, tachycardia, arrhythmias, hypertension, peripheral vasoconstriction, shock and myocardial dysfunction. Hypertension usually lasts for 4–8 hours. Hypotension which occurs in the early cholinergic phase (1–2 hours) secondary to bradycardia indicates a poor prognosis. Hypotension can also manifest during the recovery stage (48–72 hours) secondary to depletion of stored catecholamine. Pulmonary edema, another life-threatening complication, may occur due to primary myocardial dysfunction (cardiogenic) or due to acute respiratory distress syndrome (non-cardiogenic). Other rarer but fatal complications include encephalopathy, disseminated intravasculars coagulation (DIC), hemolysis, hemiplegia and pancreatitis.

MANAGEMENT

Local pain is managed with ice compression, paracetamol and regional nerve block using low concentration of lidocaine (without epinephrine). Antiemetics may be needed, if vomiting is severe. Seizures are managed with benzodiazepine.

Profuse diaphoresis and vomiting can cause fluid loss. If the cardiopulmonary assessment suggests that the child is stable but dehydrated, the hydration status is corrected by fluid replacement. Prazosin is administered orally in the prescribed dose.

PRAZOSIN

Prazosin suppresses the sympathetic outflow and activates venom-inhibited potassium channels. It blocks the postsynaptic alpha-1 receptors and also prevents prostagladin production. It reduces cardiac preload, afterload, blood pressure and CNS sympathetic stimulation without causing an increase in heart rate or cardiac output (cardio-output effect). Thus, it prevents hypertensive stress on the myocardium. Its mechanism of action seems to counter the activity of the scorpion venom.

Prazosin is available as 1 mg (scored) tablet. Sustained release tablets are not recommended in this condition, The dose recommended is 30 µg/kg/dose.

Prazosin is administered only when features of, autonomic storm exist. In hemodynamically unstable patients, the priority remains in stabilization of the airway, breathing and circulation. It seems intuitive to correct shock and BP prior to administration of prazosin.

The drug should not be given prophylactically in the absence of symptoms of autonomic storm. If the child is unable to swallow, it may be administered through a nasogastric tube. The mother should be instructed to keep the child in the supine position to avoid 'first dose hypotension' due to prazosin.

Rapid cardiopulmonary assessment should be performed every 30 minutes for next 6 hours and later every 4 hours till improvement. Prazosin is repeated in the same dose at the end of the 3 hours, later every 6 hours till extremities are warm and dry. Not more than 4 doses are usually required in children.

MANAGEMENT OF COMPLICATIONS

If the cardiopulmonary assessment suggests shock, isotonic fluid bolus is given. Since the risk of myocardial dysfunction exists, it would be wise to correct with smaller boluses of 10 mL/kg up to a maximum of 30-40 mL/kg. If shock improves, further fluids may be stopped. If shock does not improve inotropes should be considered. Dobutamine may be used, if BP is high or low normal. Severe myocardial dysfunction manifested by hypotension may be treated with ephinephrine infusion.

In case of pulmonary edema or cardiogenic shock, early intubation is indicated for provision of PEEP. Vasodilators, such as sodium nitroprusside (0.3–1 µg/kg/min) infusion or nitroglycerine (5 µg/kg/min) infusate have been used in patients with cold shock with high or normal blood pressure. Close monitoring of CVP is needed to adjust fluid therapy. Prazosin should be given one hour before termination of sodium nitroprusside.

If sodium nitroprusside is not available, isosorbide dinitrate—10 mg may be used every 10 minutes sublingually as an emergency measure. Arrhythmias are managed appropriately.

Signs of recovery are normal heart rate, appearance of warm peripheries, dilated peripheral veins, reappearance of pain and recovery of mental status.

PROGNOSIS

Pain and age greater than 6 years are good prognostic signs. Delay in initiation of prazosin therapy, pulmonary edema, arrhythmias, encephalopathy and age less than 6 years indicate a bad prognosis.

Scorpion sting may be fatal, if not treated early. Children presenting with scorpion sting envenomation should be observed for at least 24 hours even if asymptomatic. The outcomes have improved with early identification and management of pulmonary edema and shock. The early use of prazosin also seems to have improved the speed of recovery.

BIBLIOGRAPHY

1. Bawaskar HS, Bawaskar PH. Efficacy and safety of scorpion antivenom plus prazosin compared with prazosin alone for venomous scorpion (Mesobuthus tamulus sting: randomised open label clinical trial. BMJ. 2011;341:c7136.
2. Bawaskar HS, Bawaskar PH. Prazosin in management of cardiovascular manifestations of scorpion sting. Lancet. 1986;1(8479):510-1.

12.2 Diabetic Ketoacidosis: Thinking Beyond Insulin

V Poovazhagi

Reviewers: *P Ramachandran, NC Gowrishankar, Hemchand K Prasad*

INTRODUCTION

Diabetic ketoacidosis (DKA) is an acute life-threatening medical emergency encountered in children with diabetes mellitus. Management of DKA is predominantly addressed towards fluid electrolyte therapy and insulin. Management of the precipitating factors and complications need to be addressed as well. Airway, breathing and circulation is the priority in DKA management. Monitoring for complications such as cerebral edema is of paramount importance. Mortality in DKA is reported to be 3–11% in developing countries. Prevention of DKA is the best strategy to reduce mortality.

MANAGEMENT

Management of DKA comprises of initial assessment, fluid therapy, insulin therapy, treatment of precipitating factors, monitoring, prevention of complications and recurrence.

INITIAL ASSESSMENT

Initial assessment should include both clinical and biochemical parameters. Clinical evaluation includes vital signs, neurological assessment, signs of dehydration and associated features of infection. Biochemical assessment includes blood glucose, electrolytes, urea, creatinine blood ketones or urine ketones (if blood ketones are not available) and blood gases. Airway, breathing and circulation should be the priority inmanagement. Draw samples for evaluation and secure two IV access in children with DKA. Children with mild DKA may not need fluids or infusion of insulin and can be managed with oral fluids and subcutaneous insulin therapy. Routine central venous access is avoided in children with DKA. Bladder catheterization is not necessary unless the child is in altered sensorium, shock or is unable to void on demand.

FLUID THERAPY

Calculated amount of fluid is infused in children with DKA to correct dehydration along with maintenance fluids. Boluses of fluid is advised only for shock. Small volume boluses are preferred to be given slowly in children with DKA and shock. Boluses more than 30 mL/kg should be given only under supervision of the consultant. Presence of hypotensive shock should alert about coexistent sepsis other than severe dehydration in DKA. In such situations, inotropes will be started much earlier instead of infusing large volumes of fluid.

Fluid therapy in DKA is calculated to meet the replacement of the existing dehydration and the maintenance requirement. Dehydration in a child with DKA with shock is considered to be 10% and in children with no hemodynamic compromise it is taken as 8–8.5%. Dehydration correction is undertaken over 48 hours. Total fluid for correction is the sum of deficit for dehydration along with 48 hours maintenance fluids. Children with DKA should be weighed and this should be used for calculation of fluids. For example, if the child weighs 20 kg, presenting with DKA and shock, the fluid calculation will be as follows.

Total fluid deficit + 48 hours maintenance fluid is the total amount of fluids to be given over 48 hours.

20 kg × 10% dehydration + 3000 mL as maintenance for 48 hours

20 kg × 100 mL + 3000 mL = 2000 + 3000 mL = 5000 mL, i.e. 104 mL/hr

If the child received fluid boluses for resuscitation the same need not be reduced from the calculated fluids up to 20 mL/kg, however any volume of fluid used for resuscitation beyond 20 mL/kg will be reduced from the calculated fluids for rehydration. The time taken for fluid resuscitation will be appropriately reduced from the calculated 48 hours. Normal saline is the preferred fluid along with potassium replacement according to the serum potassium levels. There is no need to replace the urine loss during therapy of DKA. On an average, the total fluid calculated should not exceed the infusion rate of 1.5–2 times the regular maintenance fluid.

The calculated fluid for 48 hours need to be continued until child tolerates oral feeds. In children with signs of recovery, IV fluids can be discontinued by simultaneously introducing oral fluids, ensuring that the sum of oral and IV not exceeding the calculated fluid rate. Normal saline with potassium is the fluid of choice until the blood glucose falls to 250 mg/dL, after which the fluids can be changed over to 5% dextrose with half normal saline. However recent guidelines suggest that normal saline can be continued for the entire duration of hydration. The optimal rate of glucose decline is 100 mg/dL/hour. Do not allow the blood glucose level to fall below 200 mg/dL during insulin infusion. Hypoglycemia may develop rapidly with correction of ketoacidosis due to improved insulin sensitivity. Allowing blood glucose to drop to hypoglycemic levels is a common mistake that usually results in a rebound ketosis derived by counter-regulatory hormones. Rebound ketosis necessitates a longer duration of treatment. Cerebral edema may result with rapid correction of hyperglycemia and hyperosmolarity, as this can shift water rapidly to the hyperosmolar intracellular space.

INSULIN THERAPY

Insulin is started only after 1–2 hours of fluid therapy. Infusion of soluble insulin is recommended at 0.05–0.1u/kg/hr. (e.g. dilute 50 units Regular [soluble] insulin in 50 mL normal saline 1 unit = 1 mL). Intravenous insulin is infused at a weight-based fixed rate until ketosis has subsided. Should blood glucose fall below 250 mg/dL, 5% glucose containing 0.45 saline should be added to allow for the continuation of fixed-rate insulin infusion. Infusion is started after priming the tubing by flushing out the insulin preparation through the plastic tubing. A normal serum potassium level should be ensured prior to starting of insulin infusion in DKA. Recent evidence from developed countries favor initial insulin infusion rates of 0.05 u/kg/hr. Infusion of insulin need to be continued until resolution of ketosis as evidenced by the following parameters- Blood ketones—Beta hydroxyl butyric acid (BOHB) <1 mmol/L, closure of anion gap, pH > 7.30, bicarbonate >15 mmol/L. Insulin can be given subcutaneous after resolution of acidosis, with an overlap time of SC dose and infusion for about 60 minutes. This overlap of infusion and SC dose can be 15 minutes, if rapid analog insulins like aspart is used for subcutaneous therapy. The subcutaneous insulin requirement varies from 0.3–1 unit per kg per day depending on the age of the child. In children with mild DKA and in situations where IV infusion of insulin is not feasible subcutaneous insulin can be given as initial therapy. Initial dose SC: 0.3 unit/kg, followed 1 hour later by SC insulin lispro or aspart at 0.1 u/kg every hour, or 0.15–0.20 u/kg every 2 hour.

ROLE OF ANTIBIOTICS IN DKA

Infections are the common precipitating factor in children with DKA. Standard protocols for management of DKA do not recommend routine antibiotics. However, in countries such as India where sepsis complicating DKA is much higher in comparison to developed countries, antibiotics may be indicated until infection has been ruled out. Persistent shock, persistent acidosis, very wide anion gap and presence of fever are some of the factors that would suggest the presence of infection until lab evidence confirms the focus. Starting empiric antibiotics on suspicion of infection until culture results are available may be advisable in children with DKA.

MONITORING CHILDREN WITH DKA

Hourly monitoring of vital signs, neurological assessment and features of cerebral edema should be done. Blood glucose is monitored hourly. The 4-hourly electrolytes assessment, blood ketones, and 8 hourly urea and creatinine, are essential during therapy for DKA. Sepsis work-up samples should be drawn in children with DKA. Hyponatremia, hyperkalemia and wide anion gap metabolic acidosis, elevated urea and creatinine and elevated total counts are commonly seen in DKA at presentation.

Initial hyponatremia need not be treated as the corrected sodium values for hyperglycemia will be in the normal range. For every 100 mg of rise of blood glucose beyond hundred the serum sodium is expected to fall by 1.6 mEq/dL). However, one need to monitor rising levels of sodium with concurrent fall of blood glucose with therapy. Similarly the initial potassium values are much higher due to the extracellular shift of K due to acidosis. Since the total body potassium is much reduced in children with DKA, adequate potassium supplementation is mandatory. Potassium replacement may vary from 20 to 40 mEq/L in the maintenance fluid. To start with 20 mEq/L can be given in the calculated fluids and then modified according to the potassium levels. If the potassium level is greater than 6 mEq/L, do not administer potassium supplement in the initial few hours. If the potassium level is 4.5–6 mEq/L, administer 10 mEq/L of potassium chloride. If the potassium level is 3–4.5 mEq/L administer 20 mEq/L of potassium chloride. The correction of acidosis by using bicarbonate therapy is usually warranted only when the serum pH is less than 6.9 and/or if there is an imminent cardiac complication due to hyperkalemia. Serum phosphate levels may be low, but does not warrant acute correction. Initial raised urea and creatinine may be prerenal in majority of children with DKA, and the levels fall with adequate hydration. Persistent elevation of urea and creatinine or oligoanuria might indicate acute kidney injury in children with DKA. Elevation of creatinine in the absence high urea or oligoanuria should be interpreted with caution as ketones might interfere with laboratory evaluation of creatinine values. Serum ketones need to be monitored to identify resolution of acidosis and this will guide shifting from insulin infusion to subcutaneous insulin therapy in DKA. Persistent acidosis in DKA might indicate inadequate hydration, associated renal failure, sepsis or lactic acidosis of tissue hypoxia. Initial total cell counts may be high due to stress, and if repeated in 6 hours may show normal value. High counts in DKA do not signify infection by itself. However, presence of fever should be interpreted with caution as this is considered to be infection unless proved otherwise.

MONITORING FOR COMPLICATIONS

Common problems during therapy include cerebral edema in the first few hours of therapy. Any decline in sensorium with therapy, unexplained heart rate changes, bradypnea and hypertension may be the clinical clue. Management of DKA-associated cerebral edema is based on clinical features and one should not wait for radiological evidence. Management of this complication includes restriction of fluids to 2/3rd and avoidance of unnecessary handling of the child for suctioning to prevent spikes of rise in ICP. Mannitol or hypertonic saline can be used for reduction of raised ICP. Hypertonic saline is found to be as useful as mannitol, but without rebound rise of ICP. Hypertonic saline can be repeated in 30 minutes time, if there is no anticipated improvement. Ventilation may be supported to maintain $PaCO_2$ values at about 30–35 mm Hg.

Hypoglycemia is likely to be encountered, if the blood glucose is not maintained at about 200 mg/dL, during the course of DKA management. If the blood glucose falls below 100 mg/dL increase the glucose concentration of the intravenous fluid infusion, and if there is persisting ketosis, continue to give insulin at a dosage of least 0.05 units/kg/hour. If the blood glucose falls below 70 mg/dL, give a bolus of 2 mL/kg of 10% glucose and increase the glucose concentration of the infusion. Insulin can temporarily be reduced for 1 hour.

Blood glucose is the first lab parameter to normalize in uncomplicated DKA. Persistent acidosis would warrant continuation of insulin infusion despite fall of blood glucose. In such a scenario, increasing the dextrose content of glucose by up to 10–12.5% will prevent fall of blood glucose in the hypoglycemic range. Other rare complications include hyperkalemia, aspiration pneumonia, sepsis, renal failure, venous thrombosis, rhabdomyolysis.

PREVENTION

DKA is not only associated with increased mortality, morbidity among survivors of cerebral edema is still high. Subtle mental impairment, seizures, learning impairment, neurological sequelae in the form of motor handicaps and behavioral problems are a part of the spectrum of morbidity following DKA. Precipitating factors of DKA in children with established diabetes mellitus are poor compliance, psychological factors and associated infection. Adequate counseling, good family support and adequate encouragement from the diabetic team and knowledge about intercurrent infection management may help prevent DKA in children with established diabetes. New onset diabetes presenting with DKA can be prevented by creating awareness about diabetes among parents and school teachers. Occurrence of DKA either as new onset or among children with established diabetes is considered as a preventable healthcare failure. Prevention of DKA can be achieved by earlier diagnosis of diabetes in children with new onset disease and adequate management of intercurrent infection and ensuring good compliance to therapy among children with established diabetes. This may be the only feasible solution for minimizing mortality and morbidity in DKA in children.

KEY POINTS

- Management of Airway, breathing and circulation is the first step after assessment in DKA

- Avoid unnecessary boluses of fluids in DKA unless warranted
- Fluid therapy is calculated based on dehydration and is given over 48 hours
- Insulin infusion is started 1–2 hours after initiating fluid therapy
- Insulin is given at a rate of 0.05–0.1 u/kg/hr. until resolution of acidosis
- Sepsis work-up is mandatory in children with shock, fever or persistent acidosis
- Monitoring vital signs, neurological status, and laboratory parameters is essential in DKA management
- Look for complications like cerebral edema in the initial few hours of therapy
- Prevention of DKA is the best strategy to decrease mortality in DKA.

BIBLIOGRAPHY

1. BSPED Recommended Guideline for the Management of Children and Young People under the age of 18 years with Diabetic Ketoacidosis 2015. Available from *http://www.bsped.org.uk/clinical/docs/DKAguideline.pdf accessed on 2.2.2016.*
2. Global IDF/ISPAD Guideline for Diabetes in Childhood and Adolescence. Diabetic keto acidosis. Available from *https://www.idf.org/sites/default/files/Diabetes-in-Childhood-and-Adolescence-Guidelines.pdf accessed on 2.2.2016.*

Radiology

Reviewers: PSN Menon, Alok Gupta, R Remesh Kumar

13.1 Reading a Skiagram: Chest

S Muralinath, Mugil Varman Rajasekaran
Reviewers: *PSN Menon, Alok Gupta, R Remesh Kumar*

INTRODUCTION

Radiographs play a pivotal role in the evaluation of respiratory diseases in pediatric practice. Plain radiography is the best and the most commonly performed initial investigation having the least radiation exposure. It is unique in the sense that no other imaging modality offers a two-dimensional planar perspective of the regional anatomy under study. Added to this is the fact that the collective knowledge and cumulative wisdom accrued through decades of practice have honed the art of interpreting plain skiagrams to a state of near perfection. In the current scenario, despite the rapid advances in imaging technology and sophistication in techniques, the plain radiograph is still the first and most important imaging study utilized in the evaluation of lower respiratory tract infections. Its very simplicity and the wealth of diagnostic information that it offers have resulted in its universal acceptance.

The emphasis in this chapter is on a practical systematic approach in interpretation of a skiagram. The image should be interpreted with a sound clinical knowledge and understanding of the core pathology. The following steps are critical in interpretation of skiagrams:

- Assessing technical adequacy of the study.
- Interpretive approach to study a radiograph in a systematic manner.

TECHNICAL ADEQUACY

To begin with, look for the penetration, rotation, adequacy of inspiratory effort and motion. It should be adequately penetrated so that the pulmonary details are well brought out, which is essentially the vascular markings. When the penetration is adequate, the intervertebral disc spaces and the vessels posterior to the heart are seen well. The degree of rotation is evaluated by noting the distance between the center of the vertebral bodies and the lateral aspect of the ribs, thereby evaluating the bilateral symmetry. Classically, aeration or volume of the lungs is assessed by noting the level of the diaphragm. With adequate inspiration, the diaphragm should be at the level of the 6th rib anteriorly or the 8th rib posteriorly and evaluation of the degree of inspiration in infants often is more a matter of experience than science.

An image should always be assessed bearing these factors in mind as these can cause spurious findings which should always be interpreted with caution. For example, retrocardiac consolidation may be missed if there is poor penetration.

INTERPRETIVE APPROACH TO STUDY A RADIOGRAPH IN A SYSTEMATIC MANNER

The radiographic patterns of respiratory diseases vary with the age of the patient and with the pathogenesis and extent of the disease. Review of the entire respiratory disease in pediatrics using radiographs is beyond the scope of this chapter; hence we concentrate mainly on chest infections. Certain anatomical and functional factors that are unique in a child determine the patterns of pulmonary inflammatory disease, sequelae and the radiological appearance. This is reviewed along with the terminology used to describe pulmonary infections in children.

Thymus

The thymus is seen in the superior aspect of the anterior mediastinum. It is prominent on the chest radiograph of an infant as the thoracic cavity is relatively small; however, normal variations in radiographic appearances are common. It grows during early childhood to reach a maximum by approximately 15 years of age after which it undergoes regression. Thymus is the most common cause of widened mediastinal shadow, mistaken for mass or consolidation.

Heart

The mediastinum and cardiac contours are relatively large in an infant, and the transverse diameter of a normal heart may approach 60% of the thoracic transverse diameter.

Airways

The small airways of infants are extremely susceptible to inflammatory narrowing. The formation of bronchial tree is complete by 16th week of gestation. Airways in children remain relatively as well as absolutely smaller than in the adult. Conductance (the reciprocal of resistance) of the peripheral airways is at least five times that of the central airways in the adult, but equal to that of the central airways in the infant and young child. Air trapping or atelectasis is common.

Airspace

Alveolar development continues after birth. Alveoli add up to approximately 50–100 million at birth and 300 million in an adult. Saccular proliferation is rapid in the first few years of life, less rapid thereafter and slows after 8 years. The size of the lung acinus varies with age. It is approximately 1 mm in diameter at birth and gradually increases to 6–10 mm in diameter by early adolescence. Destructive pulmonary process or infection during infancy can alter this normal pulmonary alveolar development. Collateral ventilation in the infant is less efficient than in the adult. This is due to the relatively under-developed ventilatory channels (pores of Kohn and channels of Lambert) as well as the thick connective tissue septae and the small alveolar size.

Radiologists usually try to determine whether the disease process has primarily affected the airways or the airspaces and when parenchymal opacities are present as well as whether the abnormality is due primarily to airspace disease or interstitial disease. It is interesting to note that the appreciation of these basic patterns permits an etiologic inference to a good extent. *By and large, acute airway and interstitial disease tend to be viral in origin, whereas acute airspace disease tends to be bacterial in origin more often than not.*

Radiological Pattern and Terminology

The commonly used radiological terms include:

- Airway disease
- Airspace disease
- Airway/Airspace disease

Pneumonia

- *Airspace consolidation:* It is usually bacterial in origin. It can also be seen in viral pneumonia superadded by bacterial infection.
- *Interstitial:* It is viral in origin more often than not.

Patterns in Chest Radiographs

These are usually described as findings in airways and airspaces as shown in **Table 13.1.1**.

RADIOLOGIC FINDINGS IN AIRWAY DISEASES

Chest film may be normal or any or all of the following may be present:

- *Air trapping*
  - Can be diffuse or focal
  - May need expiratory film to assess adequately

Table 13.1.1: Patterns in chest radiographs as seen in airway and airspace

Airway	*Airspace*
• Conducting zone	• Exchange zone
• Intracellular organism	• Extracellular organism
• Infiltrative	• Exudative
• Center to periphery	• Periphery to center

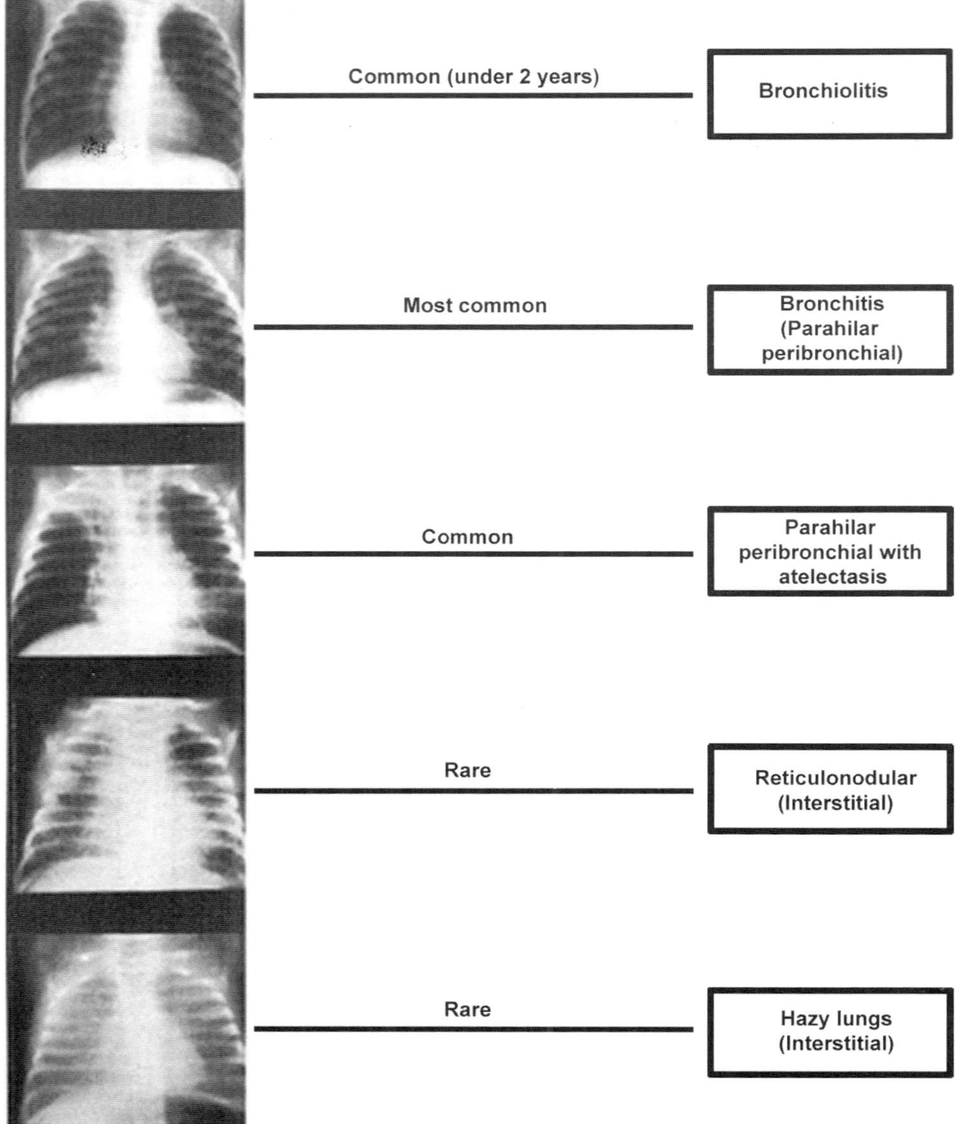

Fig. 13.1.1: Viral lower respiratory tract infections—basic radiographic spectrum

- *Bronchial wall thickening*
  - Ring and tramline shadows
- *Small nodular opacities*
- *Atelectasis*
  - May be streaky and sub-segmental
  - If lobar, right middle lobe is the most common.

Figure 13.1.1 shows the basic radiographic spectrum commonly observed in viral lower respiratory tract infections.

Round pneumonia is a form of airspace consolidation pneumonia peculiar to the pediatric age group. It presents as well-circumscribed round or oval densities. Round pneumonia is invariably bacterial in etiology and most often it is the pneumococcal infection that presents as oval or spherical masses in the early consolidative phase. When unaware of this process, it could be baffling and may mislead the clinician to think in terms of pulmonary mass or nodule. The diagnosis is rather simple once the clinical picture is taken into account. Unwarranted further evaluation for pulmonary nodule or mass is done away with once the physician is aware of this entity and appropriate antibiotic therapy will solve the issue.

RADIOLOGICAL APPROACH TO UNILATERAL HYPERLUCENCY

The first step is to identify the side of abnormality. To identify, it one has to follow the following important steps:

- *Look at the pulmonary vasculature.* The side with decreased vascularity is abnormal and the side with increased or normal vascularity is usually normal.
- *Assess the degree of variation between inspiratory and expiratory films.* The side which changes least on expiration is usually abnormal.
- *Finally look at the size of hemithorax.* The small, opaque hemithorax is usually abnormal rather than hyperlucent hemithorax, which in most cases, is due to compensatory hyperinflation **(Flow chart 13.1.1)**. In such situations, one has to again look at vascularity of the hyperlucent side which will not be decreased.

In children a unilateral hyperlucent lung is mostly due to a foreign body which should not be missed.

RADIOGRAPHS IN SUSPECTED CARDIAC DISEASE

Table 13.1.2 lists the common features to be assessed on a chest radiograph in an infant with suspected cardiac disease.

Flow chart 13.1.1: Unilateral hyperlucent hemithorax

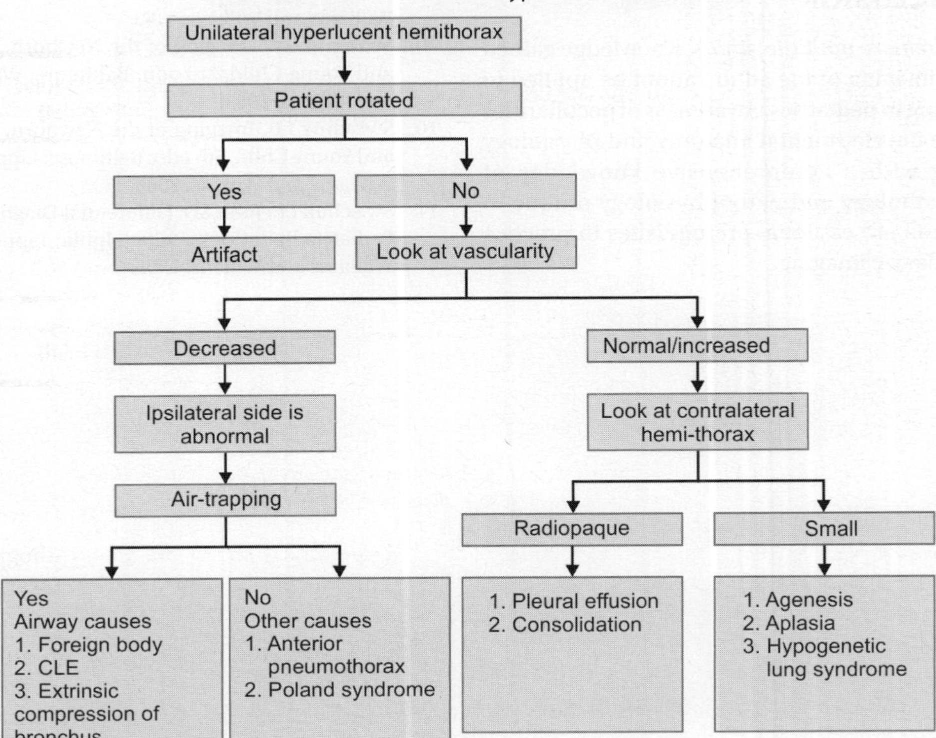

Table 13.1.2: Features to assess on chest radiograph in infant with suspected cardiac disease

Feature	*Comment*
Quality of film	Adequate inspiration Normal penetration Centered on mid-chest Non-rotation
Abdominal/ Bronchial situs	Normal/inverted/ambiguous
Aortic arch side	Left/right
Heart	Side Direction of apex Size Contour
Lung vasculature	Plethora/Oligemia/Pulmonary venous congestion
Diaphragm	Distinct Diaphragm at the side of cardiac apex should be more caudal
Lung fields	Any pathology
Musculoskeletal	Vertebral/ rib abnormalities Fracture

CONCLUSION

Children are not little adults. Knowledge gained from imaging of the adult cannot be applied to imaging in pediatrics. Awareness of peculiarities in the developmental anatomy and physiology along with a comprehensive knowledge of the pathology and pathophysiology unique to children are essential prerequisites in practice of pediatric imaging.

BIBLIOGRAPHY

1. Arthur R. Interpretation of the paediatric chest X-ray. Current Paediatrics. 2003;13:438-47.
2. Dillman JR, Sanchez R, Ladino-Torres MF, Yarram SG, Strouse PJ, Lucaya J. Expanding upon the unilateral hyperlucent hemithorax in children. Radiographics. 2011;31:723-41.
3. Garcia-Pena P, Guillerman RP. Pediatric Chest Imaging, 3rd edn. Berlin Heidelberg; Springer-Verlag, 2014.
4. Kirks DR. The pediatric ER chest: What every radiologist should know. In: Harwood-Nash DC and Pettersson H (Eds). NICER Series on Diagnostic Imaging; Pediatric Radiology. 1992. pp. 154-75.
5. Kuhn JP, Slovis TL, Haller JO. Caffey's Pediatric Diagnostic Imaging, 10th edn, Pennsylvania; Mosby, 2004.
6. Meerstadt PWD, Gyll C. Manual of Neonatal Emergency X-ray Interpretation, 2nd edn. Philadelphia; WB Saunders, 1995.
7. Rennie JM, Robertson NRC. Textbook of Neonatology, 3rd edn. Philadelphia; Elsevier Churchill Livingstone, 1999.
8. Swischuk LE. Emergency Radiology of the Acutely Ill or Injured Child, 2nd edn. Baltimore; Williams and Wilkins, 1986.
9. Swischuk LE. Imaging of the Newborn, Infant and Young Child, 3rd edn. Baltimore; Williams and Wilkins, 1989.
10. Swischuk LE. Imaging of the Newborn, Infant and Young Child, 5th edn. Baltimore; Lippincott Williams and Wilkins, 2004.
11. Swischuk LE, John SD. Differential Diagnosis in Pediatric Radiology. Philadelphia; Lippincott, Williams and Wilkins, 1995.

13.2 Practical Pediatric Nuclear Medicine

Ethiraj Prabhu, Sampath Santhosh

Reviewers: *PSN Menon, Alok Gupta, R Remesh Kumar*

INTRODUCTION

Pediatric nuclear medicine is a clinical discipline involving use of open, short-lived, medical grade radioactive substances *in vivo* or *in vitro* in the field of pediatrics for diagnosis, therapy (theragnosis) and research. These radioactive drugs (ligands) emit energy in the form of gamma rays, characteristic X-rays, beta, alpha particles and positrons for a short duration (seconds to minutes). They are administered in very minute quantities (nanogram or picogram) levels and hence are called as 'tracers'.

BACKGROUND

Pediatric nuclear medicine studies were performed as early as in 1946. Nuclear Regulatory Commission in the United States of America reports that more than 1000 nuclear medicine studies were performed on children and adolescents between 1946 and 1948. Subsequent developments were slow till the 1960s because many of the commercially available radioisotopes at that period of time had long half-lives and were also particle emitters which delivered high radiation dose to the tissues. The development of the Gamma camera between 1952 and 1958 by Hal Anger at the Donner Laboratories, California; joining of Alex Gottschalk in University of Chicago in 1962 as well as introduction of radioactive technetium (^{99m}Technetium pertechnetate) by a general surgeon, Paul Harper at the University of Chicago led to rapid development of pediatric nuclear medicine subsequently.

The Department of Nuclear Sciences and Applications of the International Atomic Energy Agency instituted Nuclear Medicine Section as a part of its Human Health Program for establishing best medical practices in nuclear medicine, appropriate use and quality management as well as sharing of expertise among various countries. A nuclear medicine database was initiated in 2007 for collecting and maintenance of updated information among its member countries. It found that on an average over 3 years, annually 25–28% of nuclear medicine studies, were bone scans, 24% were thyroid scans, 17% were renal scans and about 13% were cardiac scans in developing countries. There was a steady (25%) increase in therapeutic applications annually since 2008. During early days, significant contributions in pediatric nuclear medicine were from practitioners of adult nuclear medicine, urologists, oncologists and non-clinical scientists. However, with the current understanding of the varying physiology and strategic needs, there is significant change in the current practice of pediatric nuclear medicine.

PATIENT PREPARATION FOR NUCLEAR MEDICINE STUDIES

In a busy clinical setting, utmost importance is accorded in identification, preparation and scheduling of the patient in any pediatric nuclear medicine facility. The parents are clearly explained about the procedures involved. Support of the pediatrician is sought in terms of fixing IV access and maintenance, optimum hydration and for infant feeding tubes or urinary catheters. Extra time is allotted to complete the procedure because of several unexpected disruptions like difficulty to start an IV line, child refusing to drink adequate water, unhappy, shy and nervous children—especially when it requires undressing and voiding in front of the Gamma camera for performing voiding cysto-urethro-scintigram.

Table 13.2.1: List of various formulas in current practice

S. No.	*Method*	*Formula*
1.	Body surface area-based	(BSA m^2/1.73 m^2) × Adult dose
2.	Clark	(Weight lbs/150) × Adult dose
3.	Solomon (Fried)	(Age in months/180) × Adult dose
4.	Young	(Age in years/age in years + 12) × Adult dose
5.	Weight-based	(Weight in kg/70) × Adult dose
6.	Webster's formula	(Age + 7) adult dose/(age +1)
7.	European Association of Nuclear Medicine Pediatric Dose Card	Baseline activity multiple (based on weight and radiopharmaceutical-dependent factors)

CALCULATION OF THE RADIOPHARMACEUTICAL ACTIVITY IN PEDIATRICS

Optimum administration of radiopharmaceutical has to be ensured in order to get the best possible results in pediatric nuclear medicine practice. At the same time, ALARA (As Low as Reasonably Achievable) practice is strictly followed so as to ensure that only appropriate amount of activity is administered so that the radiation dose delivered to the patient is as low as possible.

Body surface area (BSA) is calculated by applying the following formula:

$$\text{BSA} = \text{Weight (kg)}^{0.425} \times \text{Height (cm)}^{0.725} \times 0.007184$$

Table 13.2.1 lists the various methods commonly followed across the world.

Several software ALARA-based formulas are currently available with various vendors to easily determine the safe amount of activity being administered in a busy clinical setting for pediatric patients.

SEDATION AND POSITIONING IN DIAGNOSTIC NUCLEAR MEDICINE PROCEDURES

Every nuclear medicine institution has its own policy of immobilizing the pediatric patients like the use of toys and distractions, counseling, restraints and finally sedatives as a last resort. The policies vary completely from institution to institution when compared with certain established guidelines such as the European Association of Nuclear Medicine (EANM) or Society of Nuclear Medicine (SNM) guidelines. In general, parents are made aware of the method of immobilization of the pediatric patients, possibly with some soft-padded restraints, bundling of sheets, and strategic placement of pillows, etc. failing which, informed consent is obtained and sedation is administered if required with the support of anesthesiologist.

Positioning of pediatric patients for nuclear medicine studies is highly individualized according to the physiological information sought and the purpose of the procedure. Usually positioning is comfortable and the study time is short because of smaller targets, shorter bodies; at times, it can become difficult when the patient is highly uncooperative or continuously moving.

COMMON PEDIATRIC NUCLEAR MEDICINE PROCEDURES

Tables 13.2.2 to 13.2.6 detail the various nuclear medicine studies usually performed in clinical problems related to musculoskeletal system, genitourinary system, endocrine system, gastrointestinal system, and other common systems respectively in children.

PHARMACOLOGICAL INTERVENTION STUDIES

Pharmacological intervention studies are commonly performed in nuclear medicine in order to enhance the physiology and understand

Table 13.2.2: Musculoskeletal system

S.No.	*Clinical problem*	*Nuclear medicine study*
1.	Evaluation of acute/chronic mono- or polyarthritis, stress/occult fractures, Trauma (accidental/non-accidental), primary or metastatic bone disease, Other musculoskeletal inflammation or infections, evaluating child abuse, Metabolic bone disease, Bone grafting (viability, infarcts, necrosis), Pain of suspected musculoskeletal etiology, Heterotopic calcification, juvenile rheumatoid arthritis, Any abnormal radiological, clinical finding, Osteoblastic activity evaluation for palliative bone pain therapy, Other conditions like Paget's disease, fibrous dysplasia, Langerhan's cell histiocytosis, congenital or developmental anomalies	Radionuclide bone scan ^{99m}Technetium MDP (methylene di phosphonate) or Fluorine 18-sodium fluoride (^{18}F-FDF) 1. Planar scans 2. SPECT scan 3. 3-phase bone scans 4. PET scans 5. Hybrid scans (SPECT/CT; PET/CT)
2.	Differential diagnosis of osteomyelitis and cellulitis, vascularity of bone tumor, reflex sympathetic dystrophy syndrome	Three-phase bone scan and whole body bone scan ^{99m}Tc-MDP
3.	Differential diagnosis of infection or loosening of total hip replacement prosthesis, differential diagnosis of osteomyelitis and cellulitis	Osteomyelitis study (^{99m} Tc-MDP and ^{67}Ga)
4.	Malignant bone tumor, osteogenic sarcoma, Ewing's sarcoma. Evaluate for low-back ache; sacroiliitis in systemic disease such as ankylosing spondylitis, psoriatic spondylitis, osteoarthritis, systemic lupus erythematosus (SLE), Crohn's disease, ulcerative colitis	Whole body bone scan ^{99m}Tc-MDP Quantitative sacroiliac scan (common in adults)

Table 13.2.3: Genitourinary system

S.No.	*Clinical problem*	*Nuclear medicine study*
1.	Glomerular filtration rate (GFR), quantitative renal function, urinary stone, acute renal failure, acute kidney injury, chronic kidney disease, acute and chronic rejection, neurogenic bladder, renal transplant	^{99m}Technetium – MAG3 (mercaptoacetyltriglycine), ^{99m}Tc – EC (ethylenedi-cysteine)
2.	Pyelonephritis, renal scarring, urinary tract infection (UTI), renal infarct, renal trauma, horseshoe kidney, ectopic kidney, renal cyst, renal abscess, renal tumor, relative renal function, fetal lobulation, cortical nodular hyperplasia	^{99m}Tc DMSA renal cortical study with SPECT
3.	Refractory hypertension and study for functionally significant renal artery stenosis	Captopril renogram
4.	Effective renal plasma flow (ERPF), relative renal function, obstructive uropathy, acute tubular necrosis (ATN), transplant renal function	^{99m}Tc MAG3 or ^{99m}Tc EC scan for evaluation of tubular function
5.	Scrotal varicocele, hydrocele, hernias, orchitis, epididymitis, hydrocele	^{99m}Tc RBCs scan
6.	Torsion testis evaluation and epididymo-orchitis with their DDs, hydrocele, hematocele, abscess, acute scrotal pain	$^{99m}TcO_4$ Pertechnetate testicular scan
7.	Renal tuberculosis (TB), UTI	^{67}Ga for renal tumor/inflammation survey and SPECT
8.	Bipedal edema in diabetes, filariasis, trauma, establishing the cause of swelling of lower/upper limbs, sentinel node imaging	^{99m}Tc nanoalbumin or sulfur nanocolloid injection in web space of the digits
9.	Skin viability for skin grafting, identification of suitable site, etc.	^{99m} Tc nanoalbumin intradermal injection

Table 13.2.4: Endocrine system

S. No.	*Clinical problem*	*Nuclear medicine study*
1.	Goiter, nodule goiter, hyperthyroidism, exophthalmos, Graves' disease, thyroiditis, children with thyroid disease, ectopic thyroid/sublingual thyroid	$^{99m}TcO_4$ thyroid scan – to study the trapping function of the thyroid follicle
2.	Thyroid cancer, sublingual thyroid, intrathoracic goiter, ectopic thyroid, hypothyroidism, thyroiditis, goiter, nodular goiter, hyperthyroidism, exophthalmos, Graves' disease	^{131}I thyroid uptake and low dose (50 microcurie) scan (24 hours)—to study the organification function of the thyroid follicle
3.	Detection of metastasis of thyroid cancer of papillary and follicular types following total thyroidectomy	^{131}I thyroid whole body scan (High dose – 5 millicurie) to study the presence of functioning thyroid metastasis
4.	Treatment of metastasis and thyroid cancer of papillary and follicular types, hyperthyroidism in old age	^{131}I thyroid (therapy dose 70 to 200 millicurie) treatment for differentiated carcinoma of thyroid and 6 to 10 millicurie for toxic goiter
5.	Medullary thyroid cancer, undifferentiated thyroid cancer, breast cancer, osteogenic sarcoma, cancer treatment response	^{99m}Tc (V) DMSA scan, ^{201}Tl scan, ^{68}Ga DOTATATE scan, ^{99m}Tc-SESTAMIBI scan, ^{18}F –FDG PET scan
6.	Hyperparathyroidism, hypercalcemia, parathyroid hyperplasia, parathyroid adenoma, shortened operation time after one or more previous surgical exploration	^{99m}Tc-SESTAMIBI scan for evaluation of parathyroid glands
7.	Cushing's syndrome, aldosteronism, adrenal adenoma, adrenal hyperplasia	NP59 adrenal cortical scan—rarely done in India
8.	Pheochromocytoma, extra-adrenal metastasis, medullary thyroid cancer, paraganglioma, neuroblastoma cardiac failure, lead position in cardiac resynchronization therapy	Adrenal medullary scan with ^{131}I MIBG, ^{99m}Tc HYNIC-TOC scan, ^{18}F –FDG PET scan
9.	Tumor regression and apoptosis	^{99m}Tc HYNICTOC, annexin V scan

the mechanism of dysfunction. These changes may not be obvious and easily observed under basal studies **(Table 13.2.7)**.

CONCLUSION

Pediatric nuclear medicine studies are very helpful in objectively establishing the clinical diagnosis with the help of short-lived, open, unsealed radioligands and sophisticated computerized equipment like the SPECT-CT and the PET-CT. There are significant capital investments involved in establishing a full-fledged department—although, any modern nuclear medicine department can perform almost all the relevant investigations and manage them. Few small items like colorful books, toys and appropriate environment can provide children-friendly atmosphere. Lack of availability of this facility and inadequate exposure of the practicing pediatricians, and unfound fear of radiation injury, are some of the constraints resulting in suboptimal utilization of this specialty. This specialty is now heading towards the development of personalized pediatric nuclear medicine.

Table 13.2.5: Gastrointestinal system

S. No.	*Clinical problem*	*Nuclear medicine study*
1.	Mumps, xerostomia, salivary obstruction, scleroderma, post-radiation therapy, parotid tumor	$^{99m}TcO_4$ salivary gland scintigraphy with vitamin C or lemon drops challenge
2.	Recurrent aspiration or respiratory infections, reflux esophagitis, dysphagia, motility disorders for liquids and solids	^{99m}Tc sulphur colloid dynamic esophageal transit study (Radionuclide milk scan) ^{99m}Tc mebrofenin entero-gastro-esophageal reflux study.
3.	Meckel's diverticulum, Batter's ulcer of esophagus	$^{99m}TcO_4$ Meckel's diverticulum scan
4.	GI bleeding, progressive blood loss – identification of site and quantification Hemangiomas, AV malformations in the liver and the intestines	GI bleed scan with $^{99m}TcO_4$ labeled autologous RBCs, ^{99m}Tc sulphur colloid GI bleed scans
5.	Indian childhood cirrhosis, portal hypertension, liver abscess, liver rupture, congenital anomalies of liver, focal nodular hyperplasia, space-occupying lesions in liver, splenomegaly, splenic infarcts, accessory spleen	^{99m}Tc sulphur colloid/phytate and ^{18}F-FDG PET CT of the abdomen
6.	Acute cholecystitis, biliary atresia, Caroli's disease, neonatal hepatitis, colonic transit studies, biliary leak, biliary reflux, partial liver transplantation, hepatohydrothorax	^{99m}Tc mebrofenin scans
7.	Le–Veen shunt obstruction	^{99m}Tc DTPA shunt patency study

Table 13.2.6: Other common systems in pediatric nuclear medicine

S. No.	*Clinical problem*	*Nuclear medicine study*
1.	LV ejection fraction, RV ejection fraction, left to right shunt study with quantification, heart failure, post-chemotherapy, heart transplant recipient, cardiomyopathies, valvular heart disease, aneurysms, vascular anomalies, superior vena cava obstruction, inferior vena cava obstruction, hepatoma	$^{99m}TcO_4$ RBCs radionuclide ventriculography (RNV), first pass RNV, ^{99m}Tc SESTAMIBI scans
2.	Pulmonary embolism, childhood asthma, juvenile COPD, pre-pulmonectomy evaluation, pulmonary hypertension evaluation and lung malignancies	^{99m}Tc macroaggregated albumin (MAA)
3.	Anemia, polycythemia, bone marrow distribution, bone marrow depression, leukemia, ectopic hemopoiesis, bone marrow metastasis	Bone marrow scan with I/V ^{99m}Tc nanoalbumin and ^{32}phosphorus for treatment
4.	Spleen imaging, spleen infarction, spleen abscess, accessory spleen, autosplenosis, spleen trauma, functional asplenism, spleen tumor	Heat denatured ^{99m}Tc autologous RBCs spleen scan
5.	Hodgkin's disease, non-Hodgkin's lymphoma, melanoma, lung cancer, hepatoma, leukemia, gastric cancer, esophageal cancer	^{67}Gallium whole body scan, ^{99m}Tc SESTAMIBI scan for unknown primary, ^{18}F-FDG scan for staging
6.	Seizure disorder, head injury, vasculitis, recurrent brain tumor, craniotrauma, intracerebral bleed, dementia evaluation and radiation necrosis	^{99m}Tc HMPAO, ^{99m}Tc ECD, ^{18}F-FDG scan, ^{201}Tl brain blood flow scan
7.	V–P shunt obstruction, normal pressure hydrocephalus, CSF leakage	^{9m}Tc – DTPA dynamic CSF scan
8.	Ephiphora–nasolacrymal duct function/patency evaluation	^{9m}Tc–DTPA dacryoscintigram

Table 13.2.7: Pharmacological intervention studies

S.No.	*Drug*	*Mechanism of action*	*Side effects*
Genitourinary system			
1.	Furosemide	Primarily inhibits the absorption of sodium and chloride, almost throughout the nephron	Tinnitus, allergic reactions and contraindicated in anuria
2.	Captopril/Enalapril	Prevents the conversion of angiotensin I to angiotensin II resulting in reduction of GFR	Dry cough, postural hypotension, anaphylactoid reaction, angioedema and contraindicated in pregnancy
3.	Aspirin	Inhibits prostaglandin synthesis and reduces renin secretion	Epigastric distress, nausea, GI bleed
Endocrine system			
4.	rh-TSH	Stimulates radioiodine uptake in the residual thyroid tissue as well as raises serum thyroglobulin levels	Nausea, allergic reaction and a very low risk of tumor stimulation
Gastrointestinal system (GI motility studies)			
5.	Metoclopramide	Dopamine antagonistic, stimulates GI motility, independent of vagus nerve	Nausea, diarrhea, drowsiness, fatigue, extrapyramidal symptoms, tardive dyskinesia. Contraindicated in mechanical obstruction and pheochromocytoma
6.	Erythromycin	Binds to antral and duodenal motilin receptors and initiates phase III of interdigestive motor complex	Nausea, vomiting, diarrhea, jaundice, transient deafness
Meckel's diverticulum imaging			
7.	Ranitidine	Histamine H-2 receptor blocker that inhibits secretion of $^{99m}TcO_4$ (technetium pertechnetate) by mucus and parietal cells	Headache, dizziness, diarrhea, muscular pain, hallucinations and confusions
8.	Pentagastrin	Stimulates uptake of $^{99m}TcO_4$ (technetium pertechnetate) gastric mucosa in the Meckel's diverticulum and stomach	Nausea, vomiting and tachycardia
9.	Glucagon	Reduces peristalsis which allows accumulation of tracer in the Meckel's diverticulum	Nausea, vomiting, weakness, dizziness, hypersensitivity, poor control of blood glucose, pheochromocytoma, insulinoma, glucagonoma
Hepatobiliary scintigraphy			
10.	Cholecystokinin–8	Stimulates contraction of gallbladder and simultaneously relaxes the sphincter of oddi	Abdominal pain, urge to defecate, flushing, dizziness, allergic reaction
11.	Morphine	Constricts sphincter of oddi and increases the pressure within the sphincter and the CBD	Respiratory depression, nausea, vomiting, hypotension, dysphoria, urinary retention and contraindicated in COPD and chronic liver disease
12.	Phenobarbitone	Induces the hepatic enzymes and enhances the radiotracer uptake and biliary excretion	Sedation, anxiety

BIBLIOGRAPHY

1. Blevrakis E, Partalis N, Seremeti C. Meckel's diverticulum in pediatric practice in Crete (Greece): A-10-year review. African J Pediatr Surg. 2011;8(3):279-82.
2. Conway JJ. A memoir of pediatric nuclear medicine: Part 1. Pioneers and early advances. J Nucl Med. 2006;47(4):12N-20N.
3. Gambhir S, Barai S. Radioiodine for treatment of Grave's disease in pediatric population. World J Endocr Surg. 2010;2(2):77-80.
4. Gordon I. Issues surrounding preparation, information and handling of child and parent in nuclear medicine. J Nucl Med. 1998;39:490-4.
5. Hamilton PM, Chiacchierini RP, Kaczmarek RG. A follow-up study of persons who had iodine-131 and other diagnostic procedures during childhood and adolescence. FDA 89-8276. Washington DC: Department of Health and Human Services; 1989.
6. Kim S, Salaman N, Jackson HA. PET imaging in pediatric neuroradiology: Current and future applications. Pediatr Radiol. 2010;40:82-96.
7. Pandey AK, Sharma SK, Sharma P. Development of radiopharmaceutical dose calculator in pediatric patients undergoing diagnostic nuclear medicine studies. Indian J Nucl Med. 2013;28(2):75-8.
8. Saremi F, Jadvar H, Seigel ME. Pharmacologic interventions in nuclear radiology: Indications, imaging protocols and clinical results. Radiographics. 2002;22:477-90.
9. Shulkin BL. PET in pediatric oncology. Pediatr Radiol. 2004;34:199-204.
10. Shulkin BL, Mandell GA, Cooper JA. Procedure guideline for diuretic renal scintigraphy in children. J Nucl Med Technol. 2008;36:162-8.
11. Sinha A, Bagga A, Krishna A. Revised guidelines on management of antenatal hydronephrosis. Indian Pediatr. 2013;50:215-31.
12. Zukotynski K, Grant FD, Curtis C. Skeletal scintigraphy in pediatric sports medicine. Am J Radiol. 2010;195:1212-9.

13.3 Computed Tomographic Imaging: What We Need to Know?

Kathirvelu Gopinathan, Karnan Sudha

Reviewers: *PSN Menon, Alok Gupta, R Remesh Kumar*

INTRODUCTION

The use of pediatric computed tomography (CT) scan, which is a valuable imaging tool, has been increasing rapidly. However, because of the potential for increased radiation exposure to children, pediatric CT has become a public health concern. This chapter will address the following issues:

- The basics of CT
- Role of CT in pediatric diseases
- Radiation risks of CT in children
- Strategies to minimize radiation exposure in children.

CT AS A DIAGNOSTIC TOOL

CT scanners were first introduced in 1971 with a single detector for study of brain under the leadership of Godfrey Hounsfield. From then onwards CT scanners have undergone a series of changes with increase in number of detectors and decrease in scan time. What began as single slice CT has evolved as single slice spiral, multislice spiral (2 to 320 slices), and to the present dual source CT. With the advent of multidetector CT (MDCT), scan time and motion artifacts have been reduced, which are particularly beneficial for children.

The additional benefits include that new scanners are multiphase and have better resolution; and facilitate angiography, virtual endoscopy and organ perfusion.

BASICS OF CT

Series of X-ray beams are emitted in all directions from an X-ray tube to the detectors with the subject in between. The attenuation of X-rays by various tissues is not equal. The X-rays are attenuated by different tissues in different degrees. Hence, the attenuation coefficient values are calibrated with reference to water (**Table 13.3.1**). More dense tissues appear bright and less dense tissues appear dark in CT.

CLINICAL INDICATIONS FOR CT IN CHILDREN

Head CT

Trauma: Acute subdural hematoma (SDH) appears as a crescent-shaped homogeneously hyperdense extra-axial collection that spreads diffusely over the affected hemisphere **(Fig. 13.3.1)**. Acute extradural hematoma (EDH) is biconvex in shape, and most frequently beneath the squamous part of the temporal bone **(Fig. 13.3.2)**. Subarachnoid hemorrhage (SAH) appears as hyperattenuating material filling the subarachnoid space, most commonly around the Circle of Willis due to rupture of berry aneurysms **(Fig. 13.3.3)**. CT is very useful in detecting cortical fracture and lysis.

Stroke: Acute infarct appears as cortical hypodensity with associated parenchymal swelling and resultant gyral effacement. The purpose of CT in the acute setting is to exclude intracranial hemorrhage, which precludes thrombolysis and excludes other stroke mimickers like tumors **(Fig. 13.3.4)**.

Table 13.3.1: CT density in Hounsfield units (HU) of different tissues

Tissue	*CT density (HU)*
Bone	+1000
Air	1000
Water	0 to +10
Soft tissue	+30 to +50
Fat	–30 to –50

Infections: Most infections appear as single or multiple ring-enhancing lesions; meningitis as meningeal enhancement; and ventriculitis with obstructive hydrocephalus. CT is useful in detecting the calcification related congenital and granulomatous infection more accurately.

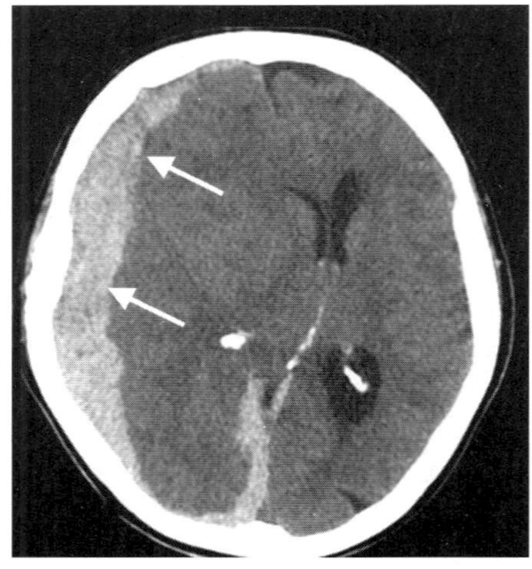

Fig. 13.3.1: Subdural hematoma. Note the crescent-shaped homogeneously hyperdense extra-axial collection of blood

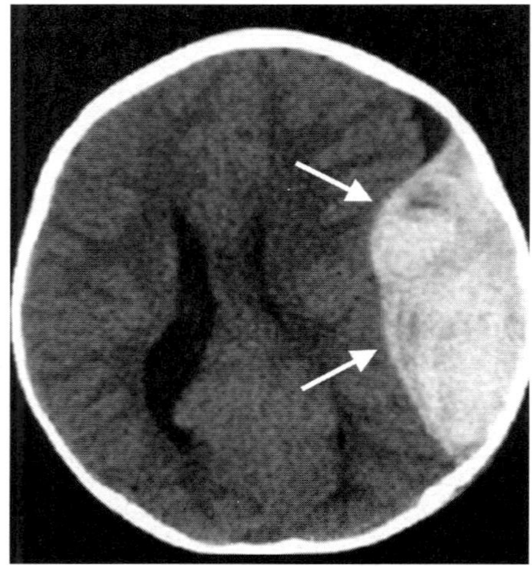

Fig. 13.3.2: Extradural hematoma. Note the biconvex shape

Ring enhancing lesions: Common causes for ring-enhancing lesions include cerebral abscess **(Fig. 13.3.5)**, tuberculoma **(Fig. 13.3.6)** and neurocysticercosis. Other causes such as metastasis, glioblastoma, subacute infarct, hemorrhage, contusion, demyelination (incomplete ring), radiation necrosis and lymphoma in an immunocompromised patient should be kept in mind.

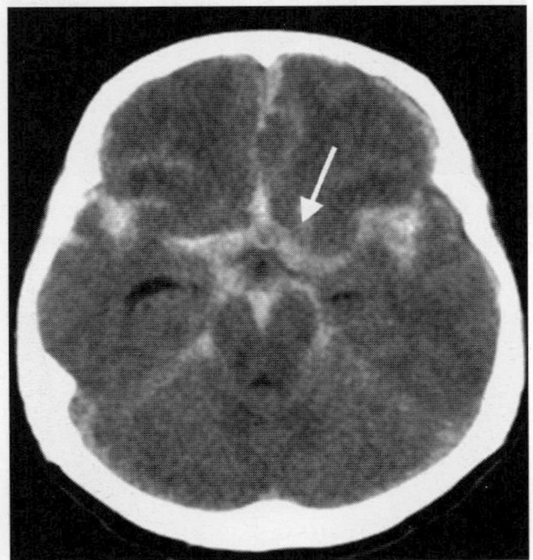

Fig. 13.3.3: Subarachnoid hemorrhage. Note the hyperdense material filling the subarachnoid space

Abdomen CT

Techniques: CT scan of abdomen is acquired in various phases like plain study, with oral contrast (positive or negative), with intravenous (IV) contrast and multiphase acquisition. Plain CT alone is useful in cases of suspected calculus and bowel perforation; in other conditions direct contrast CT is preferred to reduce the radiation dosage. Water or mannitol is used as negative oral contrast. When negative oral contrast is combined with IV contrast, there is better delineation of mucosal and mural lesions like polyps and inflammatory bowel wall thickening. Positive oral contrast gives better bowel distension and is useful in cases of bowel obstruction, malrotation, bowel perforation and anastomotic leak.

CT has a major role in pediatric acute abdomen such as acute appendicitis (**Fig. 13.3.7**), Meckel's diverticulitis, malrotation with obstruction (**Fig. 13.3.8**), peritonitis and suspected bowel perforation when ultrasonography (USG) is inconclusive.

CT abdomen is indicated in the abdominal trauma when USG shows significant free fluid and in cases of polytrauma **(Fig. 13.3.9)**.

Cross-sectional imaging is especially used in characterization of abdominal mass and

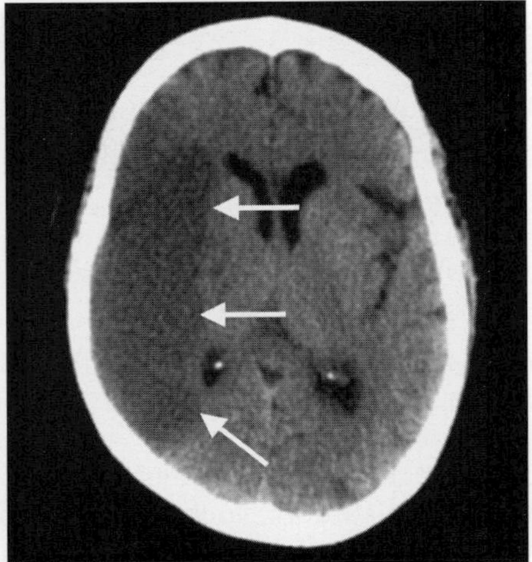

Fig. 13.3.4: Acute right middle cerebral artery territory (MCA) infarct seen as a cortical hypodensity with associated parenchymal swelling

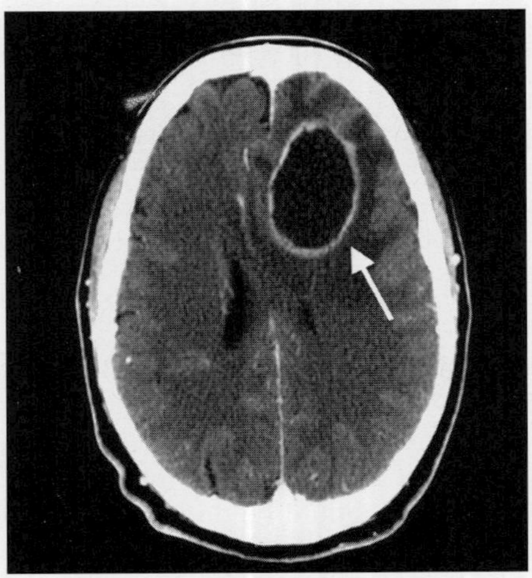

Fig. 13.3.5: Cerebral abscess: Ring-enhancing lesion

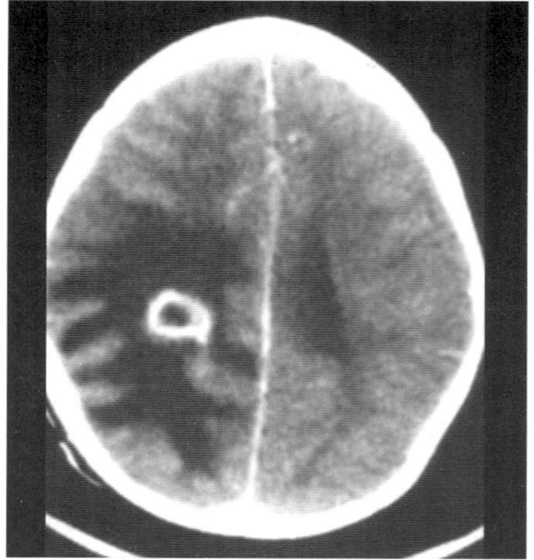

Fig. 13.3.6: Tuberculoma of brain

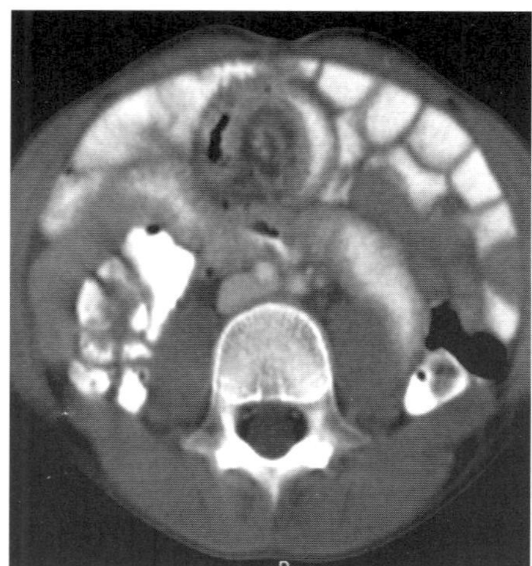

Fig. 13.3.8: Midgut volvulus: Bowel loops rotates around its mesentery – 'Whirlpool sign'

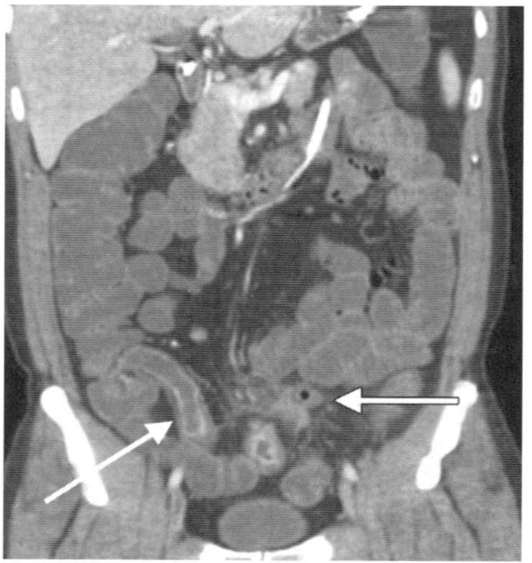

Fig. 13.3.7: Acute appendicitis: Note the dilated tubular bowel loop in right iliac fossa

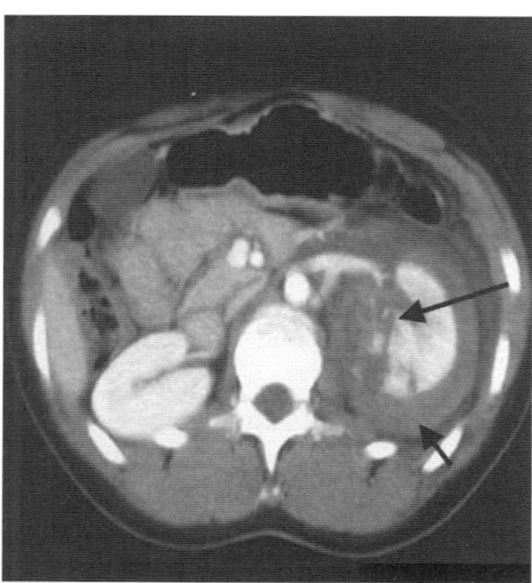

Fig. 13.3.9: Left renal laceration: Laceration extends to renal pelvis (long arrow) with perirenal hematoma (short arrow)

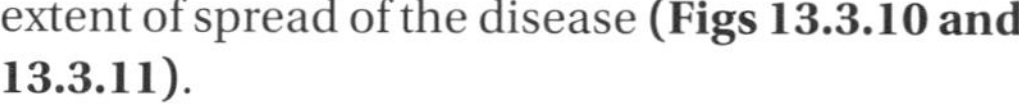

extent of spread of the disease **(Figs 13.3.10 and 13.3.11)**.

CT enteroclysis plays vital role in the initial diagnosis of inflammatory bowel disease and follow-up should be done with magnetic resonance (MR) enteroclysis **(Fig. 13.3.12)**.

Chest CT

MDCT is a valuable tool for evaluating the central airway, mediastinal structures and lung parenchyma. MDCT is more sensitive than plain radiographs in detection of structural changes within the lungs.

Chest CT is helpful in the diagnosis of congenital disorders such as congenital cystic adenomatoid malformation (CCAM) of lung and its differentiation from congenital diaphragmatic hernia; sequestration demonstrating systemic arterial supply from aorta **(Fig. 13.3.13)**; isomerism exploring the

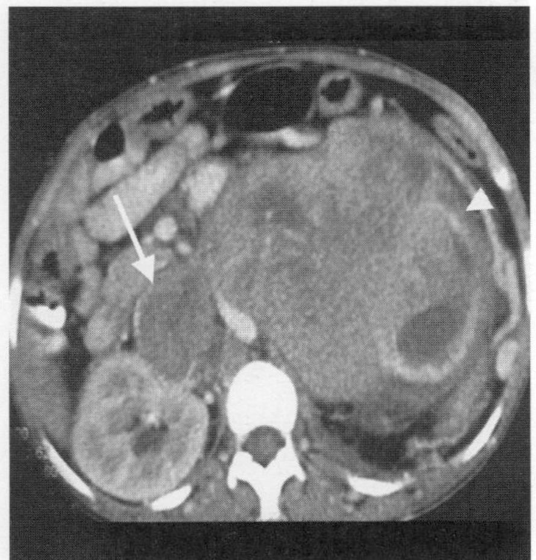

Fig. 13.3.10: Wilms tumor (arrowhead) with inferior vena cava (IVC) extension (white arrow)

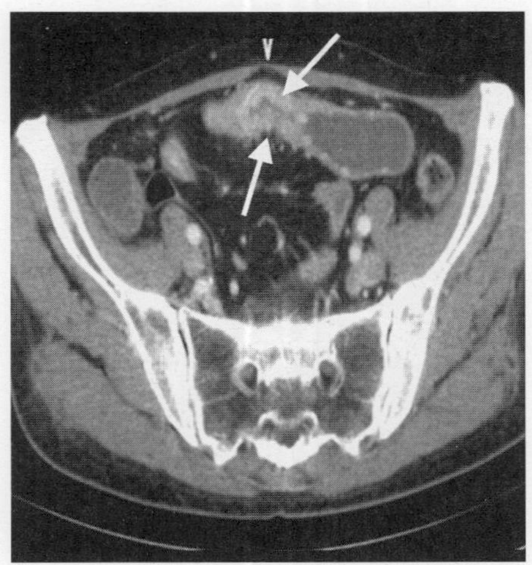

Fig. 13.3.12: Crohn's disease shows focal circumferential bowel wall thickening with enhancement and causing luminal narrowing

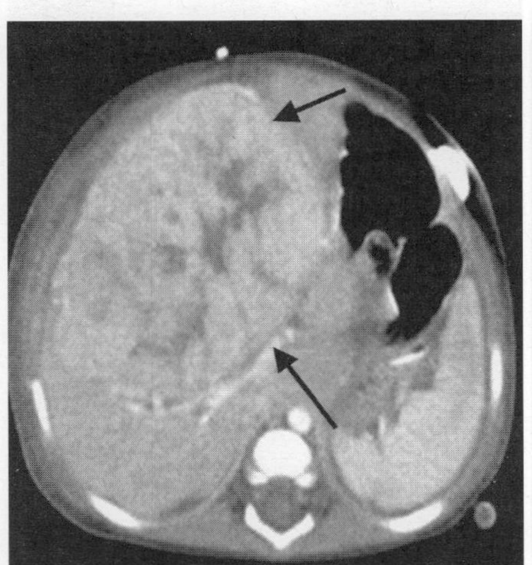

Fig. 13.3.11: Hepatoblastoma

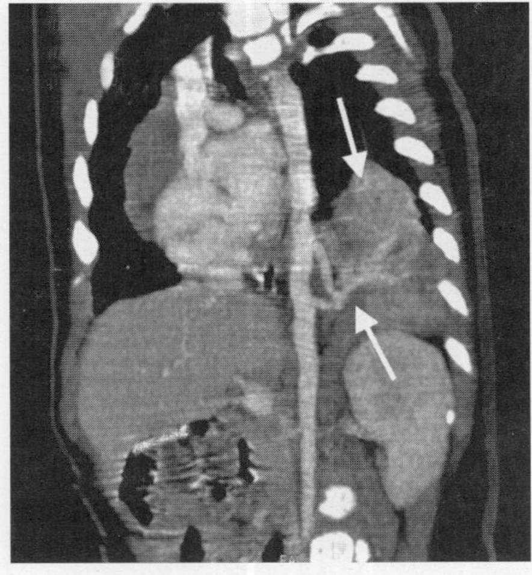

Fig. 13.3.13: Extralobar sequestration. Abnormal lung tissue in left lower lobe with supply from descending aorta

bronchial anatomy; agenesis; vascular rings compromising the airway and pulmonary arteriovenous malformations (AVM); congenital foregut duplication cysts and thymic cysts. Lung parenchymal abnormalities can have increased attenuation (as with consolidation, ground glass opacities and mosaic pattern), decreased attenuation (as in bronchiectasis, **Fig. 13.3.14**), cavitary lesions **(Fig. 13.3.15)**, lung cysts, emphysema **(Fig. 13.3.16)**, honey combing), reticular pattern and nodules (centrilobular, perilymphatic, random and tree-in-bud nodules **(Fig. 13.3.17)**. Expiratory CT is important for the diagnosis of air trapping.

CT can differentiate transudate from exudates, effusion versus empyema with thick enhancing pleura (split pleura sign, **Fig. 13.3.18**), lung parenchyma for cavitary

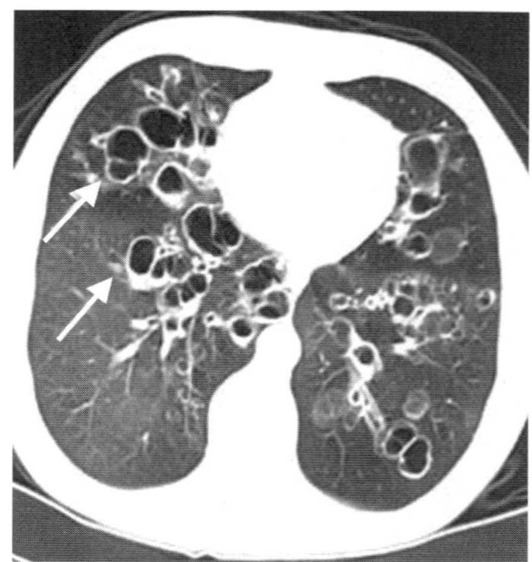

Fig. 13.3.14: Bronchiectasis: Dilated bronchus with mild wall thickening

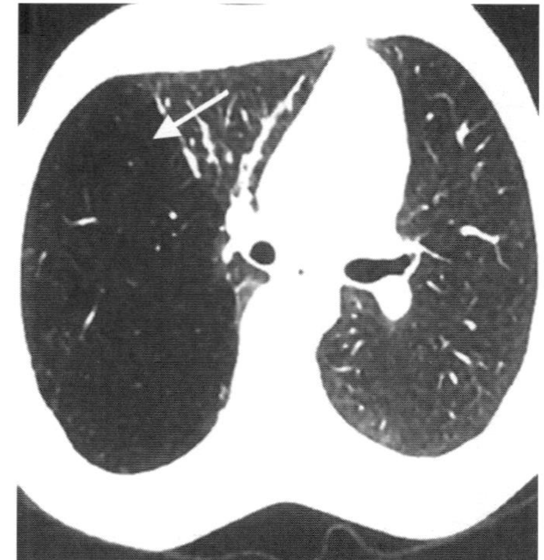

Fig. 13.3.16: Congenital lobar emphysema (CLE) shows areas of low attenuation without discernible walls in right upper lobe

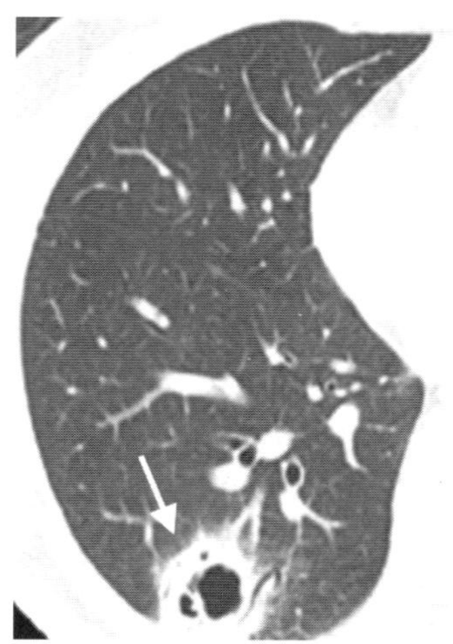

Fig. 13.3.15: Cavitary lesion of lung

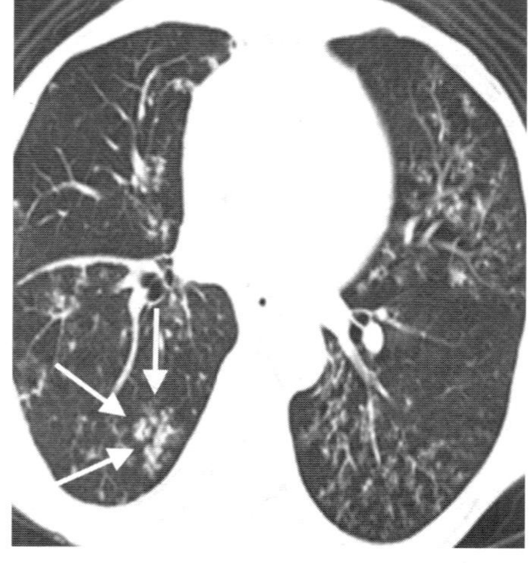

Fig. 13.3.17: Tree-in-bud nodules. Irregular nodular branching lesions predominantly along periphery

necrosis, lung abscess and confirm the position of drainage tube.

Head and Neck CT

CT should be performed as early as possible in all children with suspected acute mastoiditis which is seen as mastoid air cell opacification **(Fig. 13.3.19)**. MR imaging must be done if intracranial complications like epidural abscess, sigmoid sinus thrombosis, carotid artery spasm and petrous apicitis are suspected. This imaging approach is of great help in planning effective surgical treatment.

Thyroglossal duct cyst most commonly at infrahyoid paramedian location (**Fig. 13.3.20**) and lymphangioma are the most common congenital anomalies; complicated lymphadenitis **(Fig. 13.3.21)** is the most

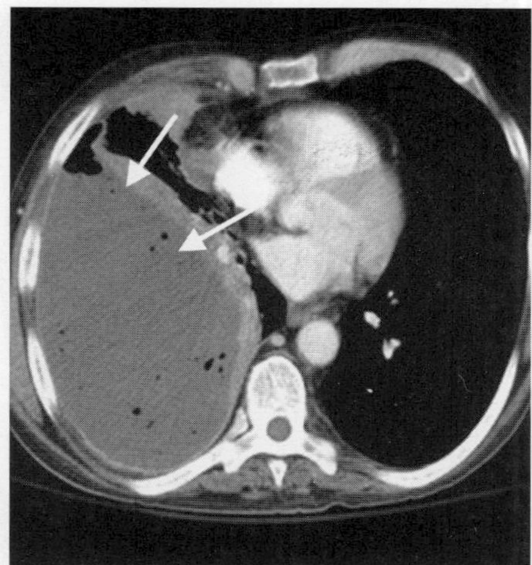

Fig. 13.3.18: Empyema shows fluid density collection with air locules in right pleural space

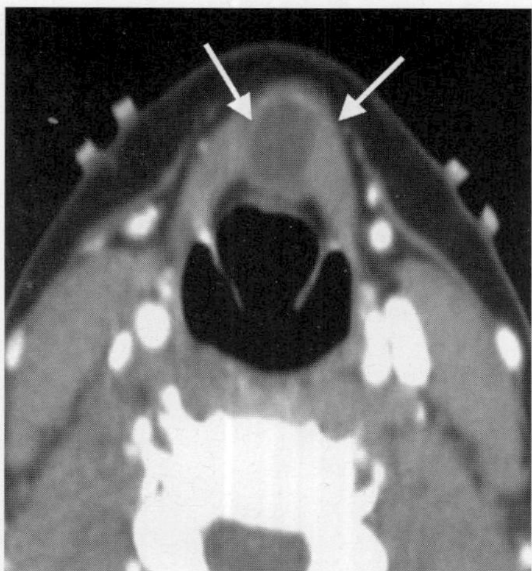

Fig. 13.3.20: Thyroglossal duct cyst shows hypodense cystic non-enhancing lesion

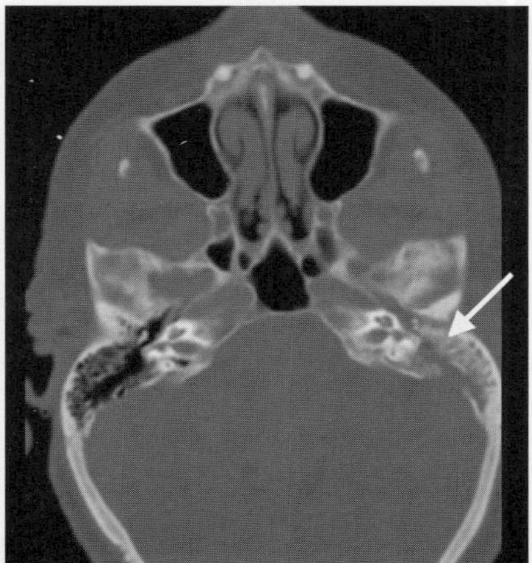

Fig. 13.3.19: Acute mastoiditis (L) shows opacification of left mastoid air cells

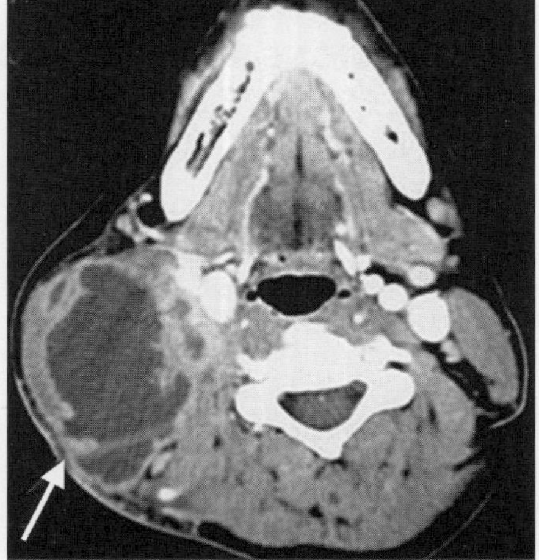

Fig. 13.3.21: Cervical necrotic lymphadenitis shows cystic lesion with peripheral enhancement in right side

common inflammatory lesion; fibromatosis colli is the most common benign tumor or tumor-like condition; and lymphoma is the most common malignant neoplasm that requires CT/MR evaluation.

RECENT ADVANCES

Three-dimensional volume rendering technique (3D-VRT) is a technique used to display 2D projection of a volume data set. Three-dimensional images integrate a series of axial CT sections into an image which is easy-to-interpret and appears similar to catheter angiograms. Volume-rendering technique (VRT) demonstrates fractures, and clearly demonstrates the relationship of the fragments to joint space and orientation of the fragments to the main components of the bone. In VRT, relationship between vessels and viscera, vascular patency, thrombus, or calcification can be well demonstrated **(Figs 13.3.22 and 13.3.23)**.

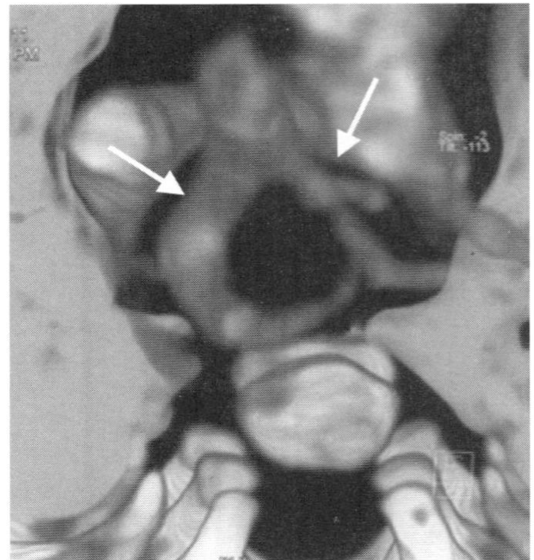

Fig. 13.3.22: 3D-VRT: Complete vascular ring (*For color version, see Plate 8*)

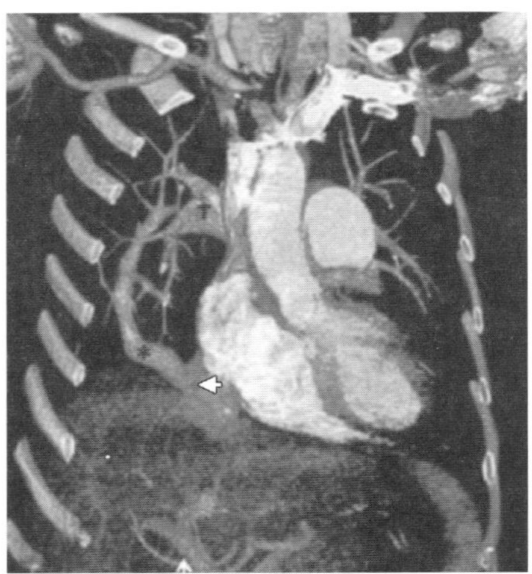

Fig. 13.3.23: 3D-VRT. Scimitar syndrome: Anomalous vein (arrowhead) draining the right lung into inferior vena cava (IVC) (*For color version, see Plate 8*)

CONSIDERATIONS FOR RADIATION EXPOSURE ESPECIALLY IN CHILDREN

The ionizing radiation doses delivered by CT are 100–500 times higher than conventional radiography and are in ranges predisposing to increased risk of cancer. Radiation effects are 10 times more for children than adults for the same dose.

Approximate effective radiation dose for a single chest X-ray is 0.1 mSv. CT abdomen and pelvis scan carry the highest radiation dose. Up to a quarter of children with a single abdomen and pelvis scan receive a dose of 20 mSv or higher.

The risks of radiation-induced leukemia and brain cancer are the highest for head scans, which are the most commonly performed CT scans in pediatrics. Although the effective dose for a head scan is relatively low, the brain and red bone marrow doses are relatively high, especially for young children, resulting in the highest risks of brain cancer and leukemia.

Though radiation exposure is a concern in both adults and children, there are some unique considerations in children.

- Children are more sensitive to radiation than adults.
- Children have a longer life expectancy than adults, resulting in a larger opportunity for expressing radiation damage.
- If CT settings are not tailored for their smaller body size, children may receive a higher radiation dose than required.

Hence, the risk of developing a radiation-related cancer can be several times higher for a young child compared with an adult exposed to a similar CT scan.

STEPS TO MINIMIZE CT RADIATION EXPOSURE IN CHILDREN

- When appropriate, other modalities like ultrasound or magnetic resonance imaging (MRI), which are nonionizing, should be considered.
- *Adjust the technical parameters for pediatric CT:*
  - Protocols based on individual size/weight parameters should be used.
  - Lower mA and/or kVp must be considered for skeletal and lung imaging, CT angiogram and follow-up scan.
- The region scanned must be limited to the smallest necessary area.

- *Image resolution:*
  - Low-resolution scans are mostly diagnostic.
  - The multiphase evaluation causes considerable increase in dose and hence used only when really necessary, especially in body (chest and abdomen) imaging.

CONCLUSION

Radiologists must consider reducing exposure as low as reasonably achievable by practicing settings customized for children. All physicians who prescribe pediatric CT should assess its use on a case-by-case basis. When used optimally, CT is one of the most valuable imaging modalities for both children and adults. The benefits of CT examinations should always outweigh the risks for an individual child.

BIBLIOGRAPHY

1. Calhoun PS, Kuszyk, BS, Heath DG, Carley JC, Fishman EK. Three-dimensional volume rendering of spiral CT data: Theory and method. Radiographics. 1999;19(3):745-64.
2. Committee to Assess Health Risks from exposure to low levels of ionizing radiation and national research council. Health risks from exposure to low levels of ionizing radiation: BEIR VII Phase 2. Washington, DC: The National Academies Press; 2006. p. 11
3. Drebin RA, Magid D, Robertson DD, Fishman EK. Fidelity of three-dimensional CT imaging for detecting fracture gaps. J Comput Assist Tomogr. 1989;13(3):487-9.
4. Miglioretti DL, Johnson E, Williams A, Greenlee RT, Weinmann S, Solberg LI, et al. The use of computed tomography in pediatrics and the associated radiation exposure and estimated cancer risk. JAMA Pediatr. 2013;167(8):700-7.
5. Preston DL, Ron E, Tokuoka S, Funamoto S, Nishi N, Soda M, et al. Solid cancer incidence in atomic bomb survivors: 1958-1998. Radiat Res. 2007;168(1):1-64.
6. Vazquez E, Castellote A, Piqueras Mauleon S, Creixell S, Pumarola F, Figueras C, et al. Imaging of complications of acute mastoiditis in children. Radiographics. 2003;23(2):359-72.
7. Vazquez E, Enriquez G, Castellote A, Lucaya L, Creixell S, Aso C, Regas J. US, CT, and MR imaging of neck lesions in children. Radiographics. 1995;15(1):105-22.

13.4 Magnetic Resonance Imaging: A Simplified Interpretation

C Amarnath

***Reviewers:** PSN Menon, Alok Gupta, R Remesh Kumar*

INTRODUCTION

Magnetic resonance imaging (MRI) is a growing modality in pediatric radiology. With radiation safety and awareness programs becoming more prevalent, the need for imaging without ionizing radiation is in high demand. As technology advances, not only sequences will continue to decrease in time but also better and faster motion insensitive sequences will become more readily available. These advances will make the use of MRI a more viable alternative to CT in pediatric population when there is a choice.

One of the biggest challenges of pediatric neuroimaging is the acquisition of high quality diagnostic images, as it requires the infant

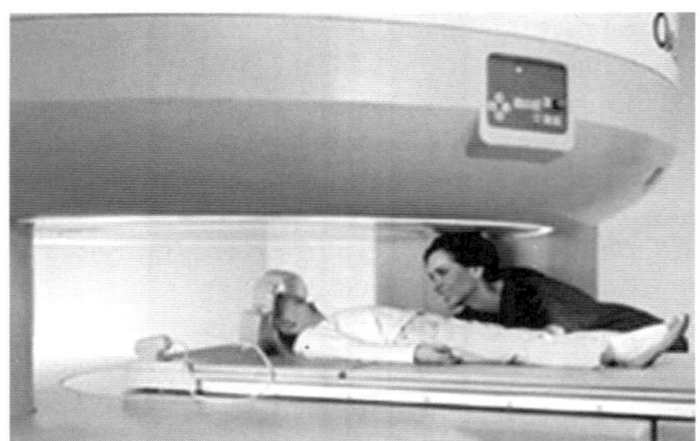

Fig. 13.4.1: Wide-bore MRI machine in which parent can accompany a child while taking imaging unlike in routine MR gantry

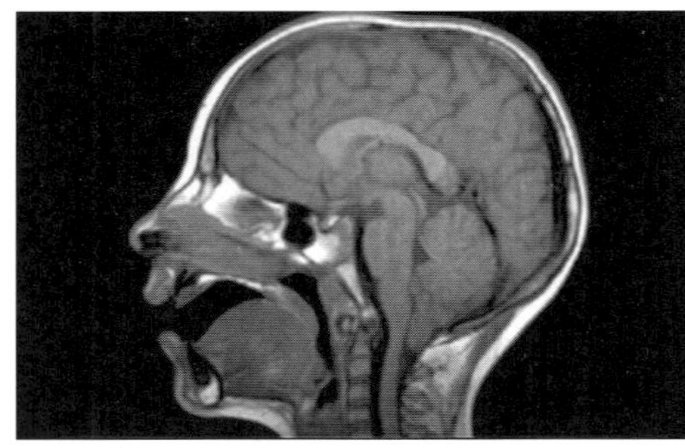

Fig. 13.4.2: Sagittal T1 WI MR shows cerebellar tonsils protruding through the foramen magnum with mild compression of the upper cervical cord

or child to keep still for a long period of time (sometimes nearly 30 minutes). The majority of neonates under 2 months of age (approximately 70%) require sedation or a general anesthetic. The wide-bore MRI has unique pediatric applications whereby the parent can now lie in the scanner with his/her child during the scan because the bore can fit both of them together (**Fig. 13.4.1**).

MRI is done to detect a variety of pathology in brain such as cysts, tumors, bleeding, swelling, developmental and structural abnormalities, infections, inflammatory conditions or problems with the blood vessels. In addition, MRI is the modality of choice for spinal imaging. Prior to ossification of the posterior elements of the spinal column, ultrasonography (US) was shown to be a valuable screening tool; however, infants with an abnormal sonogram or who have a neurological abnormality in the context of a normal sonogram, still require MR imaging for further evaluation. Few conditions require contrast administration to delineate pathology more clearly such as acute inflammation, acute infection, neurocutaneous disorders, tumors, white matter disorders, vascular anomalies and vascular disorders.

Common pediatric central nervous system (CNS) pathologies and their neuroradiological features are described in brief further.

CONGENITAL CENTRAL NERVOUS SYSTEM MALFORMATIONS

Chiari Malformations

The Chiari malformations (I–V) are a group of disorders involving mainly the posterior fossa.

Chiari type I malformation: This is defined as peg-like herniation of cerebellar tonsils into foramen magnum with vertically oriented sulci. Imaging findings in Chiari I malformation include herniation of tonsils more than 6 mm below the foramen magnum in the first decade (**Fig. 13.4.2**) and dilatation of the central spinal canal (hydromyelia). The foramen magnum looks "crowded" with small or absent cerebrospinal fluid (CSF) spaces.

The Chiari type II malformation: This is a complex set of anomalies involving cerebellum, brain and spinal cord. Virtually all patients present with meningomyelocele at birth. In this syndrome, the cerebellar tonsils and inferior vermis herniate inferiorly through the foramen magnum. The fourth ventricle is small and elongated and herniates often down to the upper cervical canal. The upper medulla kinks at the attachment with the dentate ligament; this is called a "cervico-medullary kink" and is best seen in a sagittal image (**Figs 13.4.3A and B**). The dorsal midbrain in these patients

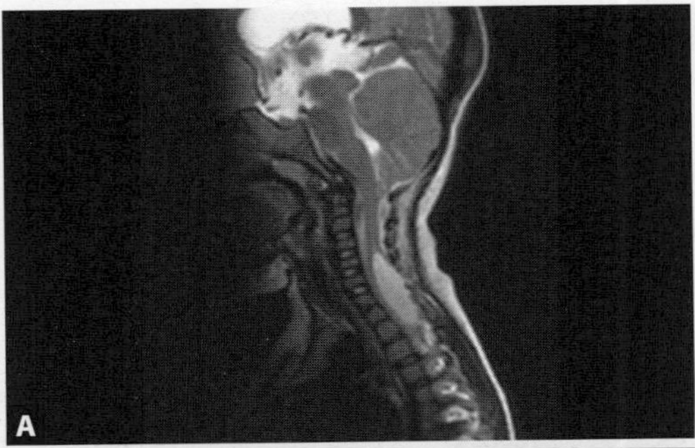

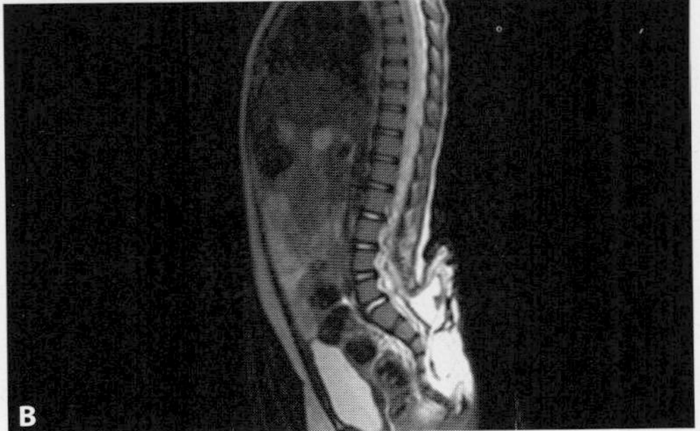

Figs 13.4.3A and B: (A) Sagittal T2WI MR cervical spine and brain shows small posterior fossa, protrusion of tissue through foramen magnum, small fourth ventricle, beaked tectum, and syringomyelia; (B) Same patient imaged at lower spinal level—myelomeningocele also is seen

demonstrates fusion of the superior and inferior colliculi making the tectum appear beaked. There are usually associated CNS malformations like corpus-callosal agenesis, interdigitated gyri following absent falx and hydrocephalus.

Chiari type III malformation: This includes cervical spina bifida and high cervical or low occipital meningoencephalocele.

Dandy-Walker Syndromes

Dandy-Walker syndromes (DWS) result from partial or complete vermian aplasia and a dilated fourth ventricle extending into the posterior fossa, as a large posterior fossa cyst that displaces the cerebellum. The inferior part of the cerebellum is upturned. There is upward displacement of the transverse sinuses, tentorium and torcular herophili (**Figs 13.4.4 A and B**). The Dandy-Walker variant, the most common form of this anomaly, demonstrates partial dysgenesis of the vermis and remnant fourth ventricle that communicates with retro-cerebellar cyst.

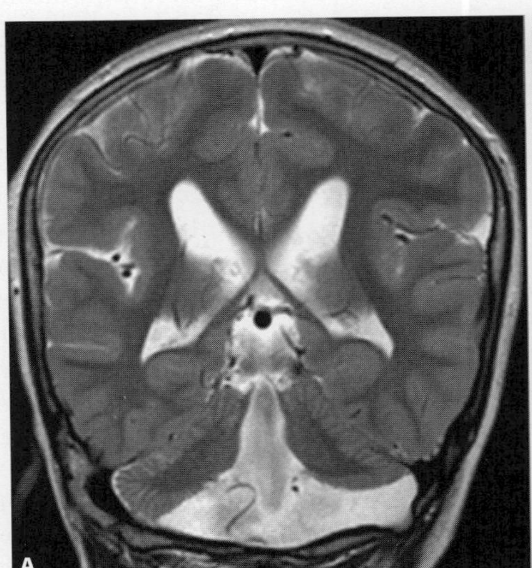

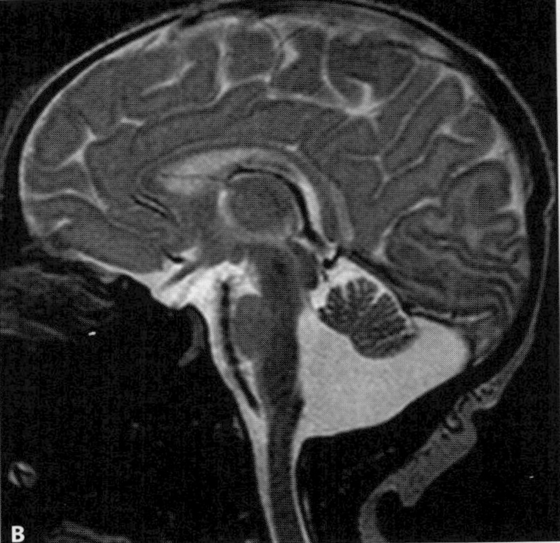

Figs 13.4.4A and B: Coronal and sagittal T2WI with Dandy–Walker malformation. (A) The fourth ventricle opens into a posterior fossa cyst. There is associated hydrocephalus; (B) The cerebellum is hypoplastic and a thin rim of cerebellar tissue is seen forming the wall of the posterior fossa cyst

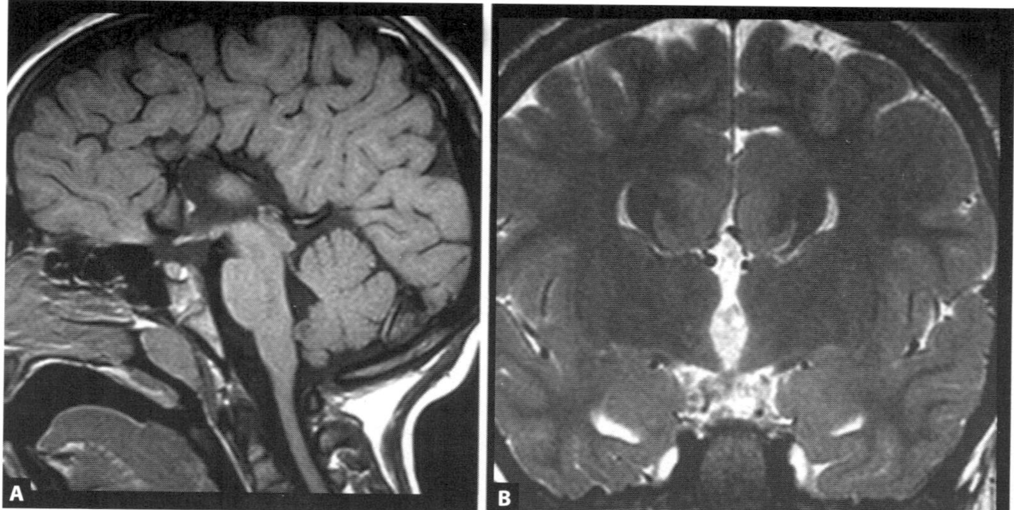

Figs 13.4.5A and B: (A) Sagittal T2WI MRI shows complete corpus callosal agenesis; (B) Coronal T2WI shows high-riding third ventricle and abnormal shape of frontal horn of lateral ventricle, and Probst bundle

Corpus Callosal Agenesis

The corpus callosum is a midline commissural fiber tract that develops from the commissural plate in the dorsal aspect of the lamina terminalis. When the corpus callosum is absent, the connections that would normally cross the midline instead turn in the interhemispheric fissure and run parallel to the fissure in the medial walls of the lateral ventricle to form the longitudinal callosal bundles of Probst (**Figs 13.4.5A and B**). Other MRI findings include the presence of parallel lateral ventricles, without the normal convergence of bodies, radial orientation of interhemispheric gyri and colpocephaly. Typically, there is a high riding third ventricle opening into the interhemispheric fissure or an interhemispheric cyst.

INTRAUTERINE CNS INFECTIONS (TORCH COMPLEX)

The stage of brain development judged by the gestational age is more important than the infecting organism in determining the pattern of CNS injury. Therefore, *in utero* infections acquired before 16–18 weeks of gestation when neurons are forming within the germinal matrix and migrating to form the cerebral cortex, produce lissencephaly and a small cerebellum. Spontaneous abortion is also a frequent outcome during this time. Between 18 and 24 weeks, when the cortical neurons are organizing, the infective insult may produce localized dysplastic cortex, polymicrogyria and porencephaly. This is seen as a smooth walled cavity, isointense to CSF on all sequences in continuity with the ventricular system and without evidence of gliosis. From the third trimester onwards the insult results in asymmetrical cerebral damage with gliosis, cystic change and calcification. **Table 13.4.1** lists the common imaging findings seen in children with various CNS infections.

NEUROCUTANEOUS SYNDROMES/ PHAKOMATOSES

The major findings on MRI of common neurocutaneous syndromes are listed in **Table 13.4.2**.

Table 13.4.1: Imaging findings in various CNS infections

Infective agent	*Imaging findings*
Cytomegalovirus (CMV)	Periventricular calcification, microcephaly, cerebellar hypoplasia, lissencephaly and polymicrogyria
Toxoplasma gondii	Microcephaly and parenchymal calcification similar to CMV infection (cerebellar hypoplasia and polymicrogyria are not seen)
Herpes simplex virus (HSV)	Diffuse white matter hyperintensity; later profound cerebral atrophy, cystic encephalomalacia and calcification
Human immunodeficiency virus (HIV) infection	Global atrophy and bilateral basal ganglia calcification are the most common imaging findings Diffuse symmetrical periventricular and deep white matter abnormalities may be present
Meningitis (The role of neuroimaging is to detect the complications and not for diagnosis)	Meningeal enhancement predominantly in basal cistern, hydrocephalus, subdural effusion, cerebritis, infarct, abscess and cortical venous thrombosis

Table 13.4.2: Phakomatoses and imaging findings

Phakomatoses	*Imaging findings*
Neurofibromatosis 1	Hamartomas, also known as 'unidentified bright objects (UBOs), in typical sites (pons, cerebellar white matter, internal capsules, basal ganglia, thalami and hippocampi), sphenoid wing dysplasia with pulsatile exophthalmos, dural ectasia with vertebral scalloping and lateral meningoceles, visual pathway gliomas, plexiform neurofibromas and cranial and peripheral nerve gliomas (**Figs 13.4.6A and B**)
Neurofibromatosis 2	MISME (multiple intracranial meningioma, schwannoma, multiple ependymoma, **Fig. 13.4.6C**)
Tuberous sclerosis	Hamartomas, subependymal nodule, cortical tubers and subependymal giant cell tumor (**Figs 13.4.7A and B**)
Sturge-Weber syndrome	Leptomeningeal angiomas seen as enhancement (unilateral, rarely bilateral), abnormal venous drainage, chronic ischemia, cortical atrophy and calcification
von Hippel-Lindau syndrome	Multiple cerebellar hemangioblastoma and spinal hemangioblastoma (cystic lesion with enhancing mural nodule)
Neurocutaneous melanosis	T1 hyperintense leptomeningeal melanosis or multiple parenchymal melanin deposits
Hypomelanosis of Ito	Hemihypertrophy, medulloblastoma, choroid plexus papilloma, polymicrogyria, heterotopias, callosal dysgenesis and vascular malformations

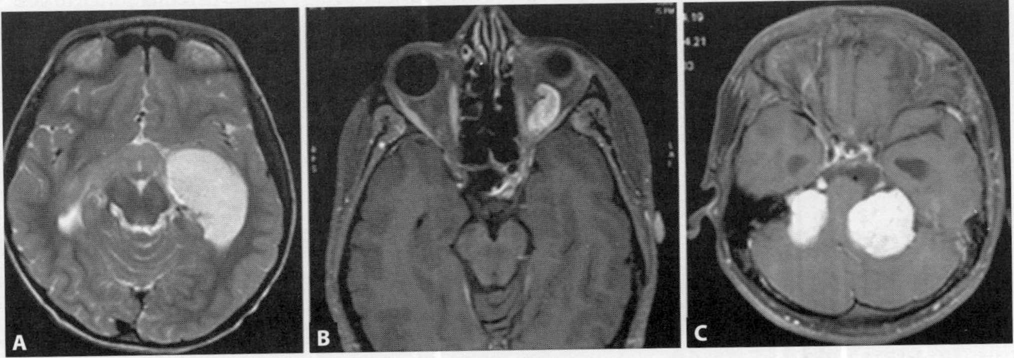

Figs 13.4.6A to C: (A and B) Show enhancing mass lesion in the left optic pathway; (C) Neurofibromatosis 2 patient with bilateral acoustic schwannoma

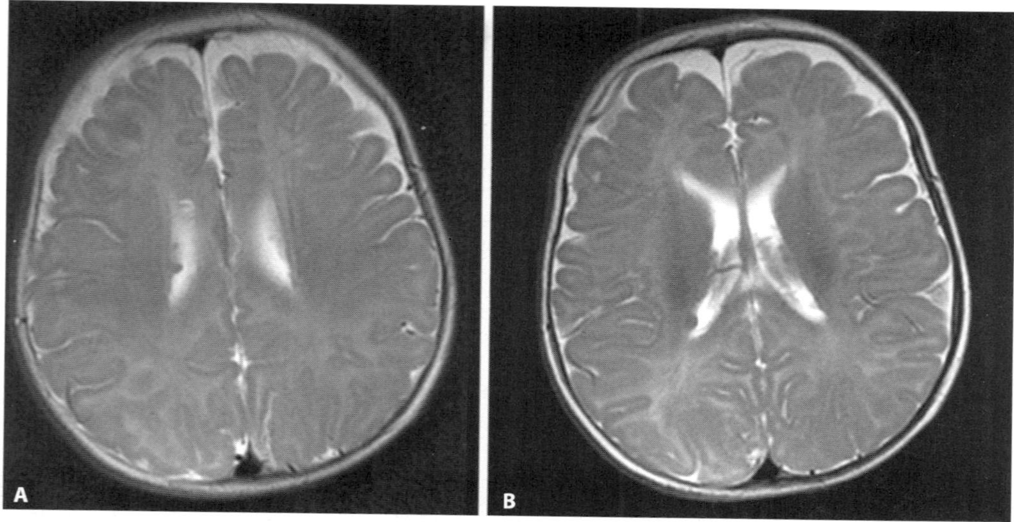

Figs 13.4.7A and B: T2W MR brain images show subependymal nodules in tuberous sclerosis

Table 13.4.3: Imaging findings in hypoxic ischemic encephalopathy (HIE)

	Hypoxemic ischemic encephalopathy (HIE)		
	Preterm	Term	Post-term (1-2 years)
Partial hypoxia	Germinal matrix, intraventricular hemorrhage, periventricular hemorrhagic infarction, white matter injury of prematurity/periventricular leukomalacia (PVL) (**Figs 13.4.8A and B**)		Cortex and subcortical white matter
Partial prolonged hypoxia	Multicystic encephalomalacia	Watershed zones in cortical and subcortical areas	
Profound hypoxia	Deep gray matter including thalami, basal ganglia, hippocampus, cerebellum, dorsal brainstem and corticospinal tracts	Deep gray matter including putamen, ventrolateral thalamus, hippocampus, dorsal brainstem and lateral geniculate nuclei Basal ganglia involvement is more severe compared to thalami The perirolandic cortex may also be affected	Basal ganglia, hippocampi, lateral geniculate body and cerebral cortex in the anterior frontal and parieto-occipital region (**Figs 13.4.9A and B**) The perirolandic cortex and thalami are typically spared

HYPOXIC ISCHEMIC ENCEPHALOPATHY

MRI is useful in detecting hypoxic ischemic injury (**Table 13.4.3**), germinal matrix and intraventricular hemorrhage, and also can be useful to distinguish other pathologies that may mimic hypoxic ischemic encephalopathy (HIE) in the neonatal period such as venous infarction, metabolic disease, infection, and congenital developmental abnormalities.

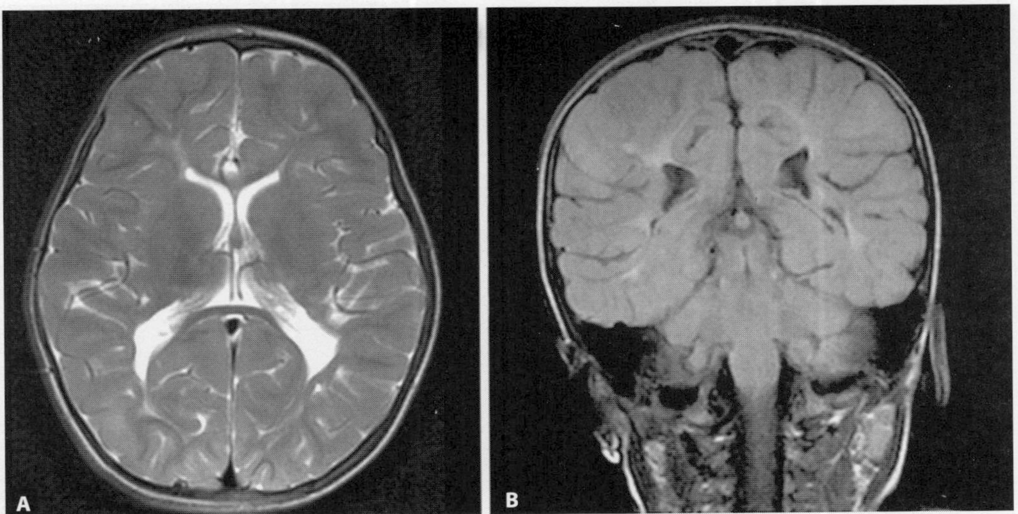

Figs 13.4.8A and B: MRI images show bilateral periventricular hyperintensity with undulating ventricular margin suggestive of periventricular leukomalacia (PVL). (A) T2 MRI brain; (B) FLAIR image

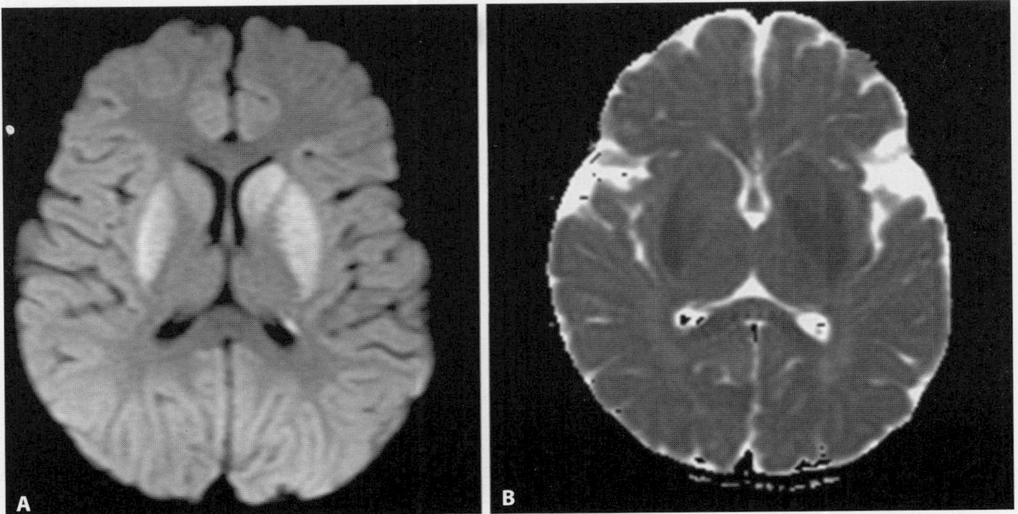

Figs 13.4.9A and B: MRI images show diffusion restriction in bilateral basal ganglia suggestive of profound hypoxic ischemic encephalopathy. (A) Diffusion weighted image (DWI); (B) Apparent diffusion coefficient (ADC) MRI brain images. Similar to T1 and T2 weighted images, DW and ADC images are the basic MR sequences to look for water diffusion in cerebral parenchyma. If there is diffusion restriction, in particular voxel of tissue, it will produce bright signal in DW image and dark signal in ADC image

TUMORS OF THE BRAIN AND SPINE

The purpose of preoperative imaging of brain tumors is to assess tumor location and type, establish whether there are single or multiple lesions, to define its relationship with vital structures and to look for any complications such as hydrocephalus (**Figs 13.4.10 and Table 13.4.4**). Contrast-enhanced T1 weighted volumetric acquisitions are also acquired for

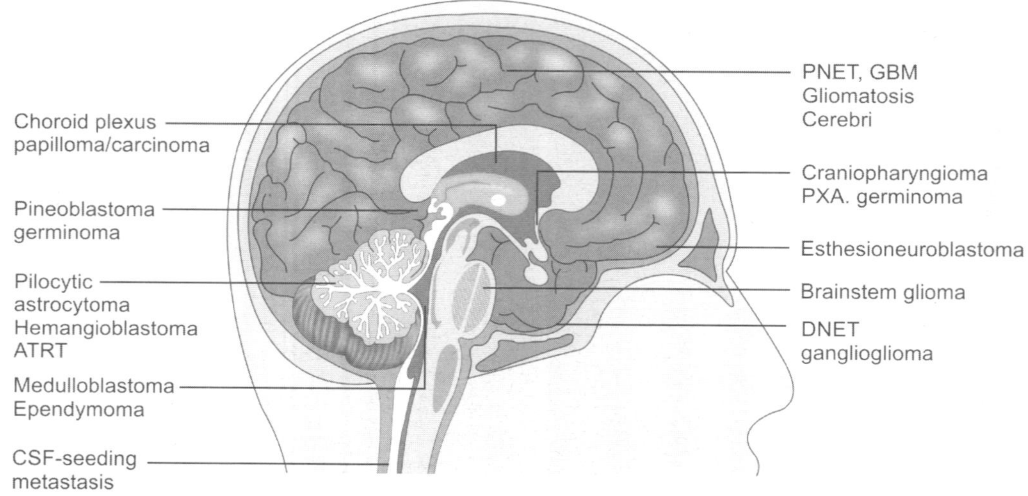

Fig. 13.4.10: Common pediatric brain tumors and their locations
Source: Robin Smithuis, Walter Montanera. Brain Tumor: Systematic Approach. Radiology Assistant; July 2, 2008.

Table 13.4.4: Common intra-axial tumors in pediatric age group

Supratentorial	*Infratentorial*
Astrocytoma	Juvenile pilocytic astrocytoma
Pleomorphic xanthoastrocytoma (PXA)	Primitive neuroectodermal tumor (PNET) – Medulloblastoma
Primitive neuroectodermal tumor (PNET)	Ependymoma
Dysembryoplastic neuroectodermal tumor (DNET)	Brainstem astrocytoma
Ganglioglioma	

Source: Robin Smithuis, Walter Montanera. Brain Tumor: Systematic Approach. Radiology Assistant July 2, 2008.

better characterization of lesion. Imaging of the spine is performed in all children with intracranial tumors to look for spinal metastasis. To avoid confusion with postoperative spinal enhancement, generally MRI brain and spine are taken before any interventional procedure like CSF tapping.

PILOCYTIC ASTROCYTOMA

Pilocytic astrocytoma (**Fig. 13.4.11**) is the most common benign brain tumor in children and occurs typically in the cerebellum, hypothalamus and optic nerves. It can also occur in the hemisphere. Pilocytic astrocytomas are associated with an excellent outcome. In the hypothalamus and in brainstem, the clinical course tends to be less favorable. These tumors rarely undergo anaplastic change. Pilocytic astrocytomas are either cystic or multicystic with a mural nodule (55%) or solid mass (45%).

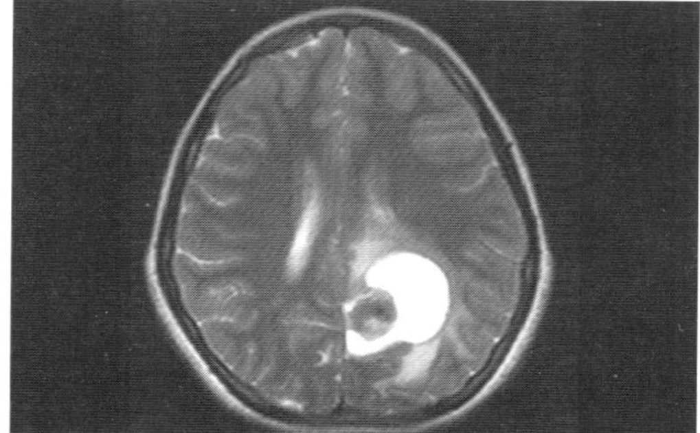

Fig. 13.4.11: Pilocytic astrocytoma. Axial T2 MR shows hyperintense left parietal mass with cystic components and mural nodule

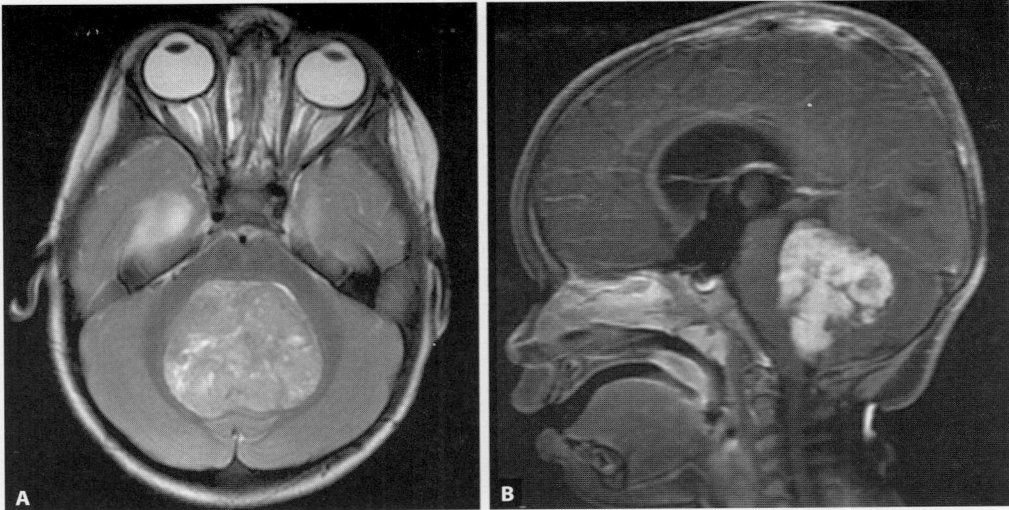

Figs 13.4.12A and B: Medulloblastoma. (A) Axial T2WI MR shows large mass filling and expanding 4th ventricle and causing obstructive hydrocephalus. Signal is only mildly heterogeneous due to small cysts and clefts in the tumor; (B) Sagittal TIC + MR show large heterogeneously enhancing primitive neuroectodermal tumor—medulloblastoma (PNET-MB) expanding fourth ventricle and uplifting posterior tectal plate. Interface with dorsal brainstem is relatively well-defined, pointing to origin of tumor from roof of 4th ventricle

The mural nodule enhances with gadolinium. The solid astrocytomas usually show heterogeneous enhancement. MR spectroscopy presents a lactate peak or elevated choline (Cho) peak.

MEDULLOBLASTOMA

Medulloblastoma (**Figs 13.4.12A and B**) is the most common posterior fossa tumor in children. Most tumors occur in the first 10 years of life. They are most commonly seen involving the cerebellar vermis and protrude into the fourth ventricle. It is the common tumor to disseminate along the CSF pathways. On CT, they are seen as an iso- to hyperdense mass with uniform enhancement. Calcification occurs in 10–20% of cases. They are usually hypo-intense on T1-weighted and heterogeneous on T2-weighted images.

BIBLIOGRAPHY

1. Barkovich AJ. Pediatric Neuroimaging. Philadelphia, Pa: Lippincott Williams and Wilkins, 2005.
2. Barkovich AJ, Lindan CE. Congenital cytomegalovirus infection of the brain: imaging analysis and embryologic considerations. Am J Neuroradiol. 1994;15(4):703-15.
3. Barkovich AJ, Sargent SK. Profound asphyxia in the premature infant: imaging findings. Am J Neuroradiol. 1995;16(9):1837-46.
4. Hatten ME. Central nervous system neuronal migration. Ann Rev Neurosci. 1999;22:511-39.
5. Nickerson JP, Richner B, Santy K, Lequin MH, Poretti A, Filippi CG, Huisman TAGM. Neuroimaging of pediatric intracranial infection—Part 2: TORCH, viral, fungal, and parasitic infections. J Neuroimaging. 2012;22: e52-e63.
6. Padget D, Lindenberg R. Inverse cerebellum morphogenetically related to the Dandy-Walker and Arnold-Chiari syndromes: bizarre malformed brain with occipital encephalocele. Johns Hopkins Med J. 1972; 131(3):228-46.
7. Pont MS, Elster AD. Lesions of skin and brain: modern imaging of the neurocutaneous syndromes. Am J Roentgenol. 1992;158(6): 1193-203.
8. Smithuis R, Montanera W. Brain tumor – Systematic approach. Radiology Assistant; July 2, 2008.

Miscellaneous

Reviewers: *P Ramachandran, NC Gowrishankar, Hemchand K Prasad, PSN Menon, Alok Gupta, R Remesh Kumar*

14.1 Timing of Surgery in Pediatric Surgical Disorders

R Velmurugan

Reviewers: *P Ramachandran, NC Gowrishankar, Hemchand K Prasad*

It is imperative for pediatricians and surgeons to be on the same page while counseling parents of children who require surgical intervention. Any dichotomy of advice to already stressed parents causes confusion and potential loss of confidence in both the pediatrician and surgeon, prompting them to seek a second opinion. In many cases, the parent decides to defer surgery altogether. This article attempts to address this conflict so that the child may benefit from timely intervention. Common surgical problems seen by the pediatrician in office practice are dealt with individually.

PHIMOSIS

It is the inability to retract the prepuce beyond the corona and is the most common problem encountered in the clinic. It is important to realize that phimosis is physiological till one year of age and simple gentle home stretching by the mother daily is enough to dilate the preputial opening. No attempt should be made to forcibly dilate the prepuce either by hand or instrument as doing, so will cause radial tears which heal by scarring that cicatrizes the prepuce and makes circumcision inevitable.

The role of steroidal creams is debatable. Applying steroids to a potential culture medium, i.e. the bag of urine in the prepuce, predisposes to balanoposthitis. It is actually the preputial stretching done while applying the cream that helps rather than the cream.

Phimosis beyond one year is pathological and requires circumcision and is ideally done at one year, but definitely by two years of age as the cerebral imprinting of sex is complete by two years and the child may perceive his penis to be abnormal otherwise.

BALANITIS XEROTICA OBLITERANS

This is a distressing condition usually in older boys, where the preputial skin and glans take the appearance and consistency of dried orange rind and is due to long standing contact dermatitis with urine. The dryness extends to the meatus as well causing meatal stenosis. It is best to avoid this problem with an early circumcision.

INGUINAL HERNIA

It is to be understood that an inguinal hernia will not resolve spontaneously and is a relative surgical emergency requiring early surgery. The inguinal canal in children lacks the obliquity seen in adults as a result of which, both the deep and superficial inguinal rings lie almost on top of each other. Therefore, simple activities of daily living like crying, coughing or straining can cause a prolapse of bowel down both rings into the scrotum which may strangulate at the narrow external ring.

This lack of canal obliquity is more pronounced in the newborn, increasing the risk of obstruction. Hence, hernias in the newborn are surgical emergencies. However, in preterm neonates, the risk of anesthesia outweighs the benefit of surgery and surgery is deferred till the baby reaches term. The baby should be observed in the ward meanwhile and discharged after hernia repair at term. Older children should undergo herniotomy as soon as feasible.

HYDROCELE

In hydrocele, the patent processus vaginalis sack is so narrow that it admits only abdominal fluid down into the scrotum and hence, usually closes by one year of age. Surgery is done for hydrocele persistent after 1–1.5 years of age. It is important to distinguish a hernia from a hydrocele as the timing of surgery differs and is best left to a surgeon to decide.

UNDESCENDED TESTIS

The understanding of pathophysiology of testicular maldescent has undergone a sea change over the past three decades and so also the timing of surgery. No surgical entity has been subject to such conflicting advice as an undescended testis (UDT).

The newborn period is the best time to record the presence or absence of the testis in the scrotum and it should be the endeavor of every neonatologist to do so. There is a postnatal testosterone surge in the first three months of life and even those testes which have mild degrees of nondescent will come down by 3–6 months of life. Any testis which is not resident in the scrotum by 6 months is unlikely to come down spontaneously and requires surgical correction. Further, irreversible histological damage sets in as early as six months and these changes are seen ominously in the contralateral descended testis also in many cases. Hence, UDT is a bilateral disease manifests unilaterally. Surgical correction of an undescended testis is mandatory by six months of age.

UMBILICAL HERNIA

Umbilical hernias are a work in progress and usually close by 1.5 years of age.

Surgery is done only if the hernia shows no sign of resolution beyond 1.5 years.

Early surgery is done if there is a history of irreducibility or if the hernia is of the proboscis type.

TONGUE TIE

This is a condition often missed on routine examination. The first word universally uttered by a child is 'TA TA' and proper phonation of that is not possible in a child with tongue tie. The child memorizes its own sound and it is important that the first words spoken should be phonetically correct. Moreover, as the child has solid food, it needs the tongue tip to clear food residue from the gingivolabial sulcus. So, tongue tie is corrected by 9 months of age before the child starts speaking.

HYPOSPADIAS

The days of staged repair of hypospadias are long past and the current recommendation is a single stage urethroplasty irrespective of the severity at 1.5 years of age. This is to ensure genital normalcy before the child is aware of its sex (which is at 2 years).

CLEFT LIP

The idea in lip surgery is to ensure soft tissue cover over the premaxilla as early as possible to prevent premaxillary protrusion and is done ideally by 3–5 months.

CLEFT PALATE

As in tongue tie, palatoplasty needs to be done before the child begins to speak and hence surgery is advised by 9 months of age.

FIRE BRIGADE EMERGENCIES

There are only three conditions in pediatric surgery where the child has to be rushed to the operating theater in minutes, i.e.:

1. Malrotation with volvulus
2. Torsion testis/painful tender testis
3. Septic arthritis of infancy.

In cases of suspected malrotation, surgeons are usually involved early and there is no dispute on its gravity or treatment.

But cases of torsion testes are invariably referred a little too late for the surgeon to salvage it from gangrene. Every case of a painful tender testis is a torsion until proved otherwise by surgical exploration. There is no investigation available currently that can exclude torsion with certainty. Hence, no time should be wasted on ultrasound or other tests and the child should be subjected to immediate scrotal exploration.

The same applies to a painful joint swelling which needs urgent decompression, failing which the articular cartilage gets destroyed. IV antibiotics and immobilization are only adjuncts to urgent surgical drainage.

CONCLUSION

The recommended timing for correction of surgical problems are as follows:

- *Inguinal hernia:* Early surgery
- *Neonatal inguinal hernia:* Emergency surgery
- *Hydrocele:* 1.5 years
- *Undescended testis:* 6 months
- *Umbilical hernia:* > 1.5 years
- *Tongue tie:* 9 months
- *Hypospadias:* 1.5 years—single stage urethroplasty
- *Cleft lip:* 3–5 months
- *Cleft palate:* 9 months
- Malrotation with volvulus, tender testis, septic arthritis: In minutes.

14.2 ROP/Cataract/Squint: When and How to Intervene?

Vasumathy Vedantham

Reviewers: *P Ramachandran, NC Gowrishankar, Hemchand K Prasad*

Childhood blindness is a pressing problem with one child going blind every minute as per the World Health Organization (*Bulletin of the World Health Organization, 2001*). The prevalence of blindness in children is around 0.3 per 1000 children, with approximately 1.4 million blind children in the world. Of all the causes of childhood blindness, retinopathy of prematurity (ROP), cataract and squint are the most important; and a bird's eye view about their management is presented in this chapter.

RETINOPATHY OF PREMATURITY

It is a blinding condition which occurs in preterm babies. The etiology is multifactorial with oxygen, light, vitamin E and genetic factors being implicated but by far the most important causative factor is prematurity itself with the resultant underdevelopment of retinal vessels.

Pathogenesis

There are twin theories in the pathogenesis of ROP:

1. *Spindle cell theory (Kretzer):* The mesenchymal spindle cells, exposed to hyperoxic extrauterine conditions, develop gap junctions. These gap junctions interfere with the normal vascular formation, triggering a neovascular response.
2. *Classical theory (Ashton):* He describes two phases—initial hyperoxic and second hypoxic phase in development of ROP. The initial hyperoxic phase of ROP results when the preterm baby stops receiving maternal insulin growth factor (IGF-1) which stimulates vessel growth. In addition, the blood oxygen concentrations are also high as the baby is placed on a ventilator or is receiving oxygen. All these lead to vasocessation and the initial hyperoxic phase of ROP. This is the reason why ROP is never

detected in the first two weeks of an infant's life. This could also explain the decreased incidence of ROP noted in the seminal study by Chow et al in Paediatrics 2003, wherein the authors noted a decreased incidence of ROP with the introduction of practices such as setting alarms for high and low oxygen levels, slow weaning of the oxygen, etc.

In the second phase, hypoxia due to withdrawal of oxygen due to improved systemic status of the baby causes vasoproliferation due to outpouring of vascular endothelial growth factor (VEGF), which leads to aberrant vasculogenesis resulting in ROP. This is again the reason why ROP is usually seen when the infant is weaned off the respirator and the rationale for the use of anti-VEGF agents in the treatment of ROP.

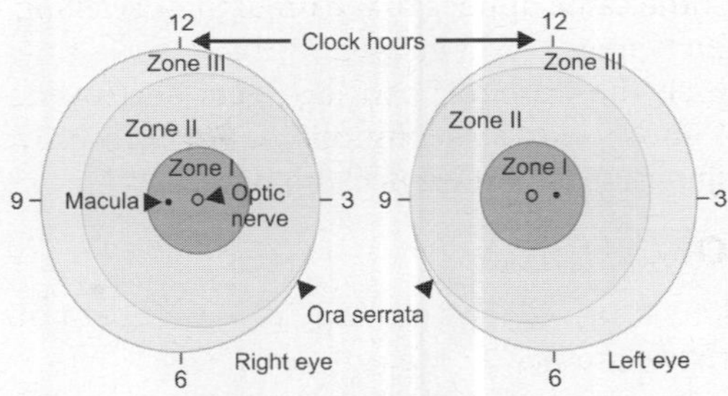

Fig. 14.2.1: Classification of ROP: Zones

Fig. 14.2.2: Stage IVB ROP
(For color version, see Plate 8)

Classification of ROP

The International classification of ROP classifies ROP based on (1) Zone, (2) Stage, (3) Extent of disease in clock hours, (4) Presence or absence of plus disease. There are also two types of ROP—the conventional ROP and AP-ROP (Agressive-posterior ROP).

The eye is divided into three zones:

Zone I: An imaginary circle centered around the optic disc with the radius twice the distance between the disc and the fovea (the center of the retina). Generally very posterior ROP such as Zone I disease are more difficult to treat and tend to progress very fast.

Zone II: A circle centered on the optic disc but straddling the ora serrata (an imaginary circle where the retina ends) nasally.

Zone III: The remaining temporal crescent of retina **(Fig. 14.2.1)**. The zoning is applicable to both types of ROP.

The several stages of conventional ROP are as follows:

Stage I: A white flat line (demarcation line) separating the vascular from the avascular retina.

Stage II: The white line becomes thicker (ridge), there might also be small white spots (early new vessels called popcorns or hot dogs).

Stage III: The ridge becomes redder and gains height due to extraretinal fibrovascular proliferation.

Stage IVA: Subtotal retinal detachment sparing the macula.

Stage IVB: Subtotal retinal detachment involving the macula **(Fig. 14.2.2)**.

Stage V: Total retinal detachment presenting with a white reflex in the pupil (Cat's eye) many a time mistaken for cataract **(Fig. 14.2.3)**.

- *Aggressive posterior (AP):* ROP or fulminant ROP however, lacks all these stages and is characterized by markedly dilated and tortuous vessels on the posterior pole and abnormally proliferating new vessels which are flat and look like nodes, bushes or hemorrhages and are usually difficult to find. In addition, many loops or collaterals are also seen. This type of ROP is usually seen in very sick and very tiny preterm babies less than 28 weeks of gestation **(Fig. 14.2.4)**.

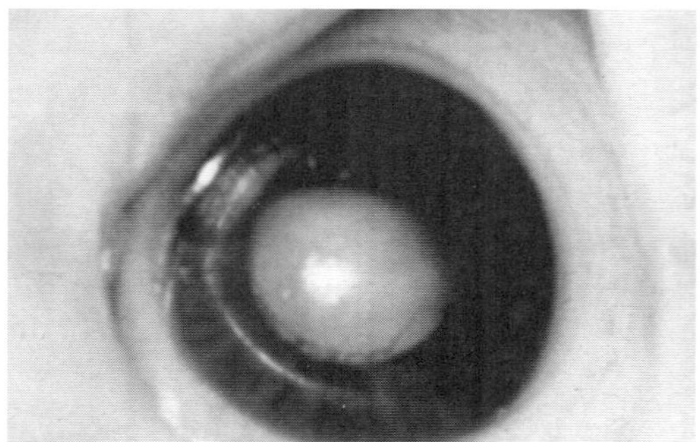

Fig. 14.2.3: Stage V ROP (*For color version, see Plate 8*)

Fig. 14.2.4: AP ROP with plus disease and collaterals (*For color version, see Plate 8*)

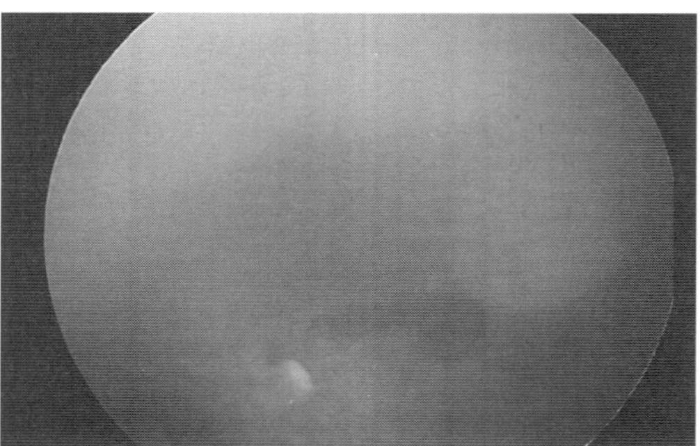

Fig. 14.2.5: Zone I ROP Stage III ROP involving all 12 clock hours with plus disease (Rush disease) (*For color version, see Plate 8*)

Plus disease is dilatation and tortuosity of both the arteries and veins akin to AV anastomoses and could easily be picked up even by a direct ophthalmoscope. Generally, presence of plus disease is an indicator of disease severity. Rush disease is Zone I ROP in very low birth weight babies with plus disease **(Fig. 14.2.5)**.

Types of ROP Requiring Treatment

- *Threshold ROP:* Stage III disease with plus disease involving 5 or more contiguous/8 or more cumulative clock hours.

  It Indicates less chance of spontaneous resolution with a 50% risk of blindness (Cryo-ROP study)
- *High-risk prethreshold ROP:* Zone I ROP, any stage with plus disease, Zone II ROP stage 2+, Zone II ROP stage 3 (<threshold clock hours) with plus disease (ETROP study)
- Aggressive posterior ROP.

Sequelae of ROP

Macular heterotopia, falciform fold, myopia, retinal detachment (RD): tractional, exudative and rhegmatogenous, squint, secondary glaucoma; generally unfavorable outcome is likely in 50% of untreated threshold ROP.

Differential diagnosis of ROP: There are many conditions, but the most important are Retinoblastoma, Norrie's disease, X-linked retinoschisis, FEVR (familial exudative vitreoretinopathy), incontinentia pigmenti, PHPV (persistent hyperplastic primary vitreous) to mention a few. Cataract and retinoblastoma also present as cat's eye reflex.

Management of ROP

ROP screening is done using either an indirect ophthalmoscope which is mounted on his/ her head by the pediatric retina specialist **(Fig. 14.2.6)** or the RETCAM wherein fundus images can be obtained by the camera and images sent by internet to the specialist for opinion.

Protocol for ROP Screening

The American Academy of Ophthalmologists (AAO) and AAP criteria for ROP screening (screen all infants with birth weight <1500 g and gestational age ≤30 weeks) cannot be extrapolated to the Indian scenario as ROP is seen in bigger and older infants in contrast to the west. The NNF recommendations are to screen all infants.

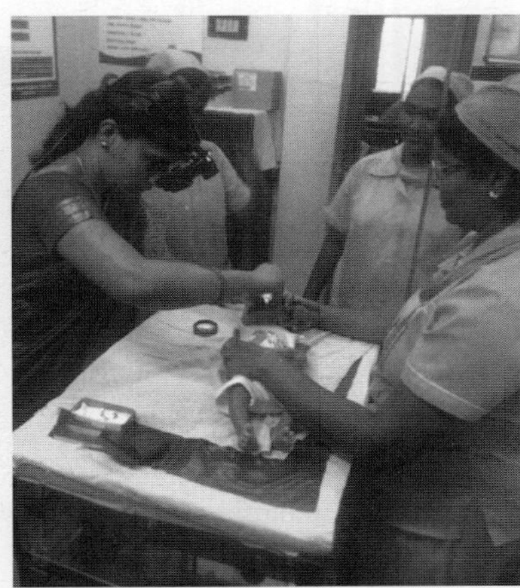

Fig. 14.2.6: ROP screening with indirect ophthalmoscope (*For color version, see Plate 9*)

- < 34 weeks gestation
- < 1750 g birth weight
- 34–36 weeks gestation or 1750–2000 g birth weight if they have risk factors for ROP *(mechanical ventilation, prolonged oxygen therapy and hemodynamic instability).*

Pediatric retina specialists in India generally screen all infants up to 2000 g birth weight and up to 35 weeks of gestational age.

The NNF also has laid down guidelines as to when to do ROP screening

- *Day 30 strategy:* The first retinal examination should be performed not later than 4 weeks of age or 30 days of life in infants born ≥28 weeks of gestational age.
- *Day 20 strategy:* Infants born <28 weeks or <1200 g birth weight should be screened early, by 2–3 weeks of age/day 20 of life, to detect AP-ROP.

Follow-up protocol:

- Normal vascularization—follow-up after 6 months
- ROP/immature vessels in zone 1 and 2—1-2 weeks follow-up until normal vascularization is achieved or threshold/HR prethreshold disease is reached
- Threshold/high-risk prethreshold disease/ AP-ROP with NVE—ablative therapy within 48–72 hours of diagnosis.

Prevention of ROP-related Blindness—Primary

- Reduce premature births
- Control O_2 concentration and variability in inspired oxygen concentration.

ROP Blindness Prevention—Secondary

- Screen for treatable ROP
- Treat avascular retina within 48–72 hours
- Retinal ablation by laser (the gold standard)/ cryo (done only in selected situations, needs general anesthesia). In laser, diode/df Nd YAG Laser is employed to photocoagulate peripheral, nonvascularized retina, and the retinal pigment epithelium (RPE) pigment absorbs the laser energy, transforming it to heat energy that thins the retina, thereby reducing the oxygen demand. The VEGF outpouring is reduced and 3 weeks later, there is regression of extraretinal neovascularization and progression of vessel growth beyond the demarcation line or ridge.

When is laser done:

- *Zone I ROP:* Any stage with plus disease
- *Zone I ROP:* Stage 3—no plus disease
- *Zone II:* Stage 2 or 3 with plus disease
- AP-ROP with new vessels.

Antivascular endothelial growth factor (anti-VEGF) injections are carried out in selected situations such as:

- Severely ill infant on an oscillating ventilator
- Hyphema, vitreous hemorrhage, severe lid edema, dense TVL (tunica vasculosa lentis) with nondilating pupils, precluding laser
- Very severe ROP/AP-ROP
- Unusual situations.

ROP Blindness Prevention—Tertiary

Prevention of ambylopia (lazy eye), squint and glaucoma by rigorous follow-up.

To summarize, ROP-related blindness can easily be prevented by a combination of energetic screening and timely treatment.

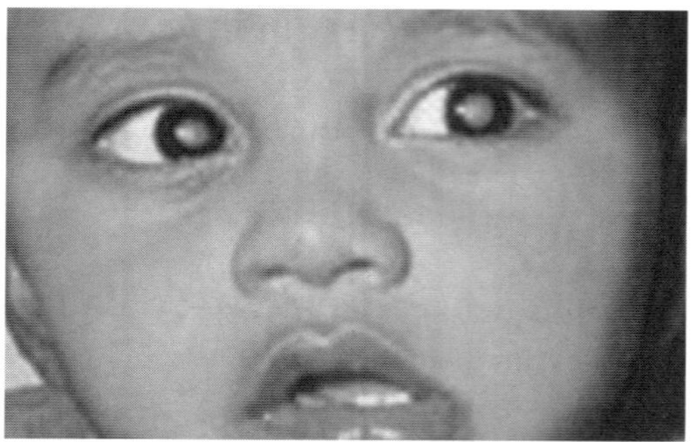

Fig. 14.2.7: Childhood cataract
(*For color version, see Plate 9*)

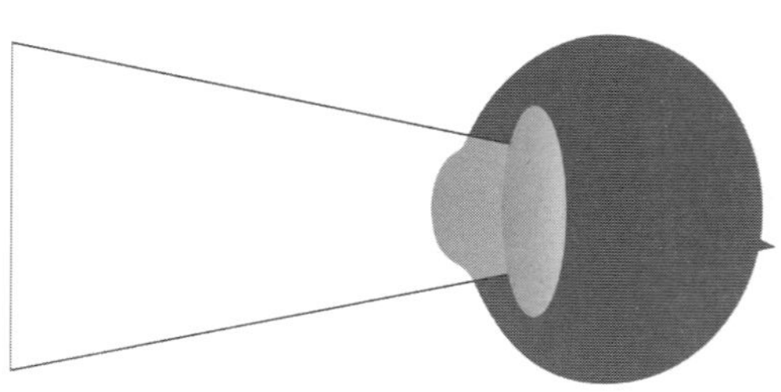

Fig. 14.2.8: Blockage of light rays by a dense cataract leading to stimulus deprivation amblyopia

CHILDHOOD CATARACT (Fig. 14.2.7)

A cataract in children not only blurs the retinal image but also disrupts the development of visual pathway in the CNS leading to amblyopia (lazy eye) **(Fig. 14.2.8)**. Therefore, in contrast to adults wherein the timing of cataract surgery is usually decided by the patients, in children, the surgery is usually not delayed, except in unusual circumstances. In addition, in terms of blind years saved, operating one childhood cataract is equivalent to operating 10 adult cataracts.

Etiology

The etiology can be established in only 60% of bilateral cataract and 40% of unilateral cataract; others are undetermined. Amongst hereditary causes, AD, AR, X-linked mode of inheritance and chromosomal anomalies are known to occur. Among non-hereditary causes intrauterine infection, maternal drugs, maternal nutrition, prematurity, radiation, photocoagulation, steroid intake and trauma are important.

Among intrauterine infections the most common cause is rubella infection in the first trimester of pregnancy. It is caused by the virus getting into the developing lens and is characterized by bilateral central nuclear cataract usually associated with microphthalmos, keratitis, microcornea, glaucoma and retinopathy. In addition, the infant has several systemic problems such as low birth weight, deafness, cardiac anomalies, hepatosplenomegaly and general delay in development.

Traumatic cataract is also more common in children as they are more prone for injuries and is usually after penetrating trauma and is associated with various degree of corneal involvement. Complicated cataract is secondary to uveitis and anterior chamber granuloma.

Differential diagnosis of childhood cataract is a veritable list and comprise the following: retinoblastoma, toxoplasmosis, toxocariasis, retinal detachment, retinopathy of prematurity (ROP), persistent hyperplastic primary vitreous (PHPV), Coat's disease, coloboma, myelinated nerve fibers, retinal dysplasia such as Norrie's disease, incontinentia pigmenti, retinoschisis and cyclitic membrane.

Management

The gold standard of management is surgical removal of the cataractous lens.

The indications of surgery are all dense cataracts (unilateral/bilateral) and partial cataracts with vision less than 6/18.

Timing of Surgery

The critical period for development of fixation reflex is between 6 weeks and 6 months of age and hence the best time for surgery is before this period to prevent stimulus-deprivation amblyopia. In dense monocular cataract, the surgery should be done as early as possible, may be on the next day after birth!

Surgical Techniques

Several surgical techniques are employed such as lensectomy, lens aspiration with intraocular lens (IOL), but the gold standard is lens aspiration with PPC (primary posterior capsulectomy), anterior vitrectomy (AV) and IOL. IOLs are generally avoided below one year of age and beyond one year of age are placed after undercorrecting their power according to the age to give allowance to the growth of the eyeball. If no IOL is implanted, contact lenses or thick aphakic spectacles are dispensed.

A rigorous follow-up involving visual acuity, visual axis, strabismus, IOP and fundus examination is carried out for all the operated children at regular intervals: up to 2 years once in 3 months, 2–5 years once in 6 months and after 5 years 6 months/yearly.

STRABISMUS (SQUINT)

Strabismus or squint is a misalignment of visual axis, wherein one eye is turned in, out, up or down. There are two types of squint:

1. *Manifest*: It is obvious at all times (Heterotropia) and
2. *Latent:* It is controlled (detected only by examination by pediatric ophthalmologist) and binocular single vision is maintained (Heterophoria).

Management of squint is carried out by the pediatric ophthalmologist by employing one of the following: correction of refractive error, prism therapy, occlusion therapy, orthoptic exercises and/or surgery **(Figs 14.2.9 and 14.2.10)**.

To summarize, ROP, cataract and squint are common causes of childhood blindness which can easily be prevented or treated by a concerted effort between the pediatrician and pediatric ophthalmologist.

SIMPLIFIED PROTOCOL FOR EYE SCREENING OF CHILDREN

- A pediatrician or family physician should examine a new born eye
- Preterm babies need to be screened before day 30 by a pediatric retina specialist
- All infants by 6 months of age should be screened for ocular health by an ophthalmologist
- By age 3 years all children should have their visual acuity estimated
- Screening at school should become a routine procedure every year in all schools.

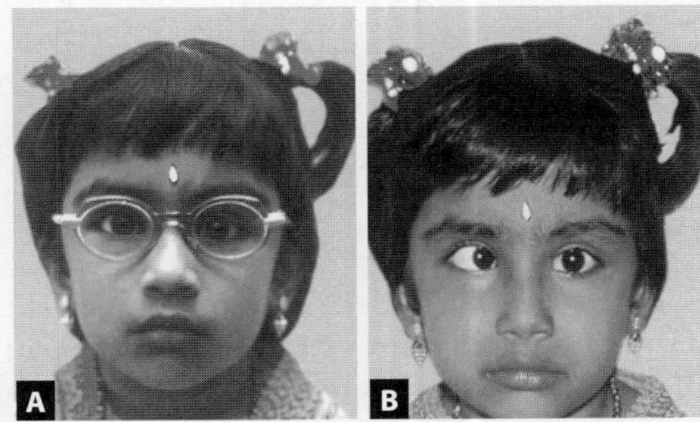

Figs 14.2.10A and B: Squint getting corrected with spectacles (*For color version, see Plate 9*)

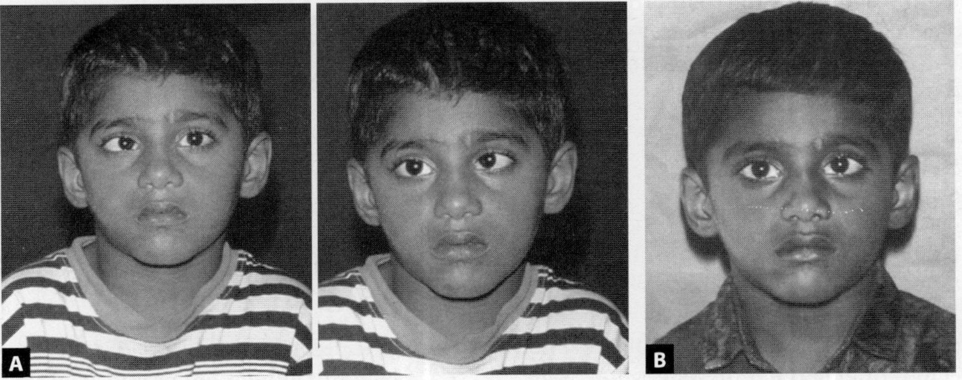

Figs 14.2.9A and B: Squint (A) Before surgery; (B) After surgery (*For color version, see Plate 9*)

BIBLIOGRAPHY

1. AAP POLICY STATEMENT. Screening Examination of Premature Infants for Retinopathy of Prematurity. Pediatrics. 2013; 131:189-95.
2. Ashton N. Oxygen and the retinal blood vessels. Trans Ophthalmol Soc UK. 1980;100:359-62.
3. Chow LC, et al. Pediatrics. 2003;111:339-45.
4. Cryotherapy for ROP Group. 3 month outcome. Arch Ophthalmol 1990;108:195-204.
5. Eckstein M, et al. Aetiology of childhood cataract in south India. Br J Ophthalmol. 1996;80(7):628-32.
6. Gunton KB, et al. Strabismus. Prim Care. 2015;42(3):393-407. doi: 10.1016/j.pop.2015.05.006. Epub 2015 Jul 7. Review.
7. Kretzer FL, Hittner HM. Retinopathy of prematurity: clinical implications of retinal development. Arch Dis Child. 1988;63:1151-67.
8. Lenhart PD, et al. Global challenges in the management of congenital cataract: proceedings of the 4th International Congenital Cataract Symposium held on March 7, 2014, New York. JAAPOS 2015 Apr;19(2):e1-8. doi: 10.1016/j.jaapos.2015.01.013.
9. Mintz-Hittner HA, Kennedy KA, Chuang AZ. BEAT-ROP cooperative group: efficacy of intravitreal bevacizumab for stage 3+ retinopathy of prematurity. N Engl J Med. 2011; 364(7):603-15.
10. Vedantham V. Retinopathy of prematurity screening in the Indian population: Its time to set our own guidelines! Editorial. Ind J Ophthalmol. 2007;55:329-30.

14.3 Skeletal Dysplasias: A Radiographic Approach

M Prabakaran

Reviewers: *PSN Menon, Alok Gupta, R Remesh Kumar*

INTRODUCTION

Skeletal dysplasias (osteochondrodysplasias) are a complex group of bone and cartilage disorders that may affect the fetal skeleton as it develops *in utero*. They occur due to genetic mutations and their phenotype continues to evolve throughout life. The word 'dysplasia' has Latin roots meaning 'bad growth'. Skeletal dysplasias include more than 380 conditions that involve abnormally developed bones and connective tissues.

DYSPLASIAS OF BONE: TERMINOLOGY

- *Dysplasia:* A disturbance in bone form or modeling intrinsic to bone.
- *Dysostosis:* A disturbance in bone form or modeling associated with a disturbance of ectodermal or other mesenchymal tissue.
- *Dystrophy:* A disturbance in bone form or modeling of nutritional or metabolic in origin.

Some dysplasias are lethal in perinatal period and are detected on antenatal ultrasound scans while the nonlethal dysplasia is present early in infancy or childhood with disproportionate short stature, failure of linear growth or with other physical deformities.

The appropriate diagnosis of a dysplasia is dependent upon the integration of clinical and family history, physical examination, radiologic examination and molecular and biochemical tests. Among these, a radiologic evaluation is an integral part of the diagnostic work-up of a dysplasia.

INTERNATIONAL CLASSIFICATION OF SKELETAL DYSPLASIA

Skeletal dysplasias are classified as:

- Defects of tubular bones and axial skeleton

- Disorganized development of cartilaginous and fibrous components of the skeleton
- Idiopathic osteolyses.

The international classification of skeletal dysplasia has provided a classification of genetic skeletal disorders with an overview of recognized diagnostic entities and groups based on clinical and radiographic features and molecular pathogenesis. A practical and useful clinical classification of the defects of tubular bones and axial skeleton are summarized in **Table 14.3.1**.

Table 14.3.1: Classification of defects of tubular bones and axial skeleton

1. Achondroplasia group
   a. Achondroplasia
   b. Pseudoachondroplasia
   c. Hypochondroplasia
2. Metatrophic dysplasia
3. Short-ribs dysplasia group (with/without polydactyly)
   a. Short-rib polydactyly syndrome (SRPS)
   b. Asphyxiating thoracic dysplasia
   c. Ellis-van Creveld dysplasia
4. Spondyloepi-metaphyseal dysplasia group
   a. Spondylo-epiphyseal dysplasia
   b. Spondylo-metaphyseal dysplasia (SMD)
   c. Dyggve melchior clausen dysplasia
5. Dysostosis multiplex group
   a. Mucopolysaccharidoses:
      i. Morquio syndrome (MPS-IV)
      ii. Hurler syndrome
6. Epiphyseal dysplasia
7. Chondrodysplasia punctata group
8. Metaphyseal dysplasia
9. Mesomelic dysplasia
10. Dysplasia with significant membranous bone involvement
    a. Cleidocranial dysplasia
11. Dysplasia with decreased bone density
    a. Osteogenesis imperfecta (several types)
    b. Mucolipidosis II
12. Dysplasia with increased bone density
    a. Osteopetrosis
    b. Pyknodysostosis
13. Disorganized development of cartilaginous and fibrous components of the skeleton
    a. Multiple cartilaginous exostoses
    b. Fibrous dysplasia

RADIOLOGICAL EVALUATION

The radiologic evaluation begins with a complete skeletal survey ideally comprising of a set of radiographs as follows:

- Skull (AP and lateral)
- Thoracolumbar spine (AP and lateral)
- Chest (AP)
- Pelvis (AP)
- One upper limb (AP)
- One lower limb (AP)
- Left hand (AP) (for bone age).

Other special X-rays may be obtained if needed. The points to be noted while reporting include the age of the child, whether the child is prepubertal or pubertal; disproportion, ossification of bone, radiodensity and presence of fractures. **Table 14.3.2** details the common body locations affected by various dysplasias which helps in their detection by radiological evaluation.

Skeletal dysplasias are characterized by disproportionate short stature and failure in linear growth. The type of short stature can be classified as rhizomelic (proximal segment—femoral or humeral shortening as in achondroplasia), mesomelic (middle segment shortening; short forearms, tibia and fibula), acromelic (distal segment shortening —forearm, fingers and toes shortening) and acromesomelic (middle and distal segment shortening). Micromelic shortening indicates disproportionate shortening of the entire leg or limb. Some examples are given in **Table 14.3.3**.

Table 14.3.2: Dysplasias with involvement of axial skeleton

Location	*Examples*
Skull	Achondroplasia Cleidocranial dysplasia
Mandible	Pyknodysostosis
Clavicle	Cleidocranial dysplasia
Ribs	Asphyxiating thoracic dysplasia Thanatophoric dysplasia
Spine	Spondyloepiphyseal dysplasia congenita Mucopolysaccharidosis
Pelvis	Achondroplasia

Table 14.3.3: Dysplasias with involvement of appendicular skeleton

Type of shortening	*Examples*	*Location of abnormality*	*Examples*
Rhizomelic	Achondroplasia Spondyloepiphyseal dysplasia congenita	Epiphyseal	Chondrodysplasia punctata Spondyloepiphyseal dysplasia
Mesomelic	Mesomelic dysplasia	Metaphyseal	Achondroplasia Chondroectodermal dysplasia
Acromelic	Acrodysostosis	Diaphyseal	Progressive diaphyseal dysplasia
Micromelic	Achondrogenesis	Combination	Spondyloepimetaphyseal dysplasia Metatropic dysplasia Mucopolysaccharidoses

ACHONDROPLASIA

Some of the important radiological features of achondroplasia **(Fig. 14.3.1A)** include the following:

- The cranial vault is large with a small skull base **(Fig. 14.3.1B)**.
- The forehead is prominent with depressed nasal bridge **(Fig. 14.3.1B)**.
- The foramen magnum is narrowed.
- The interpedicular distance gradually diminishes in the lumbar spine.
- The iliac wings are vertical **(Fig. 14.3.1C)**.
- The limbs demonstrate normal density with marked shortening of the long bones **(Fig. 14.3.1C)**.

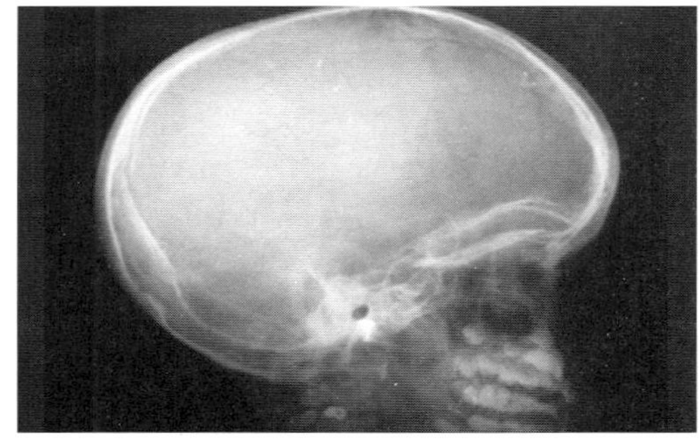

Fig. 14.3.1B: X-ray skull in achondroplasia: Note the large cranial vault, small skull base, prominent forehead, and depressed nasal bridge

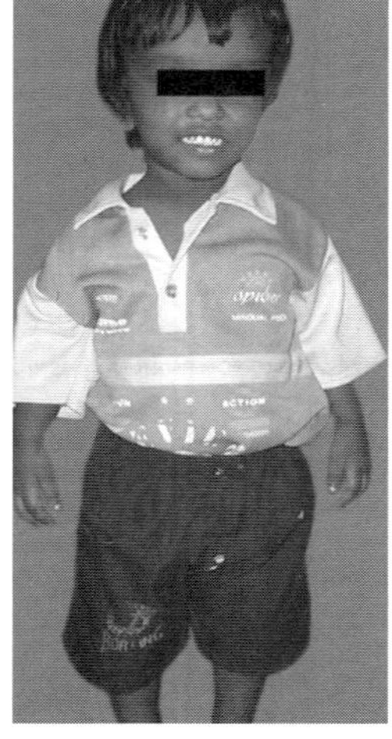

Fig. 14.3.1A: Achondroplasia showing the clinical features of rhizomelic short stature
(For color version, see Plate 10)

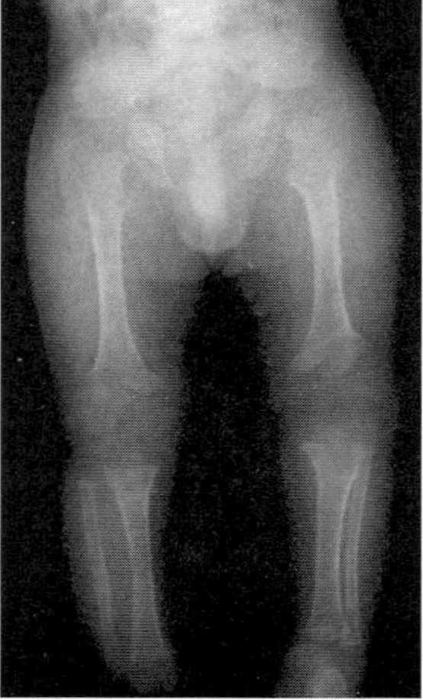

Fig. 14.3.1C: X-ray pelvis with lower extremities: Note the abnormal pelvic configuration with vertical iliac wings and marked shortening of the long bones

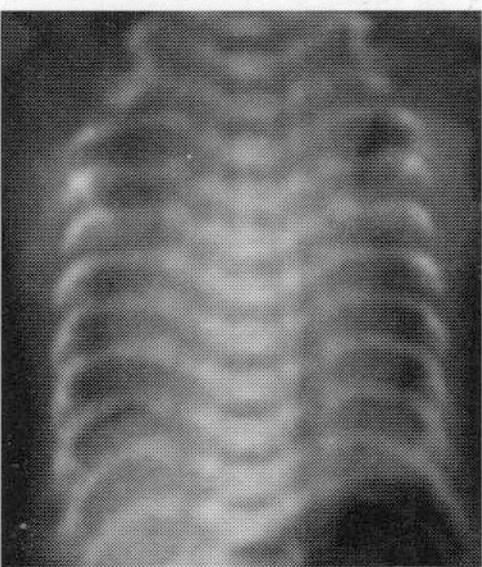

Fig. 14.3.2: X-ray chest of a child with asphyxiating thoracic dysplasia

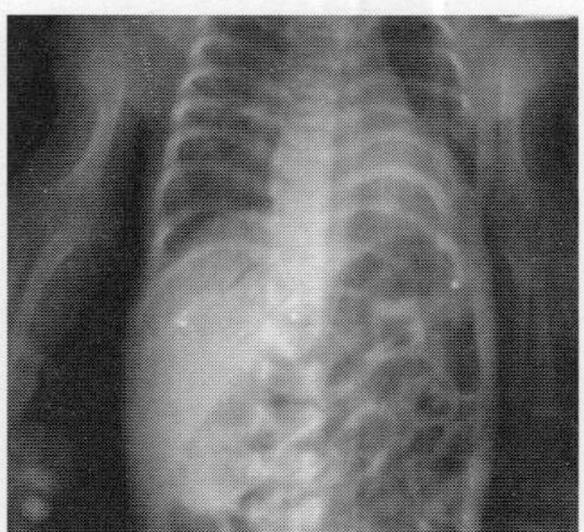

Fig. 14.3.3B: Short-rib dysplasia group: Narrowing of thorax with short ribs

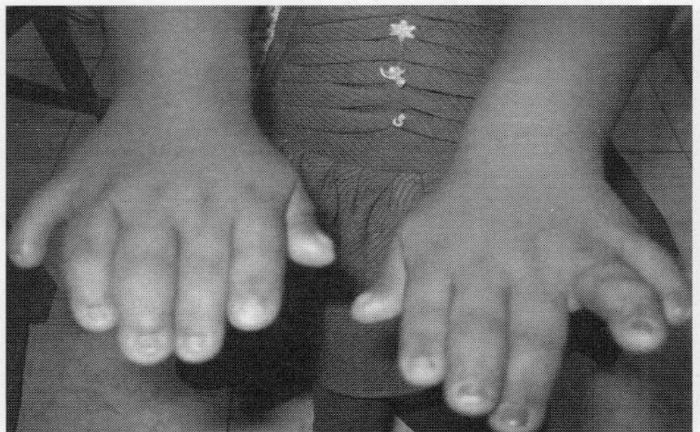

Fig. 14.3.3A: Short-rib dysplasia group with polydactyly (*For color version, see Plate 10*)

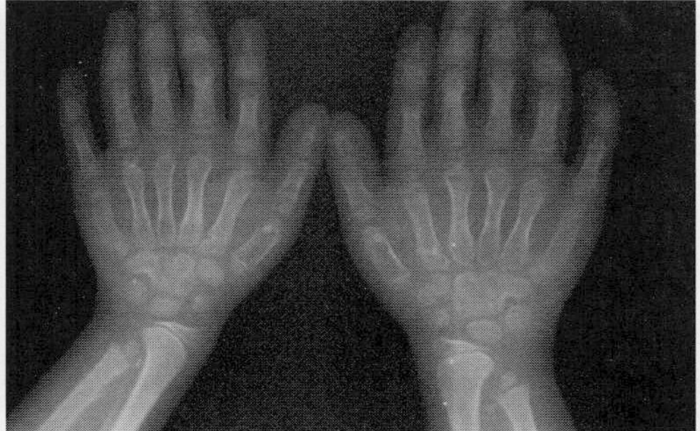

Fig. 14.3.3C: Short-rib dysplasia: Shortened long bones and polydactyly

ASPHYXIATING THORACIC DYSPLASIA: SHORT RIB DYSPLASIA GROUP (WITHOUT POLYDACTYLY)

Asphyxiating thoracic dysplasia is also known as Jeune syndrome. It is characterized by a primarily constricted long narrow thoracic cavity, short ribs with bulbous end, cycle handle bar clavicle, and small sacrosciatic notch **(Fig. 14.3.2)**.

ELLIS-VAN CREVELD SYNDROME (SHORT-RIB POLYDACTYLY SYNDROME)

Ellis-van Creveld syndrome, also known as the chondroectodermal dysplasia, is a type of mesomelic limb shortening. It is characterized by narrowing of thorax with short ribs, small and flared ilia and triradiate acetabula. Presence of polydactyly is a pointer to the clinical diagnosis **(Figs 14.3.3A to C)**.

SPONDYLOEPIMETAPHYSEAL DYSPLASIA GROUP

The term 'Spondylo' refers to spine, 'epiphyseal' refers to the growing ends of bones, and 'dysplasia' refers to abnormal growth. Spondyloepimetaphyseal dysplasia has major radiological abnormalities involving spine, epiphysis and metaphysis which are listed below **(Figs 14.3.4A to C)**:

- Flattening and fragmentation of epiphyses
- Delayed and irregular secondary ossification centers
- Flattened and squared off epiphyses
- Thinning of lateral tibial epiphysis
- Double layered patella
- Hypoplastic tibial and femoral condyles with shallow intercondylar notch
- Flattening of vertebral bodies.

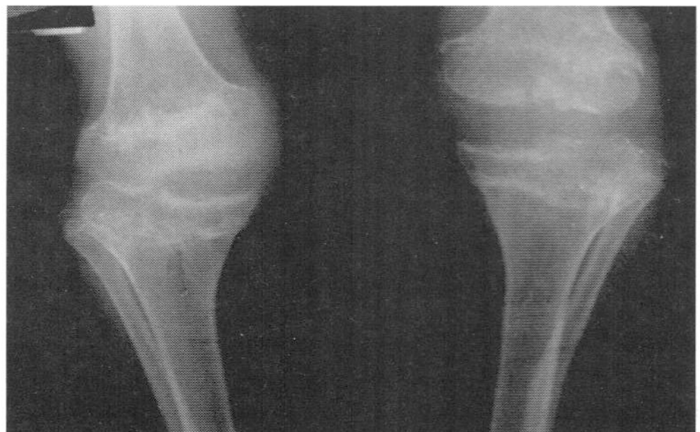

Fig. 14.3.4A: Spondyloepimetaphyseal dysplasia: Note the flattening and fragmentation of epiphyses of knee joint

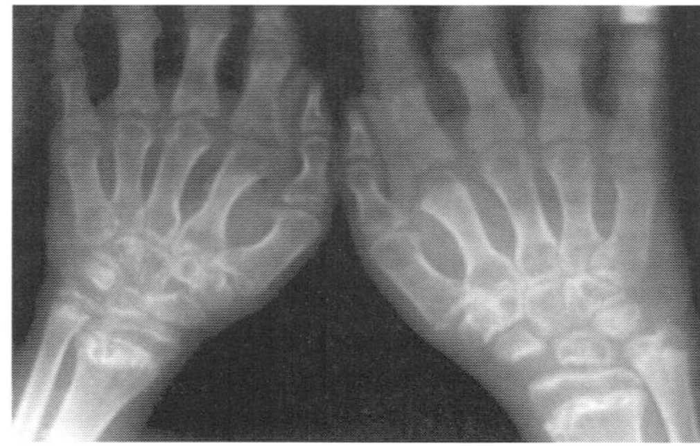

Fig. 14.3.4B: Spondyloepimetaphyseal dysplasia: Flattened, fragmented and squared off epiphyses at joints of hands and wrist with delayed and irregular secondary ossification centers

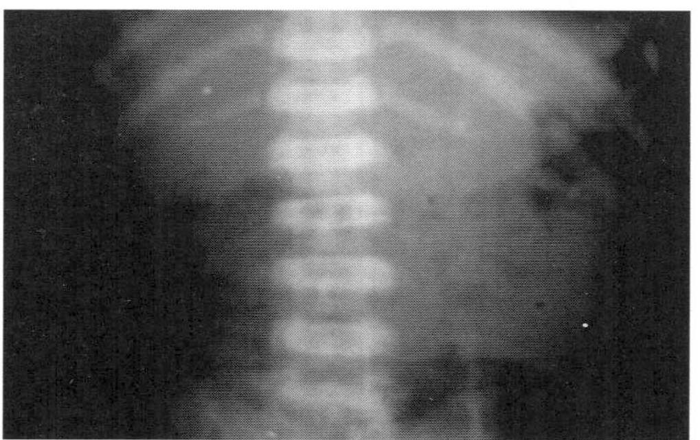

Fig. 14.3.4C: Spondyloepimetaphyseal dysplasia: Note the flattening of vertebral bodies

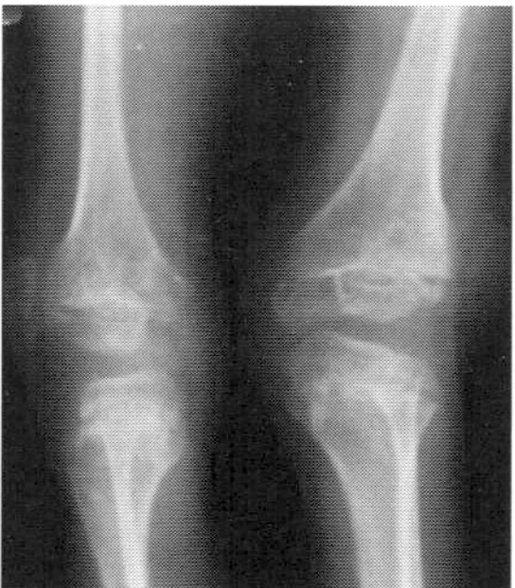

Fig. 14.3.5A: Multiple epiphyseal dysplasia

MULTIPLE EPIPHYSEAL DYSPLASIA

Multiple epiphyseal dysplasia is also known as dysplasia epiphysealis multiplex or Fairbank disease. In this dysplasia, the long bones are short with very short or even absent femoral necks. There is absent ossification of the epiphyses at of the knee at birth and absent ossification of the pubic rami. There is generalized platyspondyly **(Figs 14.3.5A and B)**.

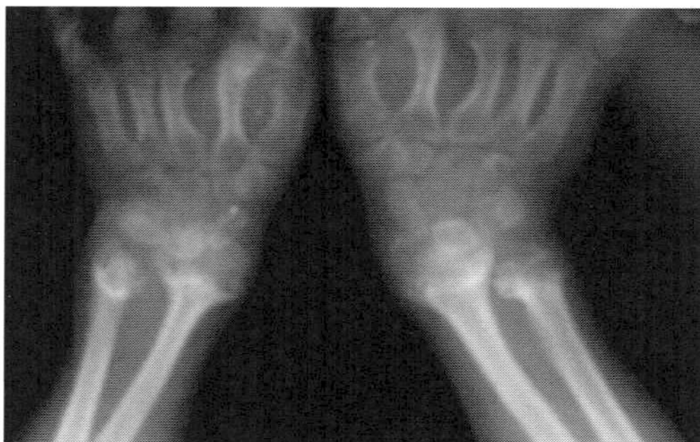

Fig. 14.3.5B: Multiple epiphyseal dysplasia

DYGGVE-MELCHIOR-CLAUSEN DYSPLASIA

Dyggve-Melchior-Clausen (DMC) syndrome is an autosomal recessive type of skeletal dysplasia, characterized by the association of progressive spondyloepimetaphyseal dysplasia (SEMD), microcephaly, mental retardation, and coarse facies. The radiographic appearance of generalized platyspondyly with double-humped end plates and the lace-like appearance of iliac crests are pathognomonic of

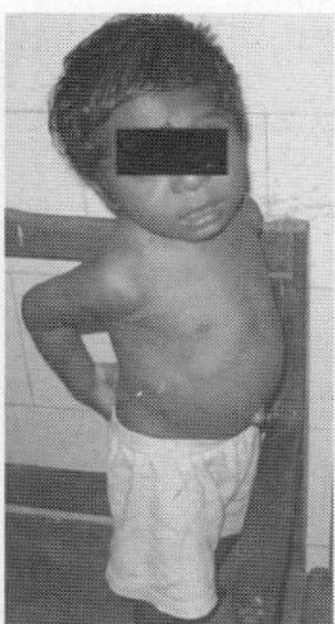

Fig. 14.3.6A: Dyggve-Melchior Clausen dysplasia (*For color version, see Plate 10*)

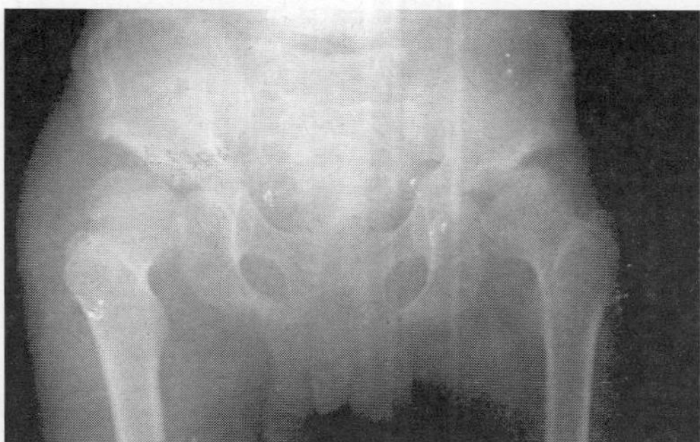

Fig. 14.3.6B: Dyggve-Melchior Clausen dysplasia: Pelvis shows the hypoplastic inferior iliac bones like mucopolysaccharidosis

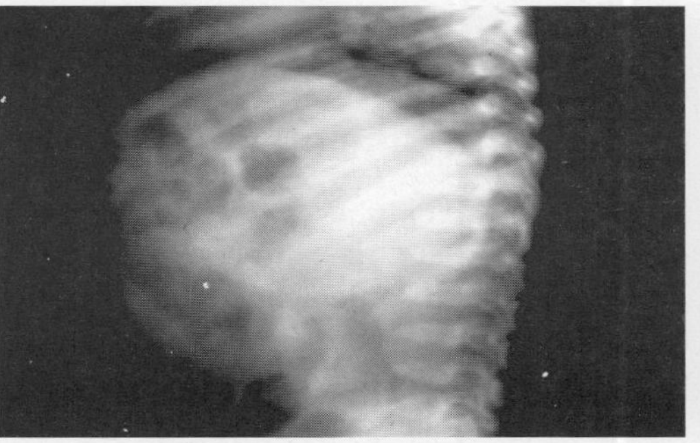

Fig. 14.3.6C: Dyggve-Melchior Clausen dysplasia

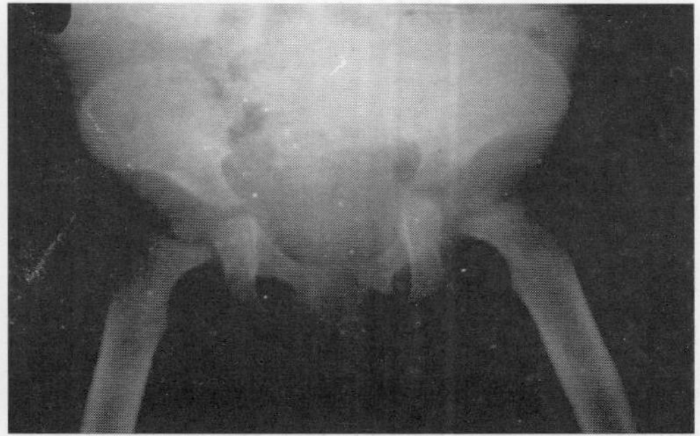

Fig. 14.3.7A: Mucopolysaccharidosis: Hip dysplasia, rounded iliac wings, inferior tapering of ileum and poorly developed acetabulum

DMC syndrome. Pelvis shows the hypoplastic inferior iliac bones like mucopolysaccharidosis **(Figs 14.3.6A to C)**. Radiographically there is severe and generalized platyspondyly, widened and irregular metaphyses of the tubular bones, coxa vara and delayed bone maturation.

MUCOPOLYSACCHARIDOSIS

Several distinctive types of mucopolysaccharidoses have been described, each with distinctive clinical and radiologic features. Hurler (MPS-IH) and Morquio syndrome (MPS-IV) are perhaps the best known radiographically. The characteristic radiological features include:

- *Pelvis:* Rounded iliac wings, inferior tapering of the ileum, hip dysplasia, poorly developed acetabulum flattening of the anterior margin of the sella (J-shaped sella) **(Fig. 14.3.7A)**.
- *Long bones:* Diaphyses are shortened and curved in the distal part; the epiphyses are slightly hypoplastic and thinned cortically with osteoporosis. Proximal pointing of the metacarpals **(Fig. 14.3.7B)**.
- *Spine:* Dorsal spine shows middle beaking in Morquio syndrome (MPS-IV) and inferior beaking at lumbar spine in Hurler syndrome (MPS-IH) **(Fig. 14.3.7C)**.

MUCOLIPIDOSIS

The radiological features depend on the age at presentation of the child. These include **(Fig. 14.3.8)**:

- *Early infancy:* Osteopenia, metaphyseal destruction, cortical bone erosion, pathological fractures, and intervertebral calcification.

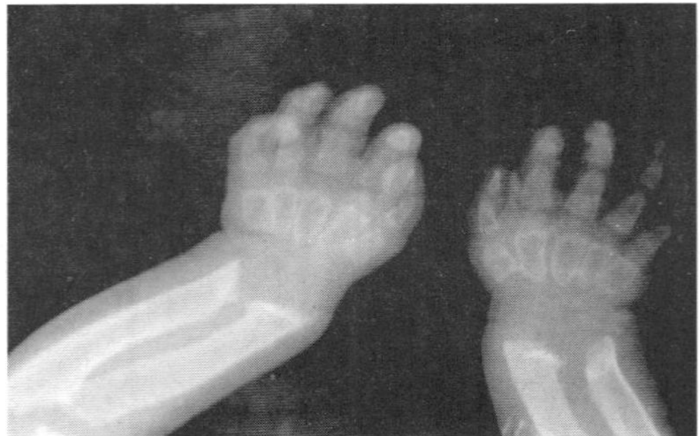

Fig. 14.3.7B: Mucopolysaccharidosis: Diaphyses are shortened and curved in the distal part; the epiphyses are slightly hypoplastic and thinned cortically with osteoporosis

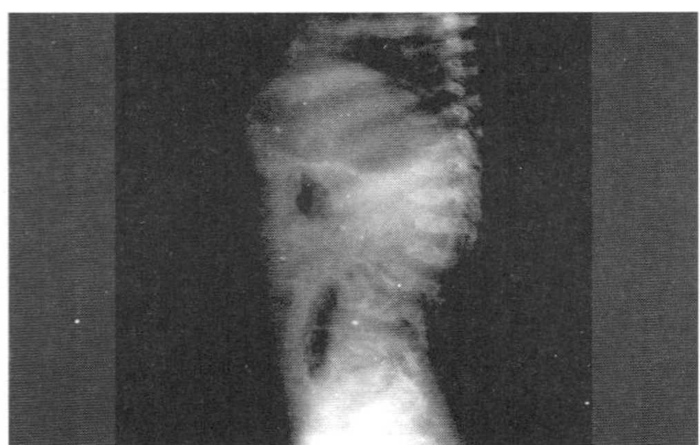

Fig. 14.3.7C: Mucopolysaccharidosis: Inferior beaking at lumbar spine in Hurler syndrome (MPS-IH)

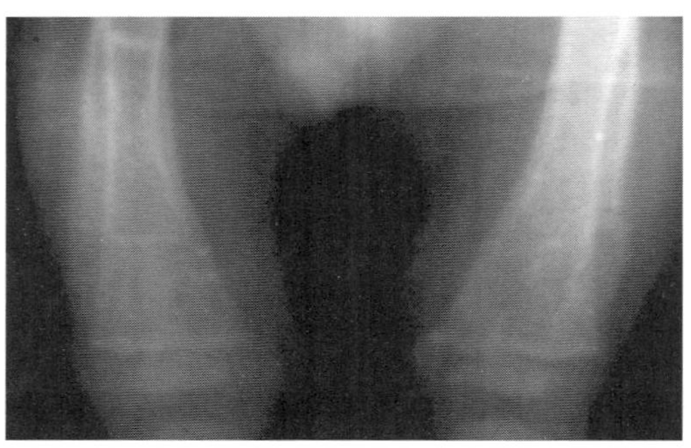

Fig. 14.3.8: Mucolipidosis: Both femurs show periosteal elevation due to mucolipidosis

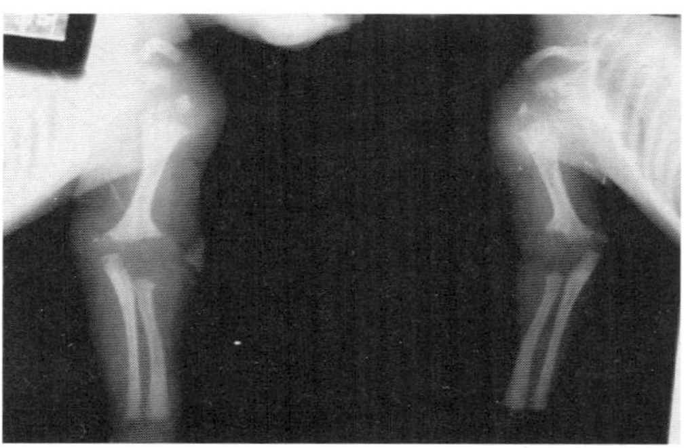

Fig. 14.3.9: Chondrodysplasia punctata: Punctate irregular epiphyses in the long bones

- *Early childhood:* Shortening of long bones, widening of metaphysis, hypoplasia of scapula, inferior beaking vertebrae, and irregularity of ossification.

CHONDRODYSPLASIA PUNCTATA GROUP OR STIPPLED EPIPHYSES

Stippling of the epiphyses is a pointer to the diagnosis **(Fig. 14.3.9)**; however it may be present in other disorders including congenital hypothyroidism (cretinism), trisomies (21 and 18), lysosomal storage disorders, multiple epiphyseal dysplasia, normal variant hypoparathyroidism, warfarin-induced embryopathy.

METAPHYSEAL DYSPLASIA

Metaphyseal dysplasia is also known as Pyle disease. It is a rare autosomal recessive disorder, characterized by flaring of the ends of long bones with relative constriction and sclerosis of the diaphysis and mild cranial sclerosis **(Figs 14.3.10A to C)**. It is one of the causes of an Erlenmeyer flask deformity. The flared metaphases are relatively lucent.

MESOMELIC DYSPLASIAS

Mesomelic dysplasia is characterized by disproportionate shortening of middle segment of long bones **(Figs 14.3.11A and B)**.

CLEIDOCRANIAL DYSPLASIA

Cleidocranial dysplasia is an autosomal dominant skeletal dysplasia with predominantly

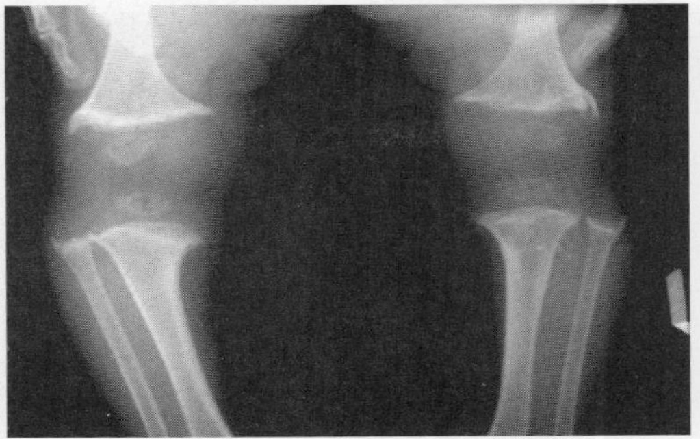

Fig. 14.3.10A: Metaphyseal dysplasia: By flaring of the ends of long bones with relative constriction and sclerosis of the diaphysis

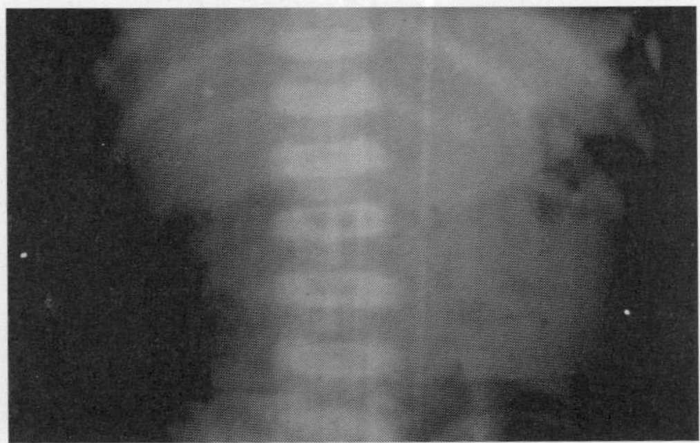

Fig. 14.3.10B: Metaphyseal dysplasia

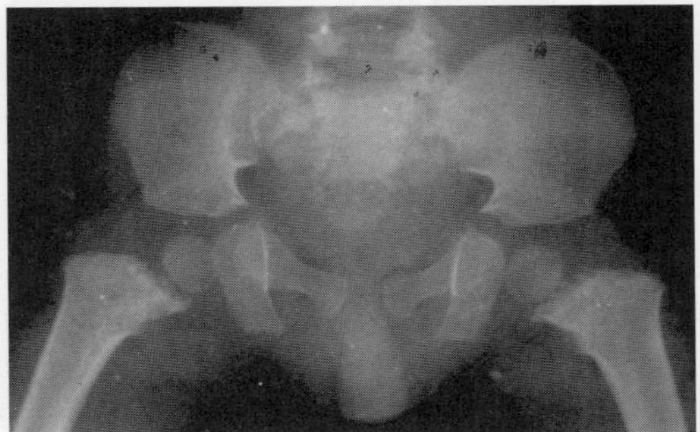

Fig. 14.3.10C: Metaphyseal dysplasia

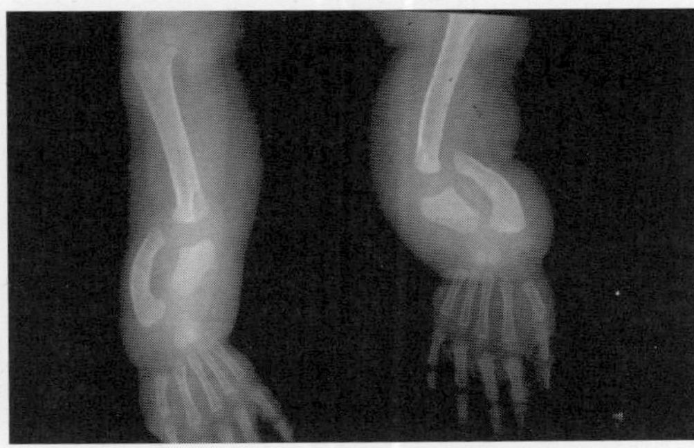

Fig. 14.3.11A: Disproportionate shortening of middle segment of long bones

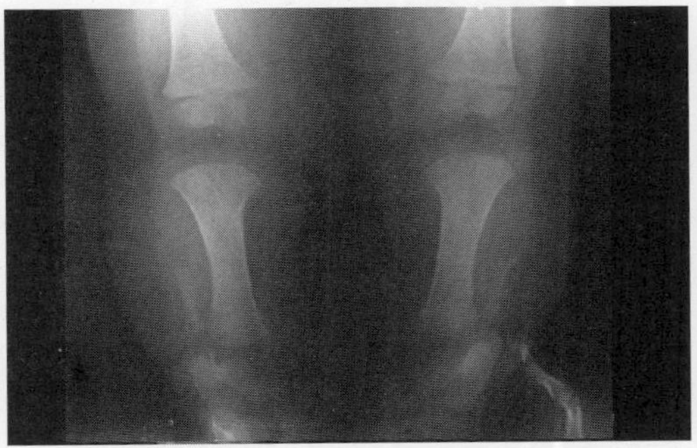

Fig. 14.3.11B: Disproportionate shortening of middle segment of long bones

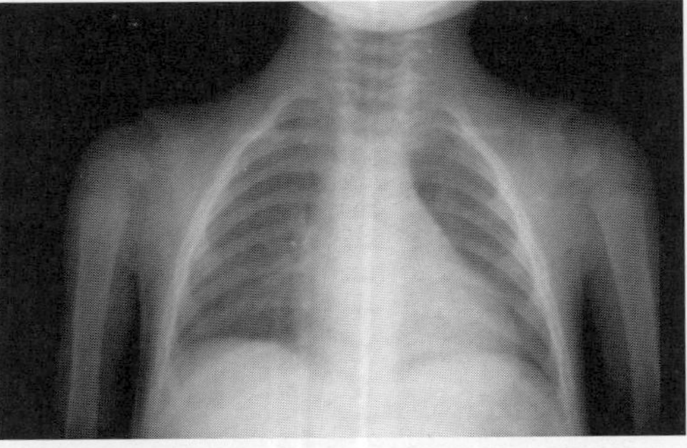

Fig. 14.3.12A: Cleidocranial dysplasia: Bilateral hypoplastic lateral 3rd clavicle

membranous bone involvement. Radiologic features include bilateral hypoplastic lateral 3rd clavicle **(Fig. 14.3.12A)** and widened symphysis pubis and ectopia vesicae **(Fig. 14.3.12B)**.

OSTEOGENESIS IMPERFECTA

The radiological features of osteogenesis imperfecta are listed further.

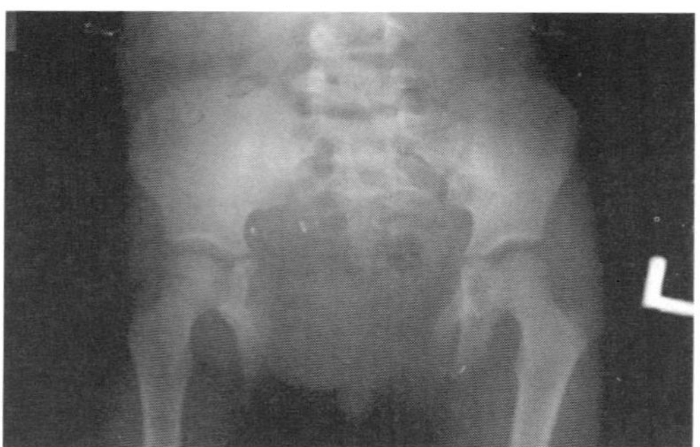

Fig. 14.3.12B: Cleidocranial dysplasia: Widened symphysis pubis and ectopia vesicae

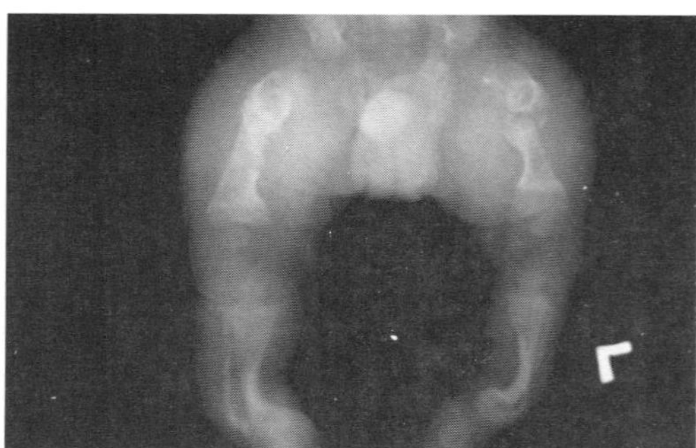

Fig. 14.3.13: Osteogenesis imperfecta: X-ray of lower limbs show shortening and multiple fractures of limbs with decreased bone density

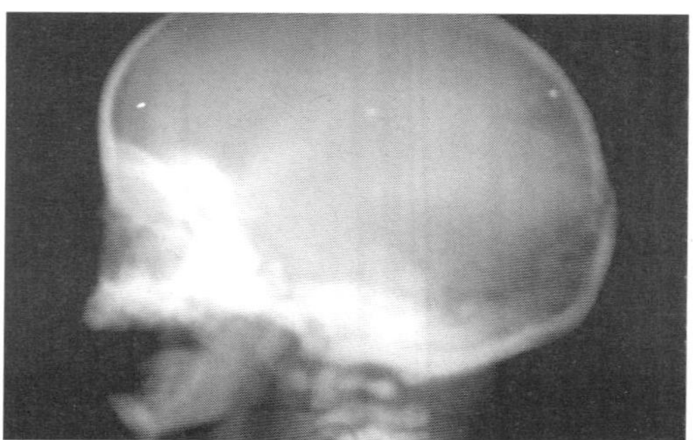

Fig. 14.3.14A: X-ray skull in osteopetrosis: Note the generalized osteosclerosis. The angle of the mandible is acute

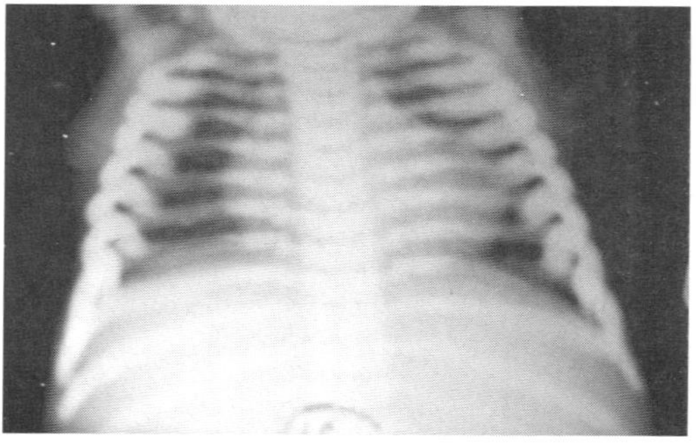

Fig. 14.3.14B: X-ray chest in osteopetrosis: Note the generalized increased density of bones

- Limited skull ossification.
- Irregular shape and fractures of the ribs.
- Shortening and fractures of the limbs with decreased bone density. Fractures may be present prenatally. Even though the fractures are common after minor trauma, they heal quickly **(Fig. 14.3.13)**.

OSTEOPETROSIS

Osteopetrosis is also known as dense bone disease or marble bone disease. The radiographs show generalized osteosclerosis which is usually diagnostic; and in some cases the disease is detected incidentally on skeletal X-rays done for some other reason **(Figs 14.3.14A and B)**.

PYKNODYSOSTOSIS

Pyknodysostosis is a rare autosomal recessive bone dysplasia, characterized by osteosclerosis with narrow medullary cavities and short stature. Long bone fractures are common. Mandibular angles are obtuse **(Fig. 14.3.15A)** with abnormal teeth. Acro-osteolysis of terminal phalanges **(Fig. 14.3.15B)** is usually present.

DIAPHYSEAL DYSPLASIA: ENGELMANN DYSPLASIA

Engelmann disease also known as progressive diaphyseal dysplasia (PDD) is an autosomal dominant sclerosing bony dysplasia, which

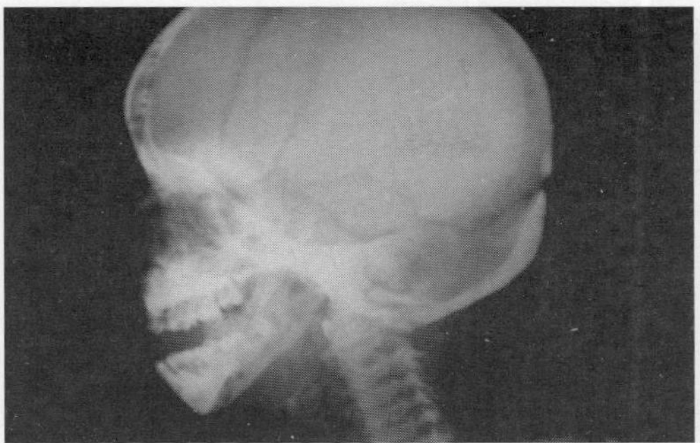

Fig. 14.3.15A: Pyknodysostosis: Mandibular angles are obtuse

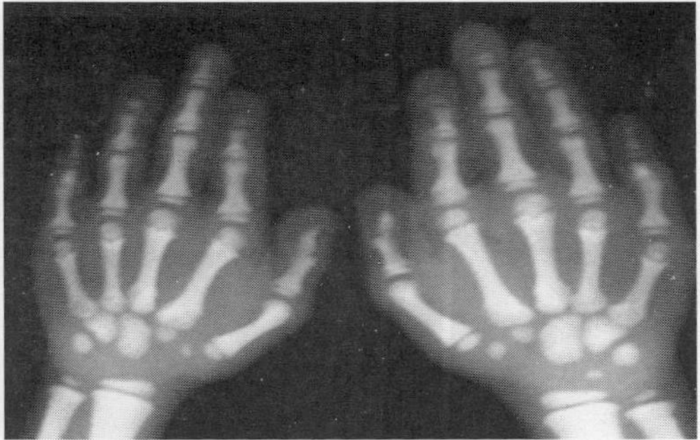

Fig.14.3.15B: Pyknodysostosis: Acro-osteolysis of terminal phalanges

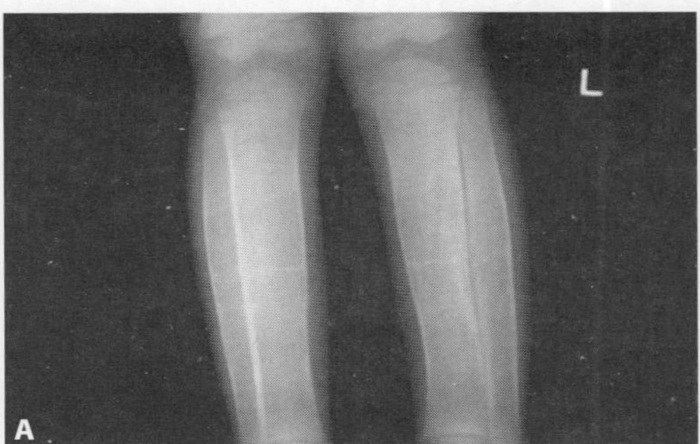

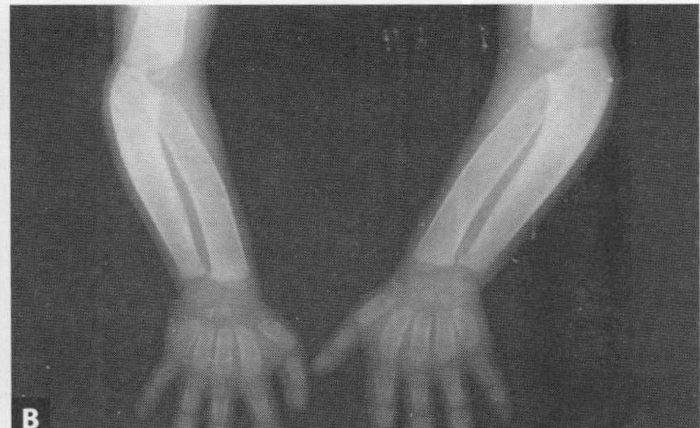

Figs 14.3.16A and B: Diaphyseal dysplasia—Engelmann dysplasia: Soft tissue thickness of extremities is less than the bone thickness

begins in childhood and follows a progressive course. Long bones show fusiform bony enlargement with sclerosis, with sparing of the epiphyses. Soft tissue thickness of extremities is less than the bone thickness **(Figs 14.3.16A and B)**.

FIBROUS DYSPLASIA

The usual appearance of fibrous dysplasia includes a lucent lesion in the diaphysis or metaphysis, with endosteal scalloping and with or without bone expansion and the absence of periosteal reaction. Classically, this finding is described as a ground-glass appearance. Eccentric expansile lytic lesion involving shaft of tibia, femur and pelvis are common **(Fig. 14.3.17)**.

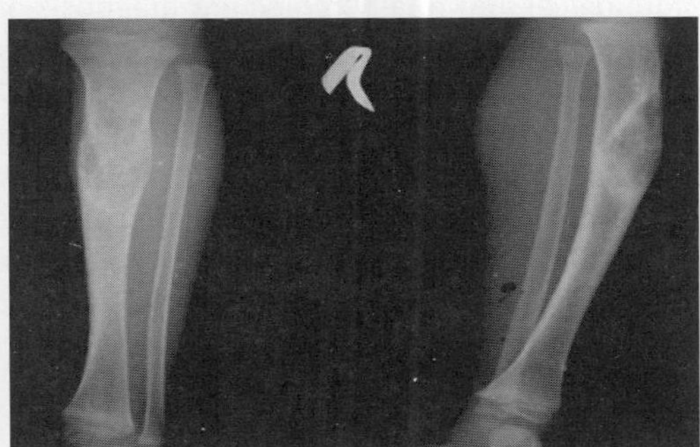

Fig. 14.3.17: Fibrous dysplasia: Eccentric expansile lytic lesion involving shaft of tibia

ECTODERMAL DYSPLASIA

Ectodermal dysplasia (ED) refers to a heterogeneous group of genetic disorders that cause abnormal ectoderm development. The effect is a nonprogressive defect in the development of two or more tissues derived from embryonic ectoderm. Absent teeth and teeth sockets is a common manifestation **(Figs 14.3.18A and B)**. When present, the teeth especially the upper incisors and cuspids are peg shaped or pointed.

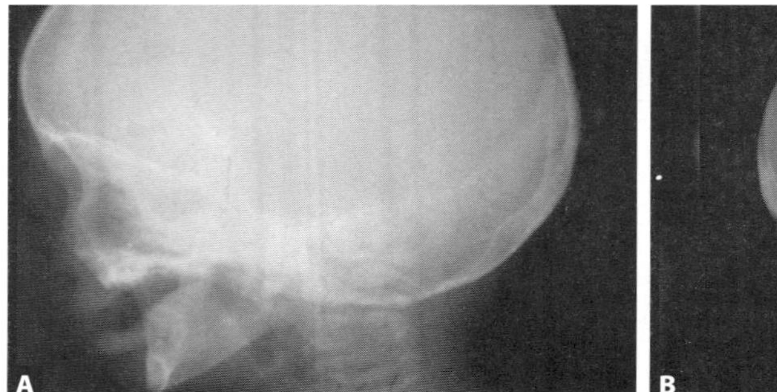

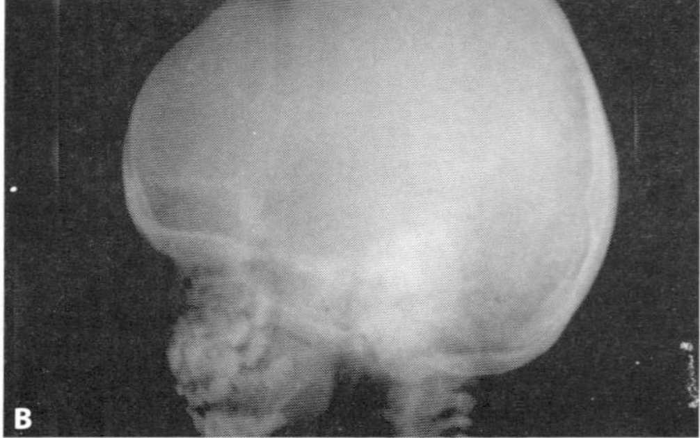

Figs 14.3.18A and B: (A) Ectodermal dysplasia: Absent teeth and teeth sockets; (B) Normal dental development

CONCLUSION

In this review, the aim was to focus on the radiological aspect of assessment of skeletal dysplasias. The outline of the basic clinical approach to a child with a suspected skeletal dysplasia is provided. The recent advances in the field of molecular pathogenetic mechanisms underlying skeletal dysplasias are beyond the scope of this review. However, we would like to emphasize that accurate clinical, radiological and finally molecular diagnosis of skeletal dysplasias is of utmost priority in this era of up to date genetic counseling, prenatal preimplantation genetic diagnoses and hopefully molecularly targeted therapeutics in the future. Correct diagnosis is important for a valid prognosis, for treatment and for genetic counseling. The diagnosis relies almost exclusively on the radiographic findings.

BIBLIOGRAPHY

1. Alianay Y, Lachman RS. A review of the principles of radiological assessment of skeletal dysplasias. J Clin Res Pediatr Endocrinol. 2011;3:163-78.
2. Krakow O, Rimolin DL. The skeletal dysplasia. Genet Med. 2010;12:327-41.
3. Lachman RS. Taybi and Lachman's radiology of syndromes, metabolic disorders and skeletal dysplasias. Mosby-Elsevier, Philadelphia; 2007.
4. Nampoothiri S, Yeshodharan D, Sainulabdin G, et al. Eight years' experience from a skeletal dysplasia referral center in a tertiary hospital in Southern India. A model for diagnosis and treatment of rare diseases in a developing country. Am J Med Genet Part A. 2014;158:1-7.
5. Vajo Z, Francomano CA, Wilkin DJ. The Molecular and genetic basis of fibroblast growth factor receptor 3 disorders: the achondroplasia family of skeletal dysplasias, muenke craniosynostosis, and Crouzon syndrome with acanthosis nigricans. Endocr Rev. 2000;21:23-39.

Index

Page numbers followed by *f* refer to figure *fc* refer to flow chart and *t* refer to table

A

D

E

F

G

L

M

N

S

T

U

V

W

X

Z